Neurophysiological Basis of Movement

MARK L. LATASH, PhD

The Pennsylvania State University

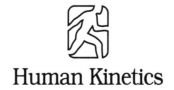

Human Kinetics

Library of Congress Cataloging-in-Publication Data

Latash, Mark L., 1953-
    Neurophysiological basis of movement / Mark L. Latash
        p.   cm.
    Includes bibliographical references and index.
    ISBN 0-88011-756-7
    1. Locomotion.   2. Neurophysiology.   3. Motor ability.
    4. Movement disorders.   I. Title.
    QP301.L364   1998
    612.7'6--dc21
                                        97-31920
                                            CIP

ISBN: 0-88011-756-7

Acquisitions Editor: Judy Patterson Wright, PhD
Managing Editor: Coree Schutter
Assistant Editor: Erin Sprague
Copyeditor: Joyce Sexton
Proofreader: Jane Hilken
Graphic Designer: Keith Blomberg
Graphic Artist: Francine Hamerski
Cover Designer: Jack Davis
Printer: Braun-Brumfield

Printed in the United States of America

10 9 8 7 6 5 4 3 2 1

Human Kinetics
Web site: http://www.humankinetics.com/

United States: Human Kinetics, P.O. Box 5076, Champaign, IL 61825-5076
1-800-747-4457
e-mail: humank@hkusa.com

Canada: Human Kinetics, Box 24040, Windsor, ON N8Y 4Y9
1-800-465-7301 (in Canada only)
e-mail: humank@hkcanada.com

Europe: Human Kinetics, P.O. Box IW14, Leeds LS16 6TR, United Kingdom
(44) 1132 781708
e-mail: humank@hkeurope.com

Australia: Human Kinetics, 57A Price Avenue, Lower Mitcham, South Australia 5062
(088) 277 1555
e-mail: humank@hkaustralia.com

New Zealand: Human Kinetics, P.O. Box 105-231, Auckland 1
(09) 523 3462
e-mail: humank@hknewz.com

CONTENTS

PREFACE

This book grew out of the sense of desperation experienced when I was preparing to teach a first-year graduate course called *Neurophysiological Basis of Movement* in the Department of Kinesiology of the Pennsylvania State University. A number of excellent textbooks existed in the areas of neurophysiology and kinesiology; however, they all emphasized a particular subarea of the field, frequently at the expense of other subareas. Thus, it was necessary to combine information from several sources to cover all the relevant levels of neurophysiological analysis. This is not surprising, because neurophysiology of movement-related structures and phenomena can hardly be considered a single field of study. Apparently, each author has his or her own vision of the state of the field and tends to stress what he or she perceives as being most important. Nevertheless, I believe that a textbook on neurophysiology of movements should provide an overview of all the relevant levels of analysis and all the relevant structures and relations. So I attempted to write such a textbook, one that would be both comprehensive and reflective of the personal views of the author.

Presently, the area of neurophysiology is too wide to allow one person to be equally competent in all its components. Moreover, this field is developing quickly, so that theories are born and die literally annually. Therefore, some of the contents of this textbook are doomed to be obsolete by the time it is available. However, I strongly believe that there is an established basis of knowledge that should be known to any person working in the area of movement studies or using movements as a tool in applied activities such as coaching and physical therapy. The purpose of this book is to outline this basic knowledge and to illustrate how it can be applied to problems at different levels of analysis of the system for movement production.

This book is very much problem oriented. It is not designed as a source of information that needs to be memorized by future students. Actually, during tests in my classes, I have always allowed the students to use books, lecture notes, and other sources of external memory to solve "mini-research" or "mini-clinical" problems. This attitude is deeply rooted in my conviction that learning should be an exercise in application of bits and pieces of information that can be taken not necessarily from one's own memory but also from books and other sources. Learning should always require an intellectual effort and carry an element of discovery—a "Wow!" factor.

In every chapter of the book, I am trying not only to explain the state of affairs in a certain area of movement neurophysiology but also to find internal logic in the way our body is designed and the way it functions. This is not an easy task, because the design and functioning of our body frequently challenge common sense and straightforward logic. However, finding this logic seems to be the most important quest for both research and education in this field.

During the work on this textbook, I was helped, directly and indirectly, by numerous colleagues. Many of them do not even know how much they helped me by writing excellent reviews, chapters, and original research papers. Discussions of problems related to teaching movement neurophysiology with Alexander Aruin, Karl Newell, Jeff Nicholas, and Vladimir Zatsiorsky were most helpful. I am also very grateful to Bruce Kay, who wrote a detailed review with numerous constructive suggestions that helped me improve the didactics of the book. Graduate students who have valiantly struggled through this course at the Penn State University provided invaluable feedback that allowed me to improve many chapters, figures, and problems. However, the most valuable support was assured by the wisdom of my father, Dr. Lev Latash, and the optimism of my daughter, Lisa.

In one of the chapters of one of the most wonderful books in human history, *The Three Musketeers* by Alexandre Dumas, Aramis is being persuaded by a couple of priests to write a dissertation that would be "both dogmatic and didactic." I honestly tried to avoid making this book dogmatic while simultaneously keeping it as didactic as possible. Did I succeed? It is now up to students and professors to pronounce the judgment.

INTRODUCTION

Our life is filled with movements. Day and night, human muscles work to assure desirable postures of the head, body, and extremities, to transfer our whole body through space, to pick up and manipulate objects, to help us interact with other human beings and animals, to exchange information with the external world, and so on. The first striking feature of all voluntary movements of healthy humans is their *meaningfulness*. They all make sense. They lead to certain goals; sometimes they may fail to achieve these goals, but more frequently they succeed. In the external physical world, with its numerous forces, unpredictable events, moving objects, and changing goals, to perform a meaningful movement is not an easy task.

The readers of this book are also going to see that the structure of the human body and some of the properties of its "motors," skeletal muscles, apparently complicate the process of control, although not without valuable gains. The complexity of the task and the presence of the complicating factors place high demands upon the supreme controller of voluntary movements, the central nervous system (CNS), which must possess versatility, resourcefulness, and a number of features that we may not even have invented appropriate words for. Therefore, I will be considering voluntary movements as both manifestations of CNS activity and a tool for understanding the CNS.

Movements are a very attractive object for study because they are readily observable and measurable, and also because there exist relatively clear relations between task and outcome (that are commonly less obvious in purely mental processes). Analysis of voluntary movements is a way of trying to understand how the brain makes decisions and how the peripheral apparatus executes them. This route leads much deeper than its obvious immediate goals of understanding how one can eat with a spoon without spilling the soup. This is a way of approaching such processes as decision making, thinking, and perceiving that create the foundation of brain functioning. It is a way to understanding of the human mind. Is there a more worthy object for study?

THE WORLDS OF HUMAN MOVEMENT

The human body is obviously a complex system. Even its subsystems are complex. Actually, a single cell is already complex enough to be considered a whole world of its own. When one deals with a complex system, the first step is always to define a set of notions that are meaningful for the chosen system or a chosen level of analysis. These sets of notions are typically selected rather arbitrarily, based on intuition, common sense, and general knowledge of physics, chemistry, and certain other disciplines. After a set of notions (an *adequate language*—a term introduced by a great mathematician, I. Gelfand) has been chosen, the system can be investigated. Within this book, several levels of complexity will be identified. Each level will require its own set of notions and methods of analysis. Identification of these levels will be rather subjective. However, their selection is not purely arbitrary. Imagine that a certain method of analysis leads to gradual penetration into the properties of a system and is successful in solving certain groups of problems. At some moment, when the same method of analysis is applied to a new group of problems, it fails completely, as if hitting an invisible wall. This is a clear sign that a *new level of complexity has been encountered that requires an intuitive, qualitative leap—the introduction of a new set of notions, that is, a new adequate language.*

Four major levels of analysis that are relevant to the generation and control of voluntary movement will be discussed. Since they have their own sets of notions and are likely to be rather independent of one another, they will be addressed as separate worlds:

- World I: Cells
- World II: Connections
- World III: Structures
- World IV: Behaviors

At the end of the book, movement pathologies will be considered as a separate world (World V: Disorders), which combines notions pertaining to all four of the other Worlds.

The reader will see that these Worlds themselves are not homogenous and that they may include objects, processes, and phenomena that require analysis at different levels of complexity. For example, processes in World IV related to the control of multi-joint movements may require a different language from the one used with respect to control of individual muscles. The language that may be appropriate for studying the simplest, monosynaptic reflexes (e.g., the well-known tendon jerk) within World II may be inappropriate when one is dealing with the more complex reflexes or reflex-type reactions that are considered later in the textbook.

THE ORGANIZATION OF THE BOOK

The organization of this textbook is straightforward. It contains 27 chapters; each chapter contains material to be covered in one extended lecture (about 1.5 hours). Each chapter starts with a set of key words and ends with a summarizing paragraph (Chapter in a Nutshell). The chapters are in an order that has been used in the course titled *Neurophysiological Basis of Movement* at the Pennsylvania State University.

Let me emphasize a few unusual features of the book. First, it contains small problems, "one-minute drills," that are scattered throughout. I have used three to five of these problems during each lecture, and they have proven effective in keeping students' attention and making sure that the number of "sleeping beauties" is minimal. These small problems range in complexity from absolutely trivial to unsolvable. However, the students should not know the difference, so that there is always a chance that some day one student will solve all the unsolvable problems. No explicit answers to the small problems are available in the textbook (although some of them are actually answered in the next paragraph of the text), because otherwise the whole purpose of presenting the problems would be lost. Besides, as I have just mentioned, some problems do not have answers!

At the end of each World, a few larger problems are offered as a means of self-testing. These problems were taken from tests given during the first two years this course was offered at the Pennsylvania State University. They require critical thinking and a degree of inventiveness in using information from previous chapters. No answers are provided, for two reasons. First, the reader is supposed to solve these problems independently. Second, some of the problems actually have a number of answers of different degrees of correctness, and it is up to each individual student to come up with an answer and be able to prove that it is correct.

Six Laboratory projects are described at the end of the textbook. Each of them actually represents a rather large research study, so that running it would probably take two to three typical lab periods (1.5 hours each period). Thus, the total number of Laboratory hours is assumed to be between 18 and 27. Certainly, the availability of equipment and time will be a major factor in actually structuring and running the Labs in each particular department. The description fits the equipment setup that we had in the Motor Control Laboratory at the Penn State University and that was used for both research and teaching purposes.

THE MAJOR PURPOSE

I see the ultimate goal of this textbook as providing enough material to teach students

- to think independently;
- to know certain basic facts about the design of our cells, muscles, neuronal structures, and the whole body;
- to have an understanding of the internal logic of the design and functioning of the system for production of voluntary movements;
- to solve problems using the basic facts;
- to design mental and actual experiments to address typical "template" research problems; and
- to read and understand research literature in the area of neurophysiology of movements.

This textbook contains material that can easily be adjusted to fit an upper-level (300 or 400) undergraduate course or a lower-level (first year) graduate course. In particular, the chapters on motor disorders and the Laboratories were written with a mature, well-prepared student in mind, while most of the earlier material can be understood by an undergraduate student. Some of the chapters within the first four Worlds contain material that may require more than one lecture for presentation to undergraduate students. On the other hand, some supporting material (in particular, elements of functional anatomy, of control theory, and of biomechanics) might be covered in other courses. It is certainly up to particular professors and particular programs to adjust the material to fit their students' backgrounds and needs.

There are no absolute prerequisites for a course based on the material in this book. However, students would definitely benefit from having had introductory courses in calculus, physics (or mechanics), chemistry, and anatomy. Then more time could be spent on really interesting things.

And now let us move through the Worlds of the neurophysiology of movements.

WORLD I

CELLS

CHAPTER 1

MEMBRANES, PARTICLES, AND POTENTIALS

Key Terms

complex system approach	**osmosis**	**Nernst equation**
biological membranes	**movement of ions**	**equilibrium potential**
movement of particles in solutions		

1.1. COMPLEX SYSTEM APPROACH

The purpose of this book is to provide basic knowledge of the mechanisms, structure, and function of the human nervous system, keeping in mind that this knowledge is going to be used for understanding how human voluntary movements are controlled. The relation between neurophysiology and motor control is not obvious and has been a controversial issue for years. There are two extreme views:

1. Function of a neural structure can be derived from properties of its elements (neural cells or neurons) and their connections. So, when researchers accumulate enough information about the structure of the central nervous system (the brain and the spinal cord), its function will become obvious. This approach is commonly called **reductionism** because it attempts to "reduce" the function of a complex system to the properties of its elements. Sometimes another fancy expression is used with respect to this approach: **ascending determinism.**

2. Function of a complex system cannot be understood on the basis of its structure and the properties of its elements. Understanding a complex system requires a special set of notions that cannot be derived from simply looking at the elements and their connections. So no matter how much information a scientist obtains about the elements of a complex system, he or she will not understand its function without forgetting about the elements, at least temporarily, and looking at the system as a whole. This approach is called the **complex system approach,** and my heart belongs to it.

If one accepts the idea that complex systems should be studied in a different way than by accumulating information about their elements, first it is necessary to realize the general properties of a complex system and to introduce an appropriate, meaningful language (set of notions). Note that systems of seemingly different complexity may be described with the same sets of notions. For example, our planetary system consists of zillions of atoms. However, the Bohr planetary model for just one atom is qualitatively rather similar to the solar planetary system (figure 1.1). Behavior of a motionless heavy rock may be much more simple and predictable than the behavior of an electron on one of the atomic orbits within the rock. This means that *a complex system does not necessarily imply a complicated description of its behavior.*

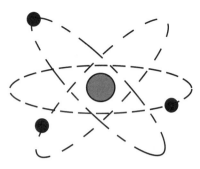

Figure 1.1 The planetary model of an atom and the structure of the solar system are quite similar. You may consider the middle circle as the sun or as the nucleus of an atom, while the black dots may be either planets or electrons.

Most of the objects surrounding us can be described with fewer parameters and simpler laws than an atomic nucleus. *This simplicity of description is in fact the most important advantage of the complex system approach.*

However, all this having been said, readers of this book will be spending a lot of time learning exactly that information about elements of the central nervous system that is likely to be helpful but insufficient for understanding how humans control voluntary movements. There are several reasons for this. First, before studying the grammar, it makes sense to study the alphabet. Neurophysiology may be considered an alphabet, a basis for any research involving the central nervous system. Second, neurophysiological studies frequently involve measuring variables that are rather directly related to movement performance, that is, to behavior, for example electrical muscle activity (electromyogram). Third, such neurophysiological indexes as the electroencephalogram (a record of the electrical field created by the brain) reflect the functioning of many elements within the system; that is, they may be considered indexes of system behavior—although not without caution and reservations, as readers will see later. Fourth, a student may eventually wish to do something different from studying control of human movements. If his or her area of interest will involve a function of the human body, knowledge of the basic neurophysiological mechanisms will be very helpful, or even vital.

Before embarking on a long and tedious trip through the straits of basic neurophysiology, let me suggest a couple of examples that I hope will make the difference between reductionism and the complex system approach obvious.

If one wanted to teach a friend how an automobile works, the worst possible route would be to start from physics of elementary particles. Although any car consists of elementary particles, its properties as a whole cannot be derived from the properties of the particles. This means that the instructor needs to make a quali-

tative leap and use a different set of notions (e.g., the angle of steering wheel rotation, pressure on the gas and brake pedals, gears, etc.). Just imagine reading a car manual that started with physics of elementary particles, then went into molecular physics, spent hundreds of pages on deriving properties of materials from molecular interactions, and so on. Such a manual might be quite helpful in many ways but not in explaining how to drive and service the car. If, on the other hand, the task is to understand the basic features of traffic within a large city, the properties of individual cars stop playing a crucial role. The traffic will be more affected by such factors as road condition, closed lanes, stop signals, traffic lights, and the like. So the basic patterns of the traffic may be the same regardless of whether the people of the city prefer driving Toyotas, Chevrolets, or BMWs.

What would be a correct approach? First, it is necessary to realize that one is dealing with a *complex system,* that is, *a system whose properties cannot be derived from and should not be searched for in the properties of its elements.* It may be said that a system is complex when it is bigger than the sum of its components. Don't misinterpret this statement; it does not mean, certainly, that any complex system can be built of any elements. The elements must possess certain properties to enable the system to function. For example, it is impossible to build a car using only oxygen molecules. However, even if it were known what molecules were used to build the car and in what proportions, this information is insufficient to enable understanding of how the car functions. The first step in studying such a system is always *to define an appropriate level of analysis,* to choose correct words that meaningfully describe the functioning of the system. In the case of the car, the shortcut is to read the manual or consult a mechanic. If, however, these solutions are inaccessible, one needs to *invent a correct language* oneself based on intuition, basic knowledge, and common sense.

All this is intuitively clear, and the reader may wonder why I am wasting time on such trivial things. They are trivial, however, only with respect to relatively simple systems that we encounter every day (cars, kitchen appliances, even computers). However, the studies of more complex systems that were not engineered by human beings quite frequently take a reductionist route, that is, use available methods for studying the system's elements and their interactions without even addressing *the first, absolutely vital step, that is, developing an adequate language for the system as a whole.*

Traditionally, complex functions of the human body are described starting from elements and going "up" in an attempt to get to the function. This kind of description creates the impression of a multimillion-piece puzzle that is supposed to come out as a nice picture. However, the box cover that shows the picture has been lost, so one is forced to manipulate the pieces without any knowledge of whether they should come out as *La Gioconda* or Westminster Abbey, in the futile hope that they will somehow fit together and the solution will emerge by itself. There is no chance for success unless the person can intuitively come up with a possible picture and proceed according to this theoretical template (plan). Trying to fit the pieces together based solely on their properties (e.g., shape) is unlikely to be successful, because each piece can be successfully attached to millions of others. The situation within any system that involves signal processing by the central nervous system is even more complicated, because the properties of any neuron (the way it processes incoming information and generates output signals) may change depending on numerous factors, including the activity of its neighbors. Imagine that pieces of the hypothetical multimillion-piece puzzle change shape when you try to attach them to each other!

Problem 1.1

Can you come up with a couple of other examples of complex systems from everyday life?

Readers of this book will study the structure and function of various elements within the nervous system, keeping in mind the limitations of the approach "from elements to function." After explaining the basics, I will try to imagine how different elements interact to give rise to a function. However, these attempts are likely to suggest how the system might have worked rather than how it actually works. The reader will see that knowledge about the structure and basic properties of the elements imposes only very soft limitations on one's imagination, so that many designs are possible.

And now, fasten your seat belts, and let us study the alphabet of the central nervous system.

1.2. THE BIOLOGICAL MEMBRANE

One of the greatest achievements of evolution (or creation) is the cellular membrane (figure 1.2). It isolates information within the cell from the external world and thus allows for its storage, it protects the contents of the cell, and it basically defines the boundary of the cell and makes the cell a unit separate from the environment. If the membrane were absolutely impermeable, the cell would not be able to interact with the world, to extract the necessary information and substances (e.g., food), and would be an alien structure rather than a part of the environment. If the membrane were permeable to ev-

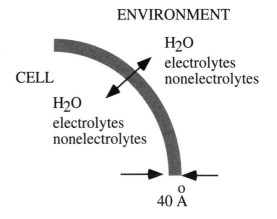

Figure 1.2 Cellular membrane is a sophisticated structure that is permeable to some substances but not others. Its selective permeability makes the membrane a unique structure that allows the cell to interact with the environment and to be separate from it.

erything, its function would be completely lost. So the most important function of the cellular membrane is **partial permeability,** which allows exchange of information with the environment while protecting the contents of the cell.

The movement of substances across the membrane is a central theme of an area of biology called **membrane physiology.** Membranes are commonly very thin (about 40 Ångstrom, or about 4 nm = $4 \cdot 10^{-9}$ m), but they control the movement of substances much more effectively than cells whose volume is relatively huge. There are three major groups of substances that can travel across the membrane and whose properties we are going to consider:

1. Solvents. The most common solvent is water; however, some substances are soluble in lipids, and this, in particular, allows them to pass through cell membranes more easily.
2. Electrolytes. These are ions (fragments of molecules) that have a non-zero electric charge.
3. Nonelectrolytes. These are molecules or fragments of molecules without a net electric charge. Many products of cellular metabolism are nonelectrolytes.

Movements of electrolytes will play a particularly important role in this book because they create electric current through the membrane. Most of the urgent information is transmitted within the nervous system (as well as within other systems of our body) with the help of electricity. So electric currents created by movements of electrolytes are vital for the information transmission that in turn underlies all the processes of the generation of commands to muscles and execution of these commands by the muscles.

1.3. MOVEMENT IN A SOLUTION

Water is a very good solvent because of the polar nature of its molecules (H_2O), that is, because this molecule has local positive and negative charges that sum up to zero. As a result, an electrolyte (e.g., a salt) dissociates in water, creating ions. Nonelectrolytes that, like water, are polar, also dissolve rather well but without breaking down to ions. Movement of water commonly occurs because of a difference in hydrostatic pressure; this so-called bulk flow or **convection** is proportional to pressure difference (figure 1.3). Bulk flow apparently carries water with all the dissolved particles.

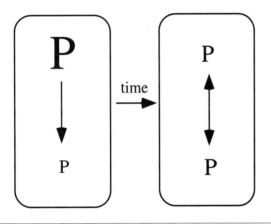

Figure 1.3   Convection is movement of a solvent (e.g., water) and solutes from an area of high pressure to an area of low pressure.

Concentration of particles of a certain kind in water defines another type of movement that is called **diffusion.** If the concentrations in two areas of a solution are different, random motion of particles (molecules or ions) in different directions leads to a net movement in a direction from the site with a higher concentration to the site with a lower concentration (figure 1.4).

As a result, *diffusion changes the concentration of particles,* leading to a decrease in the difference in concentrations at different sites. Note that relative change in concentration depends on several factors including actual difference in the number of particles and total volume of each site (compartment). The bigger the compartment, the smaller the change. While discussing diffusion of particles across cellular membrane, one typically considers extracellular space to be much larger than intracellular space so that any diffusion will lead to a change in the concentration inside the cell but not outside it. Note also that diffusion takes time, particularly when it occurs across large distances. So our body uses other means of transporting solutes over large distances, in particular, convection with the help of the circulatory system. The rate of diffusion from or into a cell depends on the surface/volume (S/V) ratio for the cell. Small cells

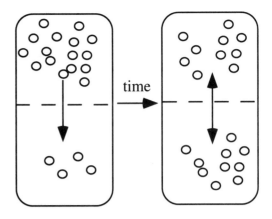

Figure 1.4   Diffusion is movement of particles dissolved in a solvent from an area of their high concentration to an area of their low concentration.

have large S/V ratios, and diffusion from or into them occurs quickly, while large cells have low S/V ratios and diffusion is slow. For a spherical cell,

$$S/V = 4\pi r^2/(4/3)\pi r^3 = 3/r$$

where r is the radius.

Electrolytes and nonelectrolytes both move with convection and diffusion. Electrolytes, however, can also move in response to an electric field. In this case, the movement of electrolytes obeys Ohm's law:

$$I = V/R$$

where I is current or change in electric charge (I = dQ/dt), V is voltage or difference of electric potentials, and R is a coefficient termed resistance (figure 1.5).

Convection, diffusion, and movement under the action of an electric field occur in a solution irrespective of the presence or absence of membranes. Let me now turn to movements of these substances across biological membranes. Membranes typically are built of lipid

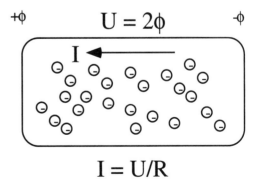

Figure 1.5   An electric field creates a difference of potentials (U) that induces a flow of charged particles (a current, I). The current is proportional to the difference of potentials. The inverse of the coefficient of proportionality is termed **resistance** (R).

layers that are quite impermeable to virtually any particle but that particularly hate to let ions through. So almost all movement of substances across membranes occurs at special sites called membrane channels. At these sites, special macromolecules let certain substances cross the membrane. For example, sodium channels use a polypeptide with an enormous molecular weight of about 260,000 daltons. The rate of movement of a substance through the membrane typically depends on the concentration gradient (as in diffusion) and on voltage gradient (if we are dealing with ions). There are substances that can cross membranes in substantial quantities without the help of channels; these are solutes that can dissolve in lipids, examples being anesthetics and some other drugs.

1.4. CONCENTRATION OF WATER: OSMOSIS

To measure concentration of all the particles in a volume of a solvent, it is necessary to know the total number of different particles in the volume. For this purpose, it is useful to borrow a special unit from electrochemistry, namely a mole. A mole is the amount of a substance for which the weight in grams is equal to the substance's molecular weight. For example, molecular hydrogen has a molecular weight of 2 (1 for each hydrogen atom); thus, 1 mole of hydrogen weighs 2 g; similarly, 1 mole of oxygen weighs 32 g (16 for each atom), and so on. Note that 1 mole of any chemical substance—for example, atom, molecule, or ion—always contains 6.02 times 10 to the power of 23 particles (Avogadro's number).

The concentration of water is measured as the total concentration of all particles. Thus, osmolarity of a solution with a nondissociating substance, for example, sucrose, will correspond to the number of molecules of this substance. So, a 1 millimolar (mM; remember that "milli" means divided by 10 to the power of 3) solution has an osmolarity of 1 mOs (milliosmole). If the substance is one that can dissociate, for example, salt, each molecule of this substance (NaCl) will produce two particles, Na^+ and Cl^-, so that a 1 mM solution of NaCl has an osmolarity of 2 mOs. Note that the concentration of a substance can change without changing its amount, that is, if the total volume of the cell changes. This can happen, for example, when a red blood cell (erythrocyte) is placed into a solution with a lower or higher concentration of salt as compared to blood plasma.

Problem 1.2

By the way, what will happen with a red blood cell in these solutions? Note that membrane surface cannot change much.

A solution is called **isoosmotic** if it has the same concentration of solute as the reference solution (plasma), **hypoosmotic** if it has a lower concentration, and **hyperosmotic** if it has a higher concentration of solute. These are nearly synonyms to the commonly used terms **isotonic, hypotonic, and hypertonic.**

Osmosis is a process of movement of the solvent (for example, water), rather than solute, across the membrane in order to obtain osmotic equilibrium. Remember that motion of ions and other particles through the membrane is typically restricted, while water can travel freely.

It is important to understand that osmotic equilibrium (a state in which water does not move from one side of a membrane to the other) is achieved only if the osmolarity of the solution on either side of the membrane is equal. So the concentration of particles inside the cell (S_i) should be equal to the concentration outside the cell (S_o). Note that concentration equals the number of particles (A) divided by volume of the site (V):

$$S = A/V. \qquad (1.1)$$

So if you take a cell from a solution with the concentration of particles S_1 and place it into a new solution with the concentration of particles S_2, cell volume will change so that osmotic equilibrium is reached (figure 1.6).

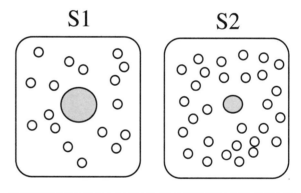

Figure 1.6 If you take a cell from a solution with a concentration of particles S_1 and place it into a new solution with a concentration of particles S_2 ($S_2 > S_1$), the cell volume will change (decrease) until a new osmotic equilibrium is achieved.

Initially, $S_{i1} = S_{o1}$. From Equation 1.1,

$$A_1/V_1 = S_{o1}.$$

In the new solution, similarly we get

$$A_2/V_2 = S_{o2}.$$

A simple transformation gives:

$$\frac{V_1}{V_2} = \frac{A_1 \cdot S_{o2}}{A_2 \cdot S_{o1}}.$$

So, in order to know how cell volume will change in a new solution, one needs to know the concentration of the solute outside and the amount of the solute inside the cell.

Problem 1.3

What will happen with the cell if it is placed in a solution containing only permeable substances?

1.5. MOVEMENT OF IONS

Ions move by both diffusion and voltage gradient (figure 1.7).

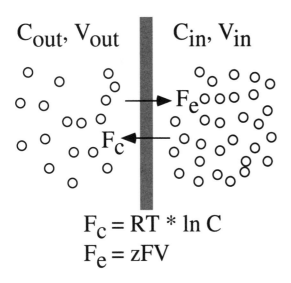

Figure 1.7 in the image:

$$C_{out}, V_{out} \qquad C_{in}, V_{in}$$

$$F_c = RT * \ln C$$
$$F_e = zFV$$

Figure 1.7 Ions move under the influence of two forces. The first is related to the concentration gradient (F_c), while the second is related to the difference of potentials (F_e).

As mentioned earlier, diffusion is driven by a concentration difference. The chemical force driving diffusion is termed **chemical potential** (F_c):

$$F_c = RT \cdot \ln C \qquad (1.2)$$

where R is the gas constant, T is absolute temperature (Kelvin scale), and C is concentration.

If there is an external electrical field, the electrical force (F_e) acting on a charged particle can be defined from:

$$F_e = z\Phi V \qquad (1.3)$$

where z is the valence (don't forget that valence can be positive or negative), F is the Faraday constant, and V is voltage. So we have the total **electrochemical force** acting on an ion:

$$F = F_c + F_e$$

If an ion is in an equilibrium, forces acting on particles of the ion on the two sides of a membrane must be equal. These forces are sometimes addressed as **electrochemical potentials:**

$$RT \cdot \ln C_{out} + z\Phi V_{out} = RT \cdot \ln C_{in} + zFV_{in}$$

From this equation, one can calculate the equilibrium potential (V_{eq}) inside the membrane with respect to the potential outside ($V_{eq} = V_{in} - V_{out}$), that is, the potential at which there is no net movement of the ions through the membrane:

$$V_{eq} = \frac{RT}{z\Phi} \ln \frac{C_{out}}{C_{in}} \qquad (1.4)$$

This is the **Nernst equation.** So equilibrium potential, by definition, is an electric potential that induces the movement of an ion across the membrane equal and in the opposite direction to movement of the ion due to the difference in concentrations (note that in figure 1.7, F_c, force due to the difference in concentrations, and F_e, force due to the difference in the electric potentials, are acting in opposite directions). Electric force acting on an ion is directly proportional to its charge; that is, it is twice as high in the case of Ca^{++} as in the case of Na^+ or K^+. It is equal in magnitude and acts in the opposite direction in the case of Cl^- as compared to Na^+.

At body temperature, RT/F is a constant, and so:

$$V_{eq} (\text{in mV}) = \frac{62 \text{ mV}}{z} \log_{10} \frac{C_{out}}{C_{in}} \qquad (1.5)$$

Note the following properties of the equilibrium potential:

1. This is a measure of the concentration ratio for an ion, which has the meaning of energy available for diffusion.
2. This is a potential when there is no net passive movement of an ion across the membrane.
3. This is actual voltage on the membrane, but only if just one ion species can move through it (e.g., if there is just one kind of channel as in squid

axon membrane, which is permeable, at rest, only to K^+).

Problem 1.4

In which direction will electric current flow across a membrane if potential inside the membrane is higher than V_{eq}? Solve for Na^+ and for Cl^-.

The direction of the current is defined by the potential on the membrane, while its magnitude is defined by Ohm's law. So, for example, electric current due to movement of K^+ ions will be:

$$I_k = g_k(V - V_k) \qquad (1.6)$$

where I is current, g_k is the conductance for K^+, V is voltage, and V_k is equilibrium voltage for K^+. Note that g is not a constant and may change quickly. Note also that the concentration gradients do not change much during brief events such as action potential. So virtually all ion movements through the membrane will be defined by Equation 1.6.

Chapter 1 in a Nutshell

Complex systems are more than an assembly of elements and should be studied with adequate sets of notions. Biological membranes are unique structures that allow cells to interact with the environment and be separate from it. Particles in solutions can move among compartments under the influence of differences in pressure, differences in concentration, and electrical field. Osmosis is a process of movement of the solvent, rather than solute, across the membrane, in order to equilibrate concentrations of all particles. Equilibrium potential is a potential on a membrane that creates an electrical force acting on charged particles, which is equal to and opposes the force due to the difference in particle concentrations.

CHAPTER 2

ACTION POTENTIAL

Action potential is the most important unit of information transmission in the bodies of higher animals. Its importance is immense. In lower animals, information within the body is transmitted mostly by diffusion and convection, that is, by bulk flow of liquids containing important chemical substances. This mechanism of information transmission is called **humoral,** and its speed is limited by the rate of liquid flow under the difference in pressure. In the process of evolution, the emergence of the ion mechanism leading to the generation and transmission of action potential signified a many-fold increase in the speed of information processing and conduction, giving species that possessed this "novelty" a significant advantage in the everlasting competition of life. The humoral mechanism of information transmission is still present in the higher animals, but all the processes that require quick decision making and quick action take advantage of the much faster, electrochemical mechanism. Some of the properties and limitations of movements of higher animals (including humans) are rather directly linked to the mechanism of generation and transmission of action potentials.

2.1. CREATION OF MEMBRANE POTENTIAL

Consider a membrane separating a volume into two halves (figure 2.1). Initially, there is no NaCl to the right of the membrane, and there is some to the left. Note that

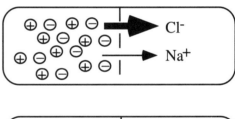
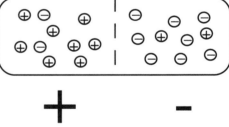

Figure 2.1 A membrane is separating two areas, with and without ions of Na$^+$ and Cl$^-$. Diffusion of these ions may occur at different speeds. As a result, a new equilibrium will be reached with different ion concentrations to the right and to the left, when the electric force will exactly compensate for the concentration gradient force.

there is no voltage across the membrane because the number of ions of Na$^+$ to the left of the membrane is exactly the same as the number of ions of Cl$^-$. Diffusion will begin because of the concentration gradient. However, different ions may move at different velocities. In our case, Cl$^-$ moves faster. Then, when the concentration of ions on both sides is equal, there will be a little bit more of Cl⁻ to the right and a little bit more of Na⁺ to the left. Thus an electric potential will emerge across the membrane, or, more precisely, a difference of potentials. Note that the potential is being created not by all the ions but only by a tiny fraction that is not balanced. For example, the extra amount of ions to create a potential of 100 mV (a typical value for membrane potentials) is only 10^{-12} M (1 picomole) for the area of membrane of 1 cm². All biological potentials are created by tiny amounts of unbalanced ions. So, to a good approximation, one can always consider the total concentration of positive ions in a solution to be equal to the total concentration of negative ions.

Problem 2.1

Find an error (an imprecise statement) in the previous paragraph.

Note that membrane behaves like an electric capacitor, that is, a physical structure able to store electric charge in the presence of an external electric field. In particular, as in regular electric capacitors, its ability to store electric charge depends on its surface but not on the volume of the solution. The net (unbalanced) charge (Q) on a membrane equals its capacitance (C) multiplied by voltage (V) across the membrane (figure 2.2):

$$Q = C \cdot V.$$

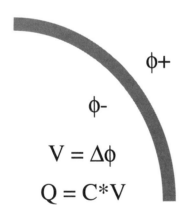

$$\phi+$$
$$\phi-$$
$$V = \Delta\phi$$
$$Q = C*V$$

Figure 2.2 A membrane may be considered a capacitor. Its charge (Q) is proportional to the difference of potentials (V) across the membrane with a coefficient termed capacitance (C).

This is a version of Coulomb's law that is also the definition for capacitance as a coefficient of proportionality between the difference of potentials and stored charge.

When the voltage changes, the charge changes as well. By definition, capacitative current is the change of charge ($I_c = dQ/dt$). So,

$$I_c = C \cdot dV/dt. \qquad (2.1)$$

Note that capacitative current is different from the current created by movement of ions through a membrane. Capacitative current is created by changing electric field, and it does not require any carriers or channels. It may play a significant role in cases of small changes in membrane potential.

There are three important ions that play special roles in the electric phenomena in neurons. These are sodium (Na⁺), potassium (K⁺), and chlorine (Cl⁻). Their concentrations inside and outside a membrane are very different (figure 2.3). Using the Nernst equation, we can calculate equilibrium potentials for these ions.

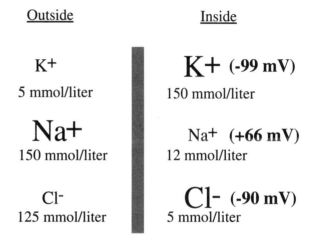

Outside	Inside
K+	K+ (-99 mV)
5 mmol/liter	150 mmol/liter
Na+	Na+ (+66 mV)
150 mmol/liter	12 mmol/liter
Cl-	Cl- (-90 mV)
125 mmol/liter	5 mmol/liter

Figure 2.3 The differences in the concentrations of three most important ions across a typical membrane. Equilibrium potentials for each ion are shown in parentheses.

Problem 2.2

Calculate (approximately) equilibrium potentials for Na⁺, K⁺, and Cl⁻.

The difference in ion concentrations inside and outside the membrane is maintained actively and this process requires energy. This mechanism is commonly called the **sodium-potassium pump.** Figure 2.4 shows schematically how the pump works in receiving energy from adenosinetriphosphate (ATP) stored in mitochondria and breaking it down to adenosinediphosphate (ADP).

Let us imagine that a number of ions, for example K⁺, Na⁺, and Cl⁻, can cross a membrane through the same channels and thus are in competition. Membrane potential will be defined according to Equation 1.5:

$$V = 62 \text{ mV} \cdot \log_{10} \frac{P_K C_{Kout} + P_{Na} C_{Naout} + P_{Cl} C_{Clin}}{P_K C_{Kin} + P_{Na} C_{Nain} + P_{Cl} C_{Clout}} \qquad (2.2)$$

Outside   Inside

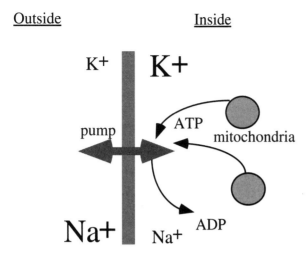

Figure 2.4 Maintaining the ion concentration gradients across the membrane requires energy, which is provided by chemical processes that transform ATP (stored in mitochondria) into ADP. This mechanism is called the sodium-potassium pump.

where P is permeability of membrane for, and C is concentration of, an ion (note the subscripts K, Na, and Cl) in and out of the cell. This is the **Goldman-Hodgkin-Katz equation.**

If the channels are perfectly selective, the equation will look like this:

$$V = \frac{g_{Na}E_{Na} + g_K E_K + g_{Cl}E_{Cl}}{g_{Na} + g_K + g_{Cl}} \qquad (2.3)$$

where g is conductance and E is equilibrium potential for a given ion. You may consider g as the number of open channels for a particular ion. Then, the more channels that are open, the bigger the contribution of the equilibrium potential of this ion to the total potential on the membrane. Equation 2.3 is a decent approximation, since membrane channels are rather specific. However, note that it is not applicable during fast changes in membrane potential, for example, during the action potential.

Problem 2.3

Why is Equation 2.3 inadequate during fast changes in membrane potential? What has not been taken into account? Why, in Equation 2.2, are members for Cl⁻ represented differently than those for K⁺ and for Na⁺?

2.2. BASIC FEATURES OF ACTION POTENTIAL

The word "potential" has quite a few meanings. We will now consider a process, a time function of transmembrane voltage that is called "action potential." Don't confuse this with membrane potential, which is a number describing the state of a membrane at a particular instant of time.

One of the most interesting features of action potential is its threshold nature. Imagine that an electrical stimulator is placed on a membrane and that it applies short pulses of electric current through the membrane (figure 2.5). At low values of the stimulating current, the membrane will respond with a small change in its potential that will rather quickly return to the equilibrium (or resting) value. The stimulus will certainly spread, because

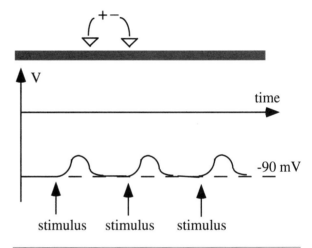

Figure 2.5 If you stimulate a membrane with relatively small electrical stimuli, its resting potential will change somewhat in response to each stimulus and then will return to its resting level.

electric field spreads, but it will not spread far because the electric field drops quickly with distance from the source of stimulation. So the maximal deviation of the membrane potential from its resting value will be seen at the site of stimulation.

If the stimulating current is increased gradually, the deviation of the membrane potential will also increase (figure 2.6), and at a certain value of the stimulus, a miracle will happen: the membrane will respond with a disproportionally huge change in its potential. The value of membrane potential at which this qualitative change occurs is termed **membrane threshold** or **stimulation threshold.** If the stimulus continues to increase, surpris-

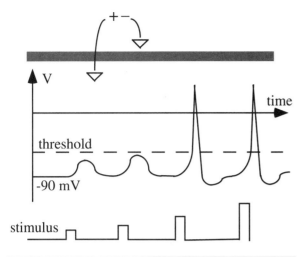

Figure 2.6 An increase in the stimulation current will lead, at low values, to a gradual increase in the deviation of the membrane potential from its resting level. At some value of the stimulus, an action potential will be generated. Further increase in the strength of the stimulation will not lead to a change in the membrane response.

ingly, no further change will occur. The membrane will react with exactly the same action potential. This feature of the action potential, either to be of a standard height or not to be at all, without any intermediate behavior, is termed the **law of "all-or-none."**

Problem 2.4

Suggest examples of the law of all-or-none from everyday life.

Please note that I am addressing transmembrane potentials, that is, the difference between the potential inside the membrane and the potential outside the membrane. If a couple of measuring electrodes are placed outside the membrane, they can record a difference of potentials between the electrodes but not across the membrane. Extracellular potentials are typically much smaller in amplitude than the action potential (by a factor of one thousandth!). Similarly, if a membrane is stimulated by a pair of extracellular electrodes, rather high currents are needed because the extracellular solution and the membrane effectively shield the inside of the cell from the effects of externally applied currents. You will need to keep this in mind when you do the Laboratories.

Let us perform a mental experiment and insert a very thin stimulating electrode through the membrane into a cell so that the integrity of the membrane is not violated (figure 2.7). If we now apply current that makes the voltage in the cell more negative, the change in the membrane potential will be called **hyperpolarization.** A current in the opposite direction will induce a change in the transmembrane potential called **depolarization.** Both hyperpolarization and depolarization spread electrotonically; that is, they affect neighboring areas of the membrane but quickly become smaller and disappear.

Let me now move to the mechanism of the generation of action potential.

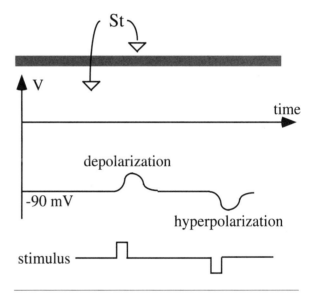

Figure 2.7 A thin electrode is inserted into the cell without breaking the membrane. Now we can apply electrical current to change the membrane resting potential.

2.3. MECHANISM OF GENERATION OF ACTION POTENTIAL

First, it is important to realize that *action potential emerges because of the dependence of membrane permeability to certain ions upon membrane potential.*

Let us consider an example (figure 2.8). There is only one ion that can move through special channels in a membrane. Each channel is being guarded by a demon who sometimes falls asleep. The probability of the demon's falling asleep depends on membrane potential so that at rest, all the demons are awake and do not let the ions cross the membrane. Short-lasting pulses of stimulation

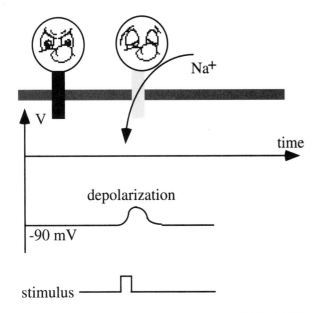

Figure 2.8   A demon is guarding each channel for Na⁺ in the membrane. Membrane depolarization makes some of the demons fall asleep, so that their channels become open. Ions will cross the membrane and increase the depolarization, putting more demons to sleep.

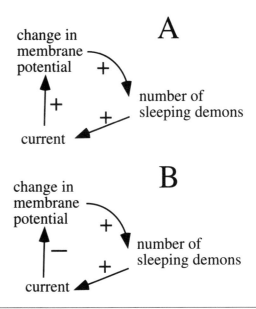

Figure 2.9   A positive feedback process (A) leads to rapid amplification of the effect, while a negative feedback process (B) quickly restores the original state.

can be applied, changing the membrane potential. A depolarizing pulse puts some of the demons to sleep so that some ions can cross the membrane. The more demons are asleep, the bigger the current created by the ions. Note, however, that *the current itself will change the membrane potential.*

There are two major possibilities:

1. The current hyperpolarizes the membrane and therefore wakes up some of the demons, who quickly start closing the gates and restoring the resting potential.

2. The current further depolarizes the membrane, that is, works in the same direction as the stimulus. Then the current puts more demons to sleep, thus opening more channels, thus increasing the current, thus putting to sleep more demons . . . and so on.

The process described in the second example is called **positive feedback** (figure 2.9), while the first possibility corresponds to **negative feedback.** Apparently, systems with positive feedback are capable of generating large signals very quickly, while systems with negative feedback generally tend to bring any "perturbing" signal down to zero.

A very similar mechanism gives rise to the all-or-none signal that propagates along a nerve: depolarization increases membrane permeability to a certain ion, while increased permeability induces membrane current that increases depolarization.

One can study the mechanisms involved in the process of generation of action potential with the voltage-clamp technique. This technique is used to keep membrane potential at a certain level with the aid of external electronics that adds charges to or removes them from the membrane, thus keeping the potential constant (like a thermostat keeping room temperature constant by adding or removing heat). These conditions do not allow the positive feedback mechanism to generate an action potential, but they allow the experimenter to study the dependence of conductance in specialized ion channels upon membrane potential.

Figure 2.10 shows the dependence of the sodium conductance (g_{Na}) upon voltage after a depolarizing voltage step is applied to the membrane. Note that g_{Na} turns off spontaneously; that is, it goes down to its original, very low value without an obvious additional external stimulus, even when the membrane voltage is kept constant artificially (shown by the "Stim" line in figure 2.10). At higher stimulation voltages, peak values of g_{Na} are much higher and the turnoffs occur faster. Note also that the time it takes g_{Na} to reach peak value is shorter for larger stimuli while for g_K it is almost unchanged. When the conductance for both major ions, Na⁺ and K⁺, is increased, one can say that the sodium-potassium pump becomes functionally disabled, and membrane potential changes are primarily defined by ion movement through the open channels.

If the voltage is turned off, that is, if the membrane potential is allowed to return to its resting value, g_{Na} goes down if it is not zero already.

There is an important phenomenon of **inactivation,** which means that after a spontaneous turnoff, g_{Na} cannot

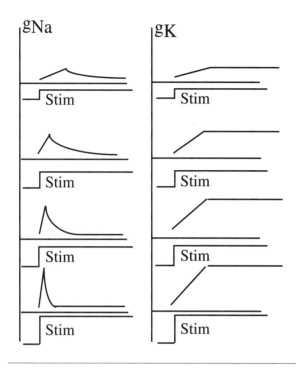

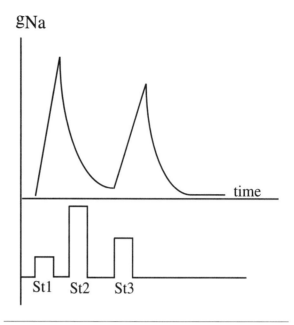

Figure 2.10 A constant depolarization is applied to the membrane. Note that Na⁺ conductance (g_{Na}) turns on and off while K⁺ conductance (g_K) changes slowly and stays at a new level. Note also that higher stimuli lead to higher values of g_{Na} achieved in shorter times.

Figure 2.11 After a stimulus (St_1) leads to an increase in g_{Na}, another stimulus is less able to turn it on for some time. For a short period of time this inactivation is absolute, i.e., g_{Na} will not respond even to a very strong stimulus (St_2, absolute refractory period). Later, a stronger-than-usual stimulus can turn g_{Na} on (St_3, relative refractory period).

be increased immediately even if you apply a very strong voltage (figure 2.11). It needs some time to recover. When the conductance cannot be increased by any external voltage, the nerve is said to be in an **absolute refractory period.** When higher-than-usual voltages are needed to increase the conductance but this can be done, the nerve is said to be in a **relative refractory period.** Refractory periods can be seen in physiological studies that you will perform in the Labs.

So, the channels can close in response to a change of membrane potential, and also "by themselves" when they get tired and require some time to recover. In the first case, one can open the channels with an external depolarizing stimulus; in the second case, the only available method is to wait.

Figure 2.10 also shows the dependence of potassium conductance (g_K) on membrane potential. Note that g_K starts to increase with depolarization but does not turn off spontaneously. It goes down to its original value only when the membrane potential returns to its resting level. This means that there is no inactivation, or no refractory period, for potassium channels. Note also that g_K increases more slowly than g_{Na}, which means that at the beginning of membrane depolarization, sodium channels will play a bigger role.

As can be seen from the figures already shown, both g_{Na} and g_K behave "smoothly" with membrane voltage;

that is, they do not show any threshold effects. In order to understand the mechanisms giving rise to the all-or-none action potential, one needs to remove the voltage clamp and allow the potential to change.

Let me note that opening channels for sodium and potassium leads to different consequences for the membrane potential because of the difference in the concentration of Na⁺ and K⁺ ions inside and outside the cell. An increase in g_K, for example, induced by a short depolarizing pulse, leads to a flow of K⁺ out of the cell. The loss of positive ions leads to a drop in the membrane potential (remember, membrane potential is measured inside the cell with respect to the outside), that is, to a decrease in depolarization or to hyperpolarization. This in turn will lead to a drop in g_K. So here is a system with a negative feedback that will quickly restore the original resting potential. An increase in g_{Na}, however, will lead to an inflow of Na⁺ inside the cell, that is, to a further depolarization. Here one deals with a system with a positive feedback that, as is well known, loves to go berserk. Different dependencies of g_{Na} and g_K on membrane potential, together with the property of sodium channels to inactivate, lead to the generation of the action potential.

Remember that the direction of flow of an ion depends on its equilibrium potential and not only on absolute potential on the membrane. So the difference between actual membrane potential and the equilibrium potential of an ion will define the direction in which the ion will flow. On the other hand, an ion with a higher permeability plays a bigger role in defining the total membrane potential than do ions with smaller permeabilities. This means that changes in g_{Na} and g_K can lead to changes in equilibrium membrane potential.

Figure 2.12 shows a diagram of action potential and the changes in g_{Na} and g_K in different phases of the potential. The sequence of events is as follows: (1) the initial depolarization (created by an external stimulus) increases g_{Na} so that the membrane potential tries to reach sodium equilibrium potential; (2) after a brief delay, g_K increases and draws membrane potential to its equilibrium potential, that is, repolarizes the membrane; (3) there is a rather long period of hyperpolarization (the afterpotential), after which membrane potential returns to its resting value.

Problem 2.5

Why does the membrane potential drop below the resting level? Can you imagine a situation in which the afterpotential will be higher than the resting potential?

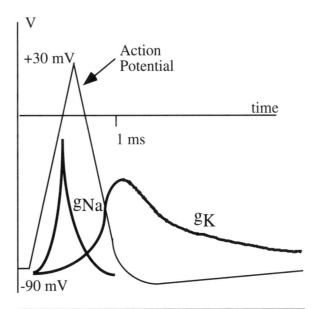

Figure 2.12   Changes in Na⁺ and K⁺ conductance during an action potential. Note that the peak of the action potential is positive, and that after the action potential the membrane remains hyperpolarized for some time.

Chapter 2 in a Nutshell

Action potential is the unit of information transmission within the bodies of higher animals. Membrane potential is created by a small number of unbalanced ions. Movement of ions through the membrane occurs at special sites called ion channels. An active molecular mechanism, a sodium-potassium pump, maintains the difference in the concentrations of sodium and potassium ions across the membrane. The dependence of the sodium ions' conductance on the membrane potential leads to the generation of an action potential when membrane depolarization reaches its threshold. After an action potential, the membrane stays in a short-lasting state of insensitivity due to inactivation of sodium channels.

CHAPTER 3

INFORMATION CONDUCTION AND TRANSMISSION

Key Terms

conduction of action
    potential

information transmission in
    the central nervous system

myelinated and
    nonmyelinated axons

neuron

synapse

synaptic transmission

neurotransmitters

temporal and spatial
    summation

As mentioned earlier, action potential is probably the most important process in our body because it is used for information transmission over considerable distances within the neuromuscular system. Its important feature is propagation; that is, an action potential never stays at one place but rather travels along nerve or muscular fibers. When speaking about a time function that travels along something, it is necessary to define precisely how to measure the velocity of this propagation. If a nerve is stimulated (I will discuss later what this means and how it can be done) at a certain point, an action potential may occur at this point. If membrane potential is recorded further down the nerve fiber (or further up, because the potential propagates in both directions), a similar time function will be seen; that is, a similar action potential will occur, although at a time delay after the first one (figure 3.1). Now, one needs to pick a well-defined point on the action potential curve—for example, time of its peak, or some other time—and measure the time interval from the moment when this point occurs at the first location to the moment when it occurs at the

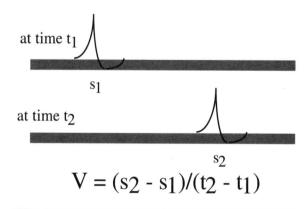

Figure 3.1 Action potential travels along a neural fiber. For calculation of the velocity of its propagation (V), it needs to be recorded at two different locations at different times.

second location: $\Delta T = T_2 - T_1$. If the distance between the two points (ΔS) is known, the average velocity of transmission can be calculated:

$$V = \Delta S / \Delta T. \qquad (3.1)$$

17

3.1. CONDUCTION OF ACTION POTENTIAL

When an action potential occurs in a certain segment of a cellular membrane, it sets up local current circuits that flow to the neighboring segments largely according to Ohm's law, that is, without any help from pumps, channels, and other sophisticated mechanisms. The charge leaks through the membrane capacitance according to Equation 2.1 in chapter 2. Figure 3.2 shows schematically a simplified electrical system simulating a membrane and the currents that flow within this system. The local currents depolarize the membrane, and if the depolarization is strong enough, another action potential, or more than one, can occur. So, strictly speaking, the action potential does not travel along a membrane of a neural fiber but rather emerges at different spots and disappears, giving rise to new potentials. However, since all the potentials look alike (remember the law of all-or-none), the process looks as if one potential were traveling along the fiber.

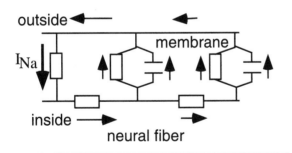

Figure 3.2   A simple electrical scheme of a membrane and the directions of local currents (shown by arrows).

Two factors are very important for the process of propagation of the action potential:

1. Inactivation of sodium channels leading to the absolute refractory period within an area of the membrane just after an action potential
2. Different density of sodium channels at different sections of a membrane

The first factor does not allow an action potential to "backfire" during its natural propagation along a fiber. That is, if an action potential appeared at point 1 in figure 3.3 at time T_1, and then disappeared giving rise to an action potential at a neighboring point 2 at T_2, the membrane at point 1 would be inactive and could not be excited by local currents created by the second action potential. So, the second action potential at point 2 could excite the membrane at point 3, but not "back" at point 1.

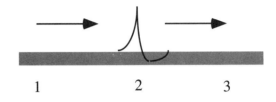

Figure 3.3   The phenomenon of inactivation of sodium channels does not allow an action potential to "backfire." If an action potential comes to point 2 from point 1, it cannot go back, and travels only forward to point 3.

The second factor makes some areas of the membrane more readily excitable and therefore favors the generation of an action potential in these particular areas.

The process of generation of a single action potential is brief, but nevertheless it takes time, while local currents spread virtually instantaneously. Let us consider two neural fibers. An action potential has just emerged in both at point A in figure 3.4. The local currents generated by the action potential spread in the surrounding tissue and decrease very quickly with distance from point A. However, the currents spread more easily and decrease at larger distances in thick fibers as compared to thin fibers. So the next most distant action potential will be generated in fiber 1 at point B and in fiber 2 at point C. Note that it will take the same time for the potential to "travel" distance B-A in fiber 1 and distance C-A in fiber 2. We have come to the conclusion that thick fibers conduct action potentials at higher velocities.

Although action potentials generally have the same shape ("all-or-none"), their width can change in certain special circumstances. Wider action potentials induce larger local currents and can bring more distant areas of the membrane to its threshold. Figure 3.5 illustrates the dependence between the pulse duration and pulse strength needed to just reach the threshold at a certain point on a

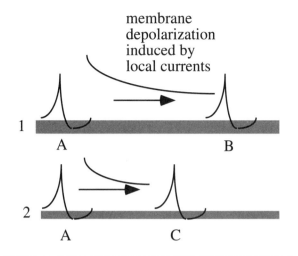

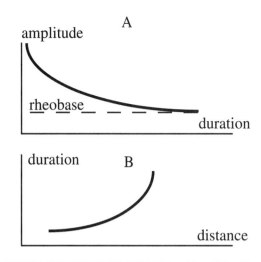

Figure 3.4 Action potentials emerged simultaneously at the same point A in fibers 1 and 2. Local currents decrease more slowly with distance in the larger fiber 1. Thus, they will bring the membrane to the threshold at a more distant point. So the next action potential will emerge at the same delay at point B in fiber 1 and point C in fiber 2.

Figure 3.5 A: The dependence between stimulus duration and its amplitude needed to just reach the threshold of the membrane. B: The dependence between stimulus duration and maximal distance at which membrane potential can reach the threshold for a constant amplitude of the stimulus.

membrane (A) and between pulse duration and maximal distance at which membrane potential can reach the threshold for a constant amplitude of the pulse (B). Note that there is the lowest strength of a stimulus (rheobase) below which an increase in the duration is unable to induce an action potential.

3.2. MYELINATED FIBERS

Some neural fibers, particularly the thickest ones, are covered with a kind of protective sheath made of **my-** elin that is built of special non-neuronal, **glial** cells. Myelin sheath has breaks that are called **Ranvier nodes** (figure 3.6). This design allows the action potential to travel at much higher speeds than in fibers without a myelin sheath. **Myelinated fibers** have two important features. First, the myelin sheath increases the distance at which local currents from an action potential are able to reach the threshold of membrane depolarization. Second, the sodium channels are concentrated in Ranvier nodes, so that their density there is much higher than "normal" and their density under the myelin sheath is much lower. As a result, if an action potential occurs at a Ranvier node, it gives rise to local currents that bring

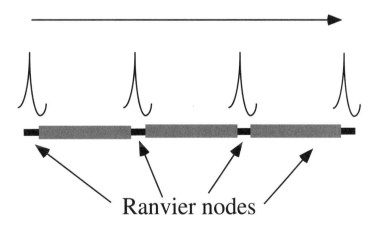

Figure 3.6 A myelinated fiber is enclosed in a sheath made of non-neural cells (glial cells). The myelin sheath has breaks (Ranvier nodes) where action potentials are generated.

the membrane to the threshold at a neighboring node, and the action potential in a sense jumps from one node to another. This leads to a considerable increase in conduction velocity. Once again, thicker fibers have larger intervals between neighboring Ranvier nodes and therefore conduct action potentials at higher velocities. There is a very simple equation relating the diameter of a myelinated fiber and the conduction velocity of action potential:

$$V = 6d \qquad (3.2)$$

where V is velocity in m/s and d is fiber diameter in microns. Note that this equation is not applicable to non-myelinated fibers.

Problem 3.3

What will happen if a myelinated fiber suddenly loses its sheath? What can you expect from such a fiber in a hot bath and in a cold bath? Note that ion diffusion proceeds much more quickly at high temperatures.

Table 3.1 compares the velocities of various processes. Note that speeds of conduction in our body are rather high, but not extremely high. Certainly they cannot be compared to the speed of light, which is equal to the speed of propagation of electromagnetic field.

Problem 3.4

The nature of action potential is electric. Why is the speed of its propagation so much lower than the speed of electric events like electric current?

Table 3.1   Characteristic Velocities of Different Processes (in meters per second)

Slow nerve conduction	0.5
Sprint	10
Speed limit (55 mph)	25
Fast nerve conduction	120
Sound in air	330
Light or electromagnetic field	300,000,000

Problem 3.5

The highest speed of neural conduction is actually comparable to the highest movement velocities observed in athletes. Does this mean that there is an upper limit for movement velocity set by action potential conduction speed?

Knowing speeds of conduction is very important for understanding many neurophysiological processes that include conduction of information from one place within the body to another. Frequently, these conduction delays dominate in the total time delay between a stimulus and a response. You will see examples in several of the Laboratory experiments you will perform.

Readers will encounter a few classifications within this textbook. One of the most helpful and commonly used is the classification of neural fibers according to their diameter and function, sensory versus motor—or, to use a different pair of terms accepted in neurophysiology, **afferent** versus **efferent.** The classification was suggested by a great physiologist, D. Lloyd, and is illustrated in table 3.2.

3.3. THE STRUCTURE OF THE NEURON

Before moving further, let me introduce certain basic notions related to the structure of a single neural cell (a neuron). Figure 3.7 shows a schematic drawing of a "typical neuron." The neuron consists of three major parts: **soma, axon,** and **dendrites.**

The **soma** or body of the neuron contains the **nucleus** (or nuclei) and other important small structures (so-called **organelles**); from these I will single out the mitochondria, which are major storage places and sources of release of molecules whose chemical transformations generate energy for the processes inside the cell, in particular for the sodium-potassium pump.

The **axon** is a long, rather thick branch that carries the output signals generated by the cell. At its end, the axon is divided into many smaller, thin branches (terminal branches) that make contacts with other cells and transduce information to these cells. These branches are commonly much shorter than the axon. Axons can be very long, up to 1 m; an example is the axon of a motoneuron—whose soma is located in the spinal cord, while it sends signals to a muscle in a foot. There are long axons of neurons within the cen-

Table 3.2 Types of Neural Fibers (Axons) and Speed of Conduction of Action Potentials

Type	Innervated structure	Fiber diameter (microns)	Conduction velocity (m/s)
Afferent or sensory (muscle nerve; classification for cutaneous nerves shown in parentheses)			
Ia (Aα)	Muscle spindle, primary endings	13-20	80-120
Ib (Aα)	Golgi tendon organ	13-20	80-120
II (Aβ)	Muscle spindle, secondary endings	6-12	40-80
III (Aδ)	Muscle deep pressure endings	1-5	5-30
IV (C)	Nociceptors (pain)	0.2-1.5	0.5-2
Efferent or motor			
Aα	Skeletal muscles	18	100
Aβ	Muscles and spindles	8	50
Aγ	Muscle spindle	5	20

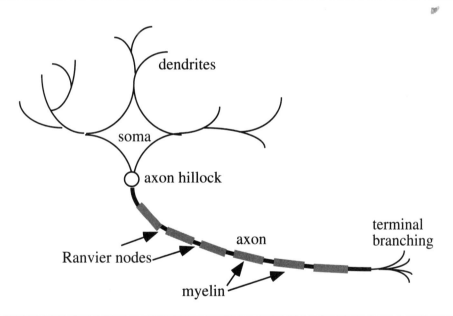

Figure 3.7 A cartoon picture of a "typical neuron."

tral nervous system as well, for example, axons of neurons in the brain that send their signals to neurons in the lower parts of the spinal cord. The place where the axon exits the soma is called the **axon hillock.** At this place the density of sodium channels is very high, so this is the place where action potentials are normally being generated.

Problem 3.6

What will happen if you stimulate an axon with a strong electrical impulse somewhere in the middle of its length? In which direction will the action potential propagate? Why?

Dendrites form a tree around the soma and serve as sites of inputs into the cell. Terminal branches of the axons of other cells make connections (**synapses**) on the dendrites as well as on the soma itself.

Basically, dendrites and soma serve as sites where information comes to the neuron from other neurons and is integrated (assessed, compared, and put together); the axon hillock is the place where action potentials are generated in response to the incoming information, and the axon serves to conduct action potentials to distant places and to transmit information to other cells.

3.4. INFORMATION CODING IN THE NERVOUS SYSTEM

Because of the law of all-or-none, individual neurons can generate only single action potentials of a relatively constant duration and amplitude. Thus, an action potential by itself transmits only 1 byte of information. It either occurs or does not occur. The only way a neuron can encode significant amounts of information is by generating sequences of action potentials. In other words, information is coded by changing the **frequency of firing.** Note that here I mean **instantaneous frequency** of neuronal firing, that is, an inverse of the time delay between two successive action potentials:

$$F_i = 1/(T_2 - T_1) \qquad (3.3)$$

where T_2 and T_1 are times of occurrence of two successive action potentials. Intervals between successive action potentials fluctuate all the time, even if the apparent input to the neuron stays constant. So neurons never fire at a constant frequency, and should be characterized either by instantaneous frequency or by average frequency of firing. Some neurons can demonstrate bursts of action potentials at a relatively high frequency separated by intervals of silence; in such cases, one number is apparently not enough to describe the behavior.

This type of information transmission is called "frequency coding" or "frequency modulation." However, if one considers groups of neurons, frequency coding loses its exclusive right as the only way to transmit information in the central nervous system. The ability of neurons to integrate incoming information (see discussion of spatial and temporal summation further on in this chapter) allows them to take into account both the timing of incoming action potentials and their number. So the firing rate (instantaneous frequency of firing) of a neuron depends on both the frequency and the magnitude of its input.

3.5. SYNAPTIC TRANSMISSION

A very important feature of neurons is the ability both to conduct information from one place to another and to transmit it to other cells. Transmission of information from one cell to another occurs at specialized sites on the membranes of the two cells. At these sites, the membranes come very close to each other and form a **synapse.** A synapse consists of three major components: **presynaptic membrane, postsynaptic membrane,** and **synaptic cleft** (figure 3.8). The presynaptic membrane belongs to the cell that transmits information (coded as a sequence of action potentials), while the postsynaptic membrane belongs to the cell that receives the information.

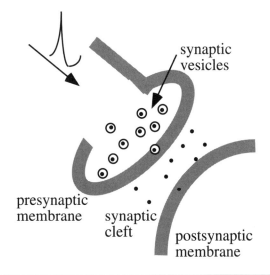

Figure 3.8 A synapse consists of a presynaptic membrane, a synaptic cleft, and a postsynaptic membrane. An action potential in a presynaptic fiber makes synaptic vesicles move to the membrane, fuse with it, and release molecules of a neurotransmitter into the cleft. The neurotransmitter acts at the postsynaptic membrane and changes its potential.

There are two major groups of synapses, **obligatory and nonobligatory.** If an action potential on the presynaptic membrane always gives rise to an action potential on the postsynaptic membrane, such a synapse is called obligatory. Typical examples of obligatory synapses are those between neural cells and muscle cells. Nonobligatory synapses are much more common within the nervous system: a single action potential on a presynaptic membrane is typically unable to induce an action potential on a postsynaptic membrane.

Neuron-to-neuron synaptic transmission uses numerous chemical substances called **neurotransmitters** or **synaptic mediators.** Neurotransmitters are normally synthesized by the presynaptic neuron and stored in special reservoirs (vesicles) close to the presynaptic membrane. The typical scheme of synaptic transmission is as follows (figure 3.8):

1. An action potential arrives to the presynaptic membrane.
2. It induces chemical changes that lead to movement of vesicles with a neurotransmitter to the presynaptic membrane, to their fusing with the membrane, and to release of the neurotransmitter molecules into the synaptic cleft. This process is called **exocytosis.**
3. The molecules of the neurotransmitter travel across the cleft by **diffusion.**
4. They act at special sites (receptors) on the postsynaptic membrane and change its potential.
5. These molecules are quickly removed from the synaptic cleft by a special chemical substance (an enzyme) or are taken back into the presynaptic membrane.

Molecules of neurotransmitters bind to receptor sites on the postsynaptic membrane and induce one of two basic effects: they can depolarize the membrane or they can hyperpolarize it (figure 3.9). In the first case, a small depolarizing potential, which is called **excitatory postsynaptic potential or EPSP,** will appear. In the second case, a small hyperpolarizing potential, which is called **inhibitory postsynaptic potential or IPSP,** will emerge. In response to a single presynaptic action potential, postsynaptic potentials last for about 15 ms and then disappear. When a number of action potentials come to presynaptic membranes that make synapses with the same postsynaptic membrane, the balance of EPSPs and IPSPs on the postsynaptic membrane will define whether the potential reaches the threshold, and whether an action potential is generated.

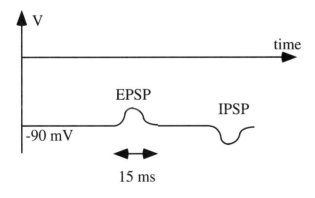

Figure 3.9 A presynaptic action potential can induce either a depolarization or a hyperpolarization of the postsynaptic membrane. These effects are called EPSP and IPSP, respectively.

3.6. NEUROTRANSMITTERS

There are three major groups of neurotransmitters: **amino acids, biogenic amines,** and **peptides.**

Amino acids are building blocks for all proteins and are very common in our bodies, and in the nervous system in particular. Not all the amino acids act as neurotransmitters. One of the most frequently encountered neurotransmitters is **gamma-aminobutyric acid,** or **GABA.** It can be found in a significant proportion of all synapses (about 25% to 40%). Among dominant excitatory neurotransmitters, let me mention **glutamic acid** and **leucine.** They depolarize the postsynaptic membrane and thus bring it closer to the threshold for generation of an action potential. **Glycine** is an inhibitory mediator found in the spinal cord in particular.

Biogenic amines are found in smaller quantities than amino acids. There are several biological amines whose role as neurotransmitters is particularly important. These are **acetylcholine, serotonin, dopamine,** and **norepinephrine.** Their action on the postsynaptic membrane is not as unambiguous as that of GABA and glutamic acid. In particular, acetylcholine commonly exerts inhibitory effects on postsynaptic neurons within the central nervous system, but it is also the most important excitatory mediator in transmission of signals from neurons to muscle fibers.

Neuropeptides are encountered in very small quantities and therefore were overlooked for many years. They generally modulate synaptic efficacy of other neurotransmitters. Typical examples are **endorphines** and **enkephalins** acting at specific receptor sites that can also be taken by certain drugs, such as opiates.

3.7. TEMPORAL AND SPATIAL SUMMATION

It has already been mentioned that neuron-neuronal synapses are mostly nonobligatory. This means that one presynaptic action potential is unable to force the postsynaptic membrane to generate an action potential. Such stimuli are called **subthreshold.** In order to generate an action potential, the postsynaptic membrane needs somehow to sum up the effects of a number of presynaptic signals. There are two basic ways of doing this.

The first way is based on the fact that most EPSPs are of a relatively long duration (about 15 ms). So if another action potential comes to the same synapse at a delay smaller than the typical duration of the EPSP, its postsynaptic effects will superimpose on the effects on the previous signal and lead to a larger EPSP (figure 3.10). This mechanism is called **temporal**

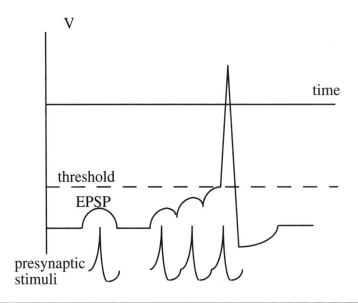

Figure 3.10 Temporal summation occurs when several action potentials arrive at a presynaptic membrane at intervals that do not allow individual EPSPs to disappear. Their effects can sum up and induce an action potential.

summation. A sequence of presynaptic action potentials may be able to bring the postsynaptic potential to the membrane threshold while a single potential is unable to do this.

Problem 3.7

What is the minimal frequency of presynaptic action potentials that can theoretically lead to temporal summation and to a postsynaptic action potential?

Another mechanism is based on the fact that a postsynaptic membrane can receive many presynaptic inputs located close to each other; it is also based on the existence of local currents through the membrane and in the surrounding media. When a presynaptic action potential induces a subthreshold EPSP (figure 3.11), the membrane depolarizes in an area that is in direct contact with the neurotransmitters released by the presynaptic membrane. Local currents spread this depolarization to neighboring areas of the postsynaptic membrane, certainly with a decrement in its amplitude. So if other synapses are located nearby (synapses 2 and 3 in figure 3.11), the postsynaptic membrane may "feel" the effects of the local currents from all the synapses (1, 2, and 3). If action potentials come simultaneously to all three synapses, the depolarization of the postsynaptic membrane in synapses will be bigger than in response to only its own action potential. This effect is called **spatial summation.**

Problem 3.8

What will happen if action potentials to synapses 1, 2, and 3 come not simultaneously but at a delay?

The mechanisms of temporal and spatial summation are examples of how postsynaptic membrane can integrate information coming from presynaptic cells. These mechanisms make it possible to transfer signals through nonobligatory synapses.

Problem 3.9

Imagine that two groups of neurons (A and B) send their signals to another group of neurons (C). Action potentials generated simultaneously by all the neurons of group A lead to a response C_1 (the number of activated neurons in group C); action potentials generated simultaneously by all the neurons of group B lead to a response C_2. What can be the magnitude of the response to action potentials in all the neurons in both groups A and B? Can it be bigger than, smaller than, or equal to $(C_1 + C_2)$? Why?

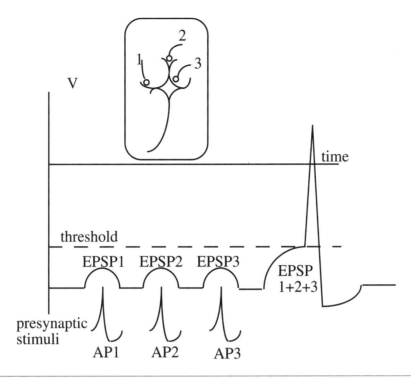

Figure 3.11 Spatial summation occurs when several action potentials AP1, AP2, and AP3 arrive simultaneously at different synapses on the same postsynaptic membrane so that their individual EPSPs sum up and can induce an action potential. The insert shows possible location of the three synapses on the target neuron.

Chapter 3 in a Nutshell

Passive spread of local currents from an action potential leads to depolarization of adjacent segments of the membrane to the threshold and to the generation of a new action potential. Speed of conduction is higher along thick neural fibers. Some fibers are covered with a special substance, myelin, that increases the speed of conduction of action potentials. Information exchange among cells occurs at special sites called synapses. The mechanism of synaptic transmission involves special chemical substances—mediators that can depolarize or hyperpolarize the postsynaptic membrane. Neural cells integrate the incoming information and generate action potentials when the effects of several synapses or several action potentials coming at a high rate are summed up.

CHAPTER 4

THE SKELETAL MUSCLE

Key Terms

skeletal muscle

myofibril

neuro-muscular synapse

excitation-contraction coupling

twitch and tetanic contractions

elements of mechanics

length- and velocity-dependence of muscle force

external regimes or muscle contraction

4.1. SKELETAL MUSCLE: STRUCTURE

Skeletal muscle is a machine (a "motor") that converts chemical energy to mechanical work and heat. It is probably the most amazing motor there is. Its ability to quickly generate power is superior to that of virtually any human-designed motor of approximately the same size. It has numerous features that may seem weird to an external observer. Some of them look rather suboptimal or even bizarre. There are two ways to look at these unique features. The first is to ask oneself: How does the central nervous system cope with (or compensate for) all the "weirdness" of the muscle design, its nonlinearities (you will learn what these are), time delays, and other features that seem terrible when they are looked at through the eyes of a 20th-century engineer? The alternative is to ask: How are the unusual features of the skeletal muscle used by the central nervous system to assure the unique properties of human movements that make them far superior to any robot's—for example, flexibility, quick learning, and the ability to handle fragile objects? I suggest readers forget about the engineering approach and look at the skeletal muscle optimistically—as a unique design created or developed by evolution, and not as a blunder of nature.

When people talk about muscles, they sometimes mean different things. For example, when a person flexes the knee, it is commonly said that the quadriceps muscle is being stretched. In this case, the word "muscle" is used to imply the whole complex of structures including muscle fibers, tendons, and ligaments. However, depending on a number of factors, the whole complex may be stretching while the muscle fibers are shortening. Within this chapter I will first discuss the "naked muscle," that is, the properties of muscle fibers irrespective of the way the force generated by the processes in muscle fibers is transferred by tendons and creates torques in joints. The role of tendons will be considered at the end of the chapter.

Whole muscle is composed of parallel fibers (muscle cells). Each fiber is a rather large cell; the fibers may be several centimeters long and from 10 to 100 μm in diameter. Muscle fibers, like any decent cell, have a membrane (**sarcolemma**); inside the sarcolemma is **sarcoplasma** containing **myofilaments** and **sarcoplasmic reticulum.** The structure of a muscle fiber is shown in figure 4.1. The lower part of the figure shows a relatively realistic three-dimensional picture of a muscle fiber, while the upper part presents a simplified two-dimensional section. The sarcolemma has many invaginations that are called T-tubules. They plunge deeply into the interior of the fiber, thus increasing the surface area by a factor of 3 to 10. T-tubules come very close to **cisternae** in sarcoplasmic reticulum. The gap there is very narrow, about 300 Å—even smaller than the typical synaptic cleft.

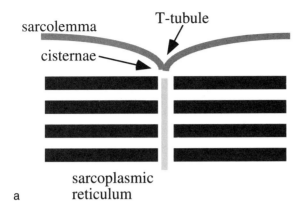

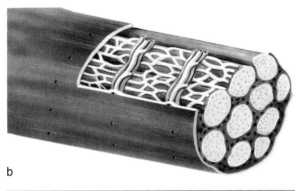

Figure 4.1   The structure of a muscle fiber. The upper part is a schematic representation of a cross section of a fiber, while the lower part shows a more realistic three-dimensional picture. Reprinted, by permission, from J.H. Wilmore and D.L. Costill, 1994, *Physiology of Sport and Exercise* (Champaign, IL: Human Kinetics), 28.

A major role in the mechanism of muscle contraction is played by Ca^{++} ions. Note that a new ion, Ca^{++}, starts to play a major biological role here. At rest, ion pumps pump Ca^{++} ions from sarcoplasma into sarcoplasmic reticulum (similar to what occurs with the sodium-potassium pump). This process, similar to that for other ion pumps, involves specialized macromolecules and requires energy. Sarcoplasmic reticulum contains a special protein that binds Ca^{++} and does not let it escape. As a result, the concentration of Ca^{++} in sarcoplasma is very low (less than 10^{-7} M). I will consider the role of calcium in muscle contraction in the next section.

4.2. MYOFILAMENTS

Myofilaments are major force-producing elements of muscle cells, consisting of two major molecules, **myosin** and **actin** (figure 4.2). Thick filaments contain mostly myosin, while thin filaments contain mostly actin. Actually, thin fibers contain two actin molecules that form a structure resembling a double helix (remember the famous DNA structure?). In order to develop force, the two

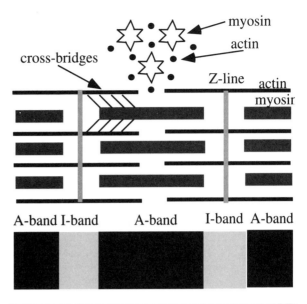

Figure 4.2   The structure of a myofibril. The lower figure shows the sequence of dark and light bands. The upper drawing shows the typical configuration of actin and myosin molecules within a myofibril.

sets of filaments, actin and myosin, must make connections between each other. These connections are called **cross-bridges.** Actin and myosin filaments are organized so that regularly arrayed myosin filaments are surrounded by six actin filaments (like a kitchen floor mosaic), while each actin molecule is in contact with three molecules of myosin. At one end, actin filaments are attached to a structure called the **Z-line.** Two sets of actin filaments and one set of myosin filaments between two Z-lines constitute a **sarcomere.** Sarcomeres are the most important functional units of myofibrils acting to produce muscle force. In order to characterize the state of a myofibril, two more terms are used: the length of the myosin filaments within a sarcomere is called the **A-band,** while the length of actin filaments that do not overlap with myosin filaments is called an **I-band.** These bands are clearly seen under a strong microscope as alternating dark (A-band) and light (I-band) zones (figure 4.2).

There are two more important protein molecules that play major roles in the mechanism of muscle contraction. The first is **tropomyosin.** Its long molecules lie along the actin molecules in thin filaments (figure 4.3). The other is **troponin.** Troponin molecules are attached at regular intervals to tropomyosin molecules, forming a complex that can change its configuration under the action of calcium ions.

4.3. NEUROMUSCULAR SYNAPSE

The **neuromuscular synapse** (or junction) is a region of contact between a single presynaptic fiber (remember that

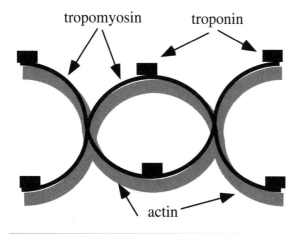

Figure 4.3 The structure of the thin filament (actin). Note long tropomyosin molecules in parallel with the actin strands. Troponin attaches to tropomyosin at regular intervals.

an axon branches, giving rise to many presynaptic fibers) and a muscle fiber. These two fibers come very close to each other so that the synaptic cleft is only about 500 Å wide, but they do not make direct contact (figure 4.4). The presynaptic axonal membrane has **active zones** that contain many synaptic vesicles with a neurotransmitter (acetylcholine) and also a high concentration of mitochondria that store and supply molecules that are metabolized to get energy.

When a decision is made by the central nervous system to induce a muscular contraction, signals eventually go to neurons in the spinal cord (or in the brainstem, for head muscles) that send their long axons to appropriate muscles or, in other words, **innervate** muscles. Action potentials travel at a high speed along these thick efferent fibers and arrive at the point of branching. There, the action potential excites each of the branches so that each delivers an action potential to a presynaptic membrane at about the same time. Neuromuscular synapses are obligatory; that is, a presynaptic action potential always induces a postsynaptic action potential and initiates the process of muscle contraction. This is achieved by an amplification of the incoming signal with chemical mechanisms. The following are the most important steps involved in the process:

Step 1: An action potential arrives at the presynaptic membrane and opens voltage-dependent Ca^{++} channels. Normally the intracellular concentration of Ca^{++} is very low. However, after an action potential arrives, the concentration of Ca^{++} increases dramatically (by a factor of 20). Intracellular Ca^{++} activates processes leading to movement of synaptic vesicles to the presynaptic membrane. The vesicles fuse with the membrane and let their contents out, into the synaptic cleft (**exocytosis**).

Step 2: The neurotransmitter (acetylcholine, ACh) released into the cleft diffuses across the short distance to the postsynaptic membrane and binds to specific molecular receptors on the postsynaptic membrane. There is a very high density of ACh-sensitive receptors on the postsynaptic membrane (up to $10,000/\mu m^2$). Acetylcholine in the synaptic cleft is quickly destroyed by a spe-

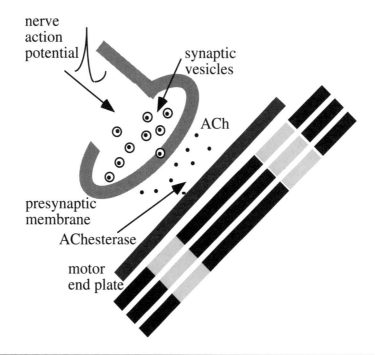

Figure 4.4 Neuromuscular synapse. A presynaptic nerve action potential induces movement of vesicles with acetylcholine to the presynaptic membrane, their fusion, and release of ACh into the cleft. ACh diffuses to the postsynaptic muscle membrane, depolarizes it, and induces an action potential.

cial enzyme, acetylcholinesterase, into two substances, acetate and choline. The presence of this enzyme makes the duration of the postsynaptic effects very brief.

Problem 4.1

Imagine that you have a muscle without acetylcholinesterase. What can you expect in response to a single presynaptic action potential?

Step 3 (figure 4.5): Acetylcholine acts on the postsynaptic membrane and induces changes in its ion permeability leading to a depolarizing potential (EPSP). In muscles, EPSPs induced by presynaptic signals are always suprathreshold, leading to the generation of an action potential on the postsynaptic membrane. Note that subthreshold depolarizing potentials may emerge spontaneously (i.e., without an apparent stimulus) at the postsynaptic muscle membrane (endplate region of muscle fiber). These potentials are about 1 mV in peak amplitude, and their functional meaning is unclear. They are called **miniature endplate potentials** or MEPPs.

Problem 4.2

A presynaptic action potential induces contraction of 20 myofibrils. Can a sequence of action potentials induce contraction of more than 20, less than 20, or exactly 20 myofibrils?

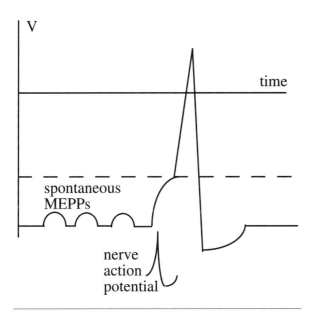

Figure 4.5 Miniature excitatory postsynaptic potentials (endplate potentials, MEPPs) spontaneously occur on the muscle postsynaptic membrane. A presynaptic nerve action potential always makes the postsynaptic membrane reach the depolarization threshold and induces a muscle action potential.

The next steps already involve events occurring in the muscle fibers, and I will address them as the mechanism of muscle contraction.

4.4. MECHANISM OF CONTRACTION

Step 4 (figure 4.6): Postsynaptic action potential travels along the muscle cell membrane (sarcolemma), entering T-tubules. There it opens Ca^{++} channels. Remember that at rest, virtually all Ca^{++} ions are stored in sarcoplasmic reticulum where they are "captured" by a special protein. Opening calcium channels leads to a massive influx of Ca^{++} ions into the sarcoplasma, increasing the concentration of these ions by a factor of 100. This increase is transient, and Ca^{++} is quickly pumped back into the sarcoplasmic reticulum.

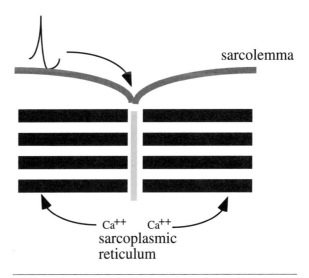

Figure 4.6 Muscle action potential travels along the sarcolemma, enters T-tubules, and leads to a release of Ca^{++} ions from the sarcoplasmic reticulum.

Step 5 (figure 4.7): This step, the **sliding-filament mechanism,** begins when calcium ions in sarcoplasma act on the troponin-tropomyosin complex. Note that at rest, tropomyosin blocks the myosin-binding site on actin, that is, a special place on an actin molecule that would eagerly attach to a special place on a myosin molecule. Calcium ions make the binding site available. If there is energy available as well (normally, ATP molecules), the myosin head binds to a site on actin and uses the energy to ratchet the filaments with respect to each other. These attachments between actin and myosin molecules are called **cross-bridges.** Then myosin releases itself from the actin site and "springs back," becoming ready to attach to the next available site and repeat the cycle (given that Ca^{++} ions and energy are still available). The

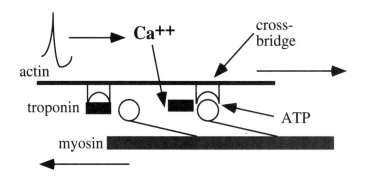

Figure 4.7   The sliding-filament theory. Ca⁺⁺ ions remove troponin and free a site for myosin to bind to actin (this process uses the energy from ATP). A rachet motion occurs, moving the filaments with respect to each other.

interaction between myosin and actin filaments occurs in three-dimensional space so that each myosin molecule simultaneously makes and breaks cross-bridges with six actin molecules. This means, specifically, that when some of the cross-bridges break, others maintain force of contraction. Force developed by a muscle fiber may be considered approximately proportional to the average number of simultaneously engaged cross-bridges.

Problem 4.3

What would happen if the troponin-tropomyosin complex were permanently inactivated?

Steps 4 and 5 are commonly addressed as **excitation-contraction coupling.**

Step 6: After excitation stops (action potentials do not arrive any more), Ca⁺⁺ is actively pumped from sarcoplasma into sarcoplasmic reticulum; the troponin-tropomyosin complex takes over all the sites of myosin binding; and the filaments slide back along each other (relaxation).

Note that the sliding-filament mechanism provides an explanation for some of the features of the dependence of muscle force upon muscle length that will be considered next.

Problem 4.4

Imagine that a muscle is developing force under a constant level of stimulation. Draw a diagram of dependence of muscle force upon muscle length based on what you already know.

4.5. TYPES OF MUSCLE CONTRACTION

Muscular contraction leads to the generation of force always directed to shortening the muscle. Further on in this book, the reader will see that a muscle can develop active force while its length is increasing (**eccentric contraction**). However, in such cases, muscle length is always changing under the action of another force, produced either by other muscles or by the environment, or because of the inertia of the muscle and body parts to which it is attached.

When a single action potential comes to a muscle fiber, it responds with a unitary contraction that is called twitch contraction or simply a **twitch** (figure 4.8). Depending on the properties of the fiber, twitch contractions last from a few tens of milliseconds to a couple of hundred milliseconds. Note, for comparison, that muscle action potential has the duration of about 10 ms. This means that the mechanical consequence of an action potential lasts much longer than the action potential itself.

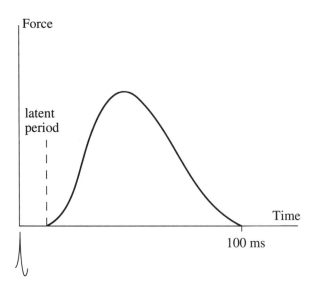

Figure 4.8   A typical twitch contraction of a muscle in response to a single stimulus.

If several fibers are stimulated simultaneously, their twitch contractions will superimpose. This superposition can lead both to an increase in the peak amplitude of the twitch contraction and to its prolongation if a muscle fiber with a long-lasting twitch is added to a group of fibers with short-lasting twitches.

If two action potentials come to the same fiber at a short interval, their mechanical effects may superimpose, as shown in figure 4.9, so that the peak force of the contraction will increase. If many action potentials come at a frequency that allows a superposition of their mechanical effects, a sustained level of contraction, called **tetanus** or tetanic contraction, is observed (figure 4.10). Tetanus may display local peaks of contraction at relatively low frequencies of action potentials (the so-called sawtooth tetanus) or lead to total fusion of individual twitches, in which case it is called **smooth tetanus.**

4.6. ELEMENTS OF MECHANICS

Let me now turn to real life and remind the reader that muscles do not exist by themselves; their action at joints

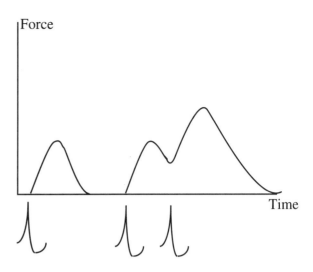

Figure 4.9   Two action potentials come at a short interval and induce two twitch contractions. Their mechanical effects superimpose, leading to a higher level of peak muscle force.

is affected by the mechanical properties of tendons and ligaments. Typical models of muscles involve at least four components (figure 4.11): a **contractile element** (force generator), which we have been considering up to now; a **damping element** (dashpot); and two **elastic elements,** one parallel and one serial. Unfortunately for investigators, most of these elements are essentially **nonlinear.**

It seems to be the proper time to introduce a little bit of physics. Elastic elements or springs resist external attempts at changing their length by developing force acting against the imposed deformation. In the most simple case of a **linear spring,** the force developed by the spring is described by **Hooke's law:**

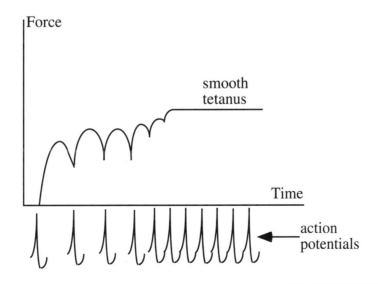

Figure 4.10   A sequence of action potentials may lead to a tetanus (a sustained contraction). At a high frequency of action potentials, individual contractions may fuse, leading to a smooth tetanus.

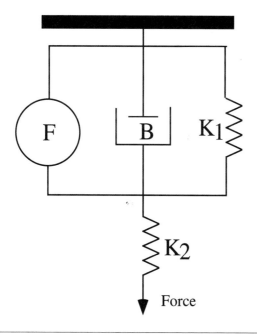

Figure 4.11 A simple mechanical model of a muscle. It contains a force generator (F), a viscous element (B), and two elastic elements, a parallel spring (K_1) and a series spring (K_2).

$$F_e = -k \cdot (x - x_0) \qquad (4.1)$$

where F_e is elastic force, x is spring length, x_0 is "zero length," that is, the length at which elastic forces are zero, and k is a coefficient termed stiffness. Note that the minus sign implies that force acts against the change in length with respect to x_0.

Damping can be defined as the ability of a system to generate force against the vector of velocity:

$$F_d = -b \cdot \frac{dx}{dt} = -b \cdot V \qquad (4.2)$$

where F_d is damping force, V is velocity of length change, and b is a coefficient. Sometimes damping is imprecisely addressed as viscosity. Note again that the minus sign implies that force acts against the velocity vector.

All material objects also have inertia, which is a coefficient between applied force and acceleration:

$$F_i = m \cdot \frac{d^2x}{dt^2} = m \cdot a \qquad (4.3)$$

where F_i is inertial force, a is acceleration, and m is a coefficient termed mass.

Equations 4.1 through 4.3 describe what are called **linear elements.** Such elements produce outputs in proportion to input signals. For example, if a force F_1 acts on a spring and induces a displacement x_1, and force F_2 produces a displacement x_2, the combined action of the two forces ($F_1 + F_2$) will produce displacement ($x_1 + x_2$).

The same rule of simple summation can be applied to damping and inertial forces. Such systems are relatively easy to analyze, and equations describing their behavior can frequently be solved analytically.

Linear systems are commonly studied in textbooks of elementary physics; however, in real life they are rare. It does not take much to make a system nonlinear. For example, if stiffness depends on spring length, this element is already nonlinear, and consequently a system with such an element is very likely to be nonlinear. Now we will return to the simple model shown in figure 4.11 and confess that all the elements of this model are nonlinear. Nonlinear systems are described with equations of motion that typically cannot be solved analytically and require complex simulation analysis.

4.7. FORCE-LENGTH AND FORCE-VELOCITY RELATIONS

A typical example of the nonlinear behavior of a whole muscle is its force-length relationship. Such a relationship can be obtained in an experiment in which muscle length is fixed at a certain value **(isometric conditions)**, a standard stimulation is applied to the muscle nerve with the aid of an external electrical stimulator, and peak muscle force is measured. Then muscle length is fixed at a different value, the same stimulation is applied, and the force is measured again. And so forth. As a result, a force-length curve similar to the ones shown in figure 4.12 is observed. It is important to remember that the measurements are performed when muscle length is not changing, which means that inertial and viscous properties do not play any role. If the parameters of the stimulation are changed and the same experiment is performed, the curve will shift to the right or to the left, nearly parallel to the length axis. So the muscle behaves like a nonlinear spring (note that its stiffness, the slope

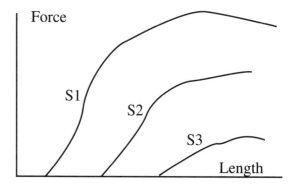

Figure 4.12 Force-length curves measured in a muscle for different levels of external stimulation (S_1, S_2, and S_3). Note that the muscle behaves like a nonlinear spring. Changing the strength of the stimulation modifies zero length of the spring.

of the curve, changes with length as well as with the level of excitation) whose zero length changes in response to a change in an incoming activation signal (stimulation).

One can measure the force-length relation in a single sarcomere, that is, inside the contractile element shown as F in figure 4.11. The active force developed by the sarcomere will show a dependence on sarcomere length that is somewhat similar to that for the whole muscle. At low values of sarcomere length, cross-bridges cannot develop force because of the lack of space; at intermediate values of length, the force is maximal; and at high values of sarcomere length, there are only a few cross-bridges that can generate force, and it drops again.

Another commonly studied relation, for a whole muscle, is the force-velocity curve. Such curves are usually studied in experiments in which a muscle performs a twitch contraction under different loads and the peak velocity of muscle shortening is measured. The curve typically looks parabolic (figure 4.13) and can be well approximated with the famous Hill equation:

$$(F + a) \cdot V = b \cdot (F - F_0) \qquad (4.4)$$

where F is force, F_0 is force at zero velocity (in isometric conditions), V is peak velocity of shortening (i.e., it is negative for a stretched muscle), and a and b are constants specific for a given muscle.

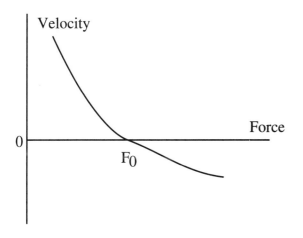

Figure 4.13 A typical force-velocity curve for a whole muscle. According to tradition, the y-axis represents velocity of muscle **shortening.** Note that the muscle develops higher forces when it is lengthening (negative velocity) than when it is shortening (positive velocity). Compare this figure with the Hill equation.

In real life, muscle length, velocity, and force change simultaneously. Figure 4.14 illustrates the behavior of a whole muscle in a range of values for all three variables. This is a rather busy figure, but it gives you an idea what to expect from a muscle when its length changes during force generation.

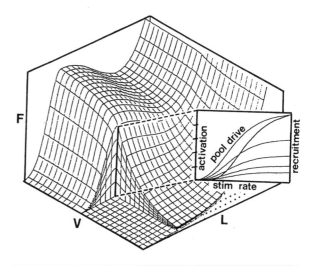

Figure 4.14 This figure combines the dependences of muscle force upon length and velocity into one three-dimensional graph. Sections of this graph at V = 0 will give a curve from figure 4.12, while sections at a constant muscle length will give curves like the one shown in figure 4.13.
Reprinted, by permission from L.D. Partridge and L.D. Partridge, 1993, *The Nervous System* (Cambridge, MA: MIT Press), 358.

4.8. EXTERNAL REGIMES OF MUSCLE CONTRACTION

We have already used the expression "isometric conditions." Let me introduce this and a couple of other terms formally. Muscle contraction in conditions preventing changes in muscle length is termed **isometric,** and a load leading to such conditions is termed an **isometric load.** When muscle contracts acting against a constant external force, such contraction and load are termed **isotonic.** If a muscle is acting against a springlike load, the load is termed **elastic.** Examples of different loading conditions are shown in figure 4.15.

The problem with these terms is that they are misleading. Consider, for example, what will happen if

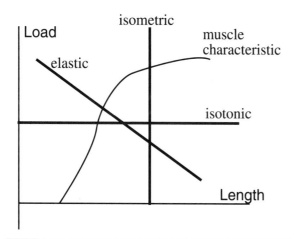

Figure 4.15 A muscle always works against a load. Three types of loads are illustrated. Isometric load prevents changes in muscle length; an isotonic load does not change; an elastic load acts like a spring. A typical muscle characteristic is shown for comparison (the thin curve).

movement in a joint is prevented (isometric conditions). If a muscle acting at this joint is activated, it will develop contractile force that will act on all the elements, including the parallel and serial elastic elements. Depending on the relative stiffness of these elements, contractile force will induce a change in their relative length even if the length of the whole complex (muscle+tendon) is kept constant. Note that a relaxed muscle is usually less stiff than its tendon, while activated muscle is usually more stiff than the tendon. Thus, muscle fiber length will change in isometric conditions as well.

Problem 4.9

What will happen with the relative length of muscle fibers and with the tendon under activation in isometric conditions?

Chapter 4 in a Nutshell

Muscle contractions are produced by an interaction of two types of molecules, actin and myosin, inside muscle cells. Muscle cells are excited through neuromuscular synapses with the help of a mediator, ACh. Action potentials lead to release of calcium ions that make cross-bridge formation between actin and myosin molecules possible. In response to a single stimulus, muscle fibers generate a single twitch contraction. A number of stimuli coming at a high frequency lead to the summation of individual twitches and the generation of a tetanic contraction. Muscle force increases with muscle length and decreases with the velocity of muscle shortening. Muscle always acts against external loads, typical examples being isometric, isotonic, and elastic loads.

CHAPTER 5

RECEPTORS

Key Terms

classification of receptors

Weber-Fechner law

muscle spindles

fusimotor innervation

Golgi tendon organs

articular receptors

skin and subcutaneous receptors

5.1. GENERAL CLASSIFICATION AND PROPERTIES OF RECEPTORS

Receptors are specialized cells or subcellular structures that change their properties in response to stimuli (sources of energy) of a special type or modality. Thus, different receptor systems enable human beings to differentiate among different sources of energy (e.g., light, sound, and mechanical energy) that is being absorbed by the body. Receptors of a certain type are typically rather specific; that is, they ignore alien stimuli, although many of them can be forced to fire with an electrical stimulation or even with a strong mechanical stimulus. The reader probably knows that a hard hit in an eye can lead to a whole bunch of sparks, that is, to visual images induced by the activity of visual receptors in the eye. Interestingly, although many of our receptors react to electrical stimulation and transduce information using electrical phenomena, humans do not have a developed system for sensing electromagnetic field outside the visible light range.

The obvious function of receptors is to make information about particular types of stimuli available to other neurons within the central nervous system. Some of this information is related to the environment, while other information is related to the state of the body itself. There are three major groups of receptors:

1. **Interoceptors** transduce information from within the body.

2. **Exteroceptors** transduce information from the environment.

3. **Proprioceptors** transduce information about the relative configuration of body segments.

Receptors within each group can be sensitive to stimuli of different modalities; on the other hand, receptors belonging to different groups may react to energy of the same kind. For example, there are mechanoreceptors, that is, receptors that react to mechanical stimuli in each of the three groups. Receptors sensitive to certain chemicals (**chemoreceptors**) are rather widespread. Some of them are located on membranes and are sensitive to certain neurotransmitters. As already described, these receptors play a major role in synaptic transmission of information. On the other hand, the activity of chemoreceptors in your mouth and nose plays an extremely important role in human life, creating the senses of taste and smell.

Before moving to the mechanisms and function of specific groups of receptors, let me mention a law that is applicable to **conscious perception** of signals from many of the receptor systems. This law states that perceived **sensation** is related to stimulus magnitude by a logarithmic function. The reader can study this by changing the magnitude of a stimulus of a certain modality and asking a subject to report how strong the stimulus feels on a scale from 0 to 10. The law is called the Weber-Fechner law:

$$P = k \cdot \log \left(\frac{M}{M_0} \right) \qquad (5.1)$$

where P is the magnitude of perception, M is the magnitude of your stimulus, M_0 is the magnitude of your stimulus when the subject just feels it (the **threshold stimulus**), and k is a constant. This law is an example of so-called psychophysical functions that relate dimensions measured directly by an experimenter to perceived dimensions reported by the subject.

Problem 5.1

Give an example of a receptor system that does not obey the Weber-Fechner law.

Now we will consider proprioceptors whose activity is closely tied to the motor function.

A typical **proprioceptor** is a specialized neural cell whose body is located in a special place, a **ganglion,** close to the spinal cord (figure 5.1). These neurons are rather unusual in their structure; they do not receive inputs from other neurons and do not have a typical dendritic tree. Their axons serve both as an input to the neuron and as its output. The axon of such a neuron is termed an **afferent axon** or **afferent fiber;** it has a characteristic **T shape.** An afferent axon splits into two branches very close to the neuron body. One of the branches goes to a peripheral site in the body where it ends with a specialized ending (**sensory ending**) whose membrane can

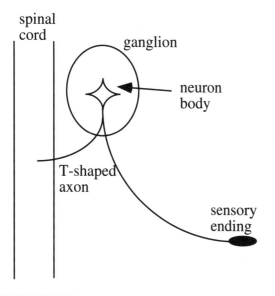

Figure 5.1 The body of a sensory neuron is located in a ganglion near the spinal cord. One branch of its T-shaped axon goes to the peripheral sensory ending, while the other branch goes through the dorsal roots into the spinal cord.

be depolarized to the threshold by a stimulus of a certain strength and modality. The other branch goes through the back (dorsal) portion of the spinal canal (through the dorsal roots) into the spinal cord where it can make connections with many different neurons, leading to different effects.

5.2. MUSCLE SPINDLES

The muscle spindle is one of the most amazing inventions of nature. The lower part of figure 5.2 illustrates the location of a muscle spindle within a muscle, while the upper part shows its internal design in more detail. These structures with their very sophisticated design let other neurons within the central nervous system know the length and velocity of muscle fibers. Muscle spindles have an elongated shape (they are commonly about 1 cm long) with a thicker area in the middle that makes them look like regular spindles. They are scattered among muscle fibers in large quantities.

Each spindle contains specialized muscle fibers (termed **intrafusal fibers**) that are oriented parallel to the regular, power-producing **extrafusal** muscle fibers. The middle part of a spindle is covered with a capsule made of connective tissue. At both ends, intrafusal muscle fibers are connected either to extrafusal fibers or to tendinous ligaments. So when the extrafusal fibers change their length, the intrafusal fibers are stretched or shortened correspondingly.

Spindles contain two major types of intrafusal fibers, called **bag fibers** and **chain fibers.** These names reflect the distribution of nuclei within a fiber—clustered as in a bag, or chainlike. In turn, bag fibers are of two subtypes, static and dynamic. Two types of sensory endings can be found in muscle spindles. They are located mostly in the middle (equator) portion of the spindle. Endings of the first type, called **primary spindle endings,** are seen on virtually all intrafusal fibers, including both bag and chain fibers; endings of the second type, called **secondary spindle endings,** are rarely seen on dynamic bag fibers but are common in static bag and in chain fibers. A spindle ending, like any sensory ending of a proprioceptive neuron, is located at the end of the axon of a neuron whose body is in a spinal ganglion. Axons of primary endings belong to afferent fiber group Ia, while axons of secondary endings belong to afferent fiber group II.

Primary sensory endings are sensitive to both muscle length and velocity. Figure 5.3 shows a typical response of a primary ending to an externally imposed muscle stretch at different velocities. Note that the frequency of firing of the ending is higher after the stretch than before, which means that the ending is **sensitive to muscle length** itself. However, during stretching, the frequency of firing of the ending is higher for faster stretches, which means that the ending is **sensitive to velocity** as well.

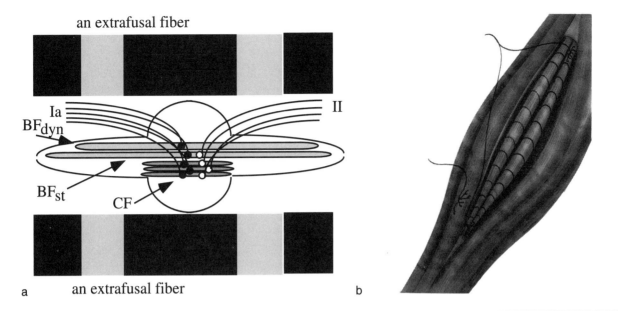

an extrafusal fiber

Ia

BF$_{dyn}$

II

BF$_{st}$

CF

a   an extrafusal fiber   b

Figure 5.2 A muscle spindle is oriented parallel to extrafusal muscle fibers. It is covered with a capsule and contains two types of intrafusal muscle fibers, the bag fibers (BF) and the chain fibers (CF). Two types of sensory endings can be found in muscle spindles, primary (Ia) and secondary (II). Primary endings are typically seen in virtually all intrafusal fibers, while secondary endings are seen in CF and static BF, but not dynamic BF. The lower part of the figure shows a more realistic picture of a muscle spindle surrounded by extrafusal muscle fibers.

Reprinted, by permission, from J.H. Wilmore and D.L. Costill, 1994, *Physiology of Sport and Exercise* (Champaign, IL: Human Kinetics), 61.

Note that the velocity sensitivity of primary spindle endings leads to an increase in the frequency of their firing during stretches and to a decrease during muscle shortening. Primary afferent axons are among the fastest neural fibers. They are myelinated, with diameters ranging from 12 to 20 μm, which corresponds to action potential velocity of up to 120 m/s.

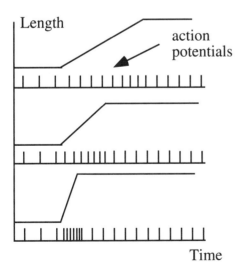

Figure 5.3 Typical responses of a primary spindle ending to an externally imposed muscle stretch at different velocities. Note that the response increases with muscle length and with the velocity of stretch.

Problem 5.2

Can the frequency of firing of a primary ending be higher or lower than that shown in figure 5.3 before the muscle stretch for the same muscle length?

Secondary endings are sensitive only to muscle length, not to velocity. Figure 5.4 shows the response of a typical secondary ending to muscle stretching and shortening. Secondary ending axons are smaller and the speed of conduction is also lower, ranging from 20 to 60 m/s.

Problem 5.3

Draw a graph of time changes in firing frequency for a primary ending and for a secondary ending if muscle length changes as a sine function.

Problem 5.4

Draw a graph of length changes for a muscle whose typical primary spindle ending shows a ramplike increase in the firing frequency with time from a certain steady level to another, higher, steady level, followed by a ramplike decline in the firing frequency to a level somewhat higher than the original one.

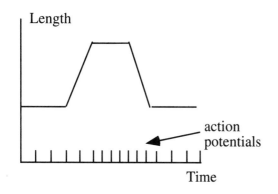

Figure 5.4 A typical response of a secondary spindle ending to an externally imposed muscle stretch and shortening. Note that the response increases with muscle length and does not depend on velocity.

Endings in muscle spindles have very high sensitivity to low-amplitude changes in muscle length, particularly if these changes occur at a high frequency. This is especially true for primary spindle endings, which can be forced to fire in response to every cycle of a high-frequency vibration (on the order of 100 Hz) when the amplitude of the vibration is 1 mm and the vibration is applied to the skin over the muscle belly or the tendon. If a vibrator is attached directly to muscle fibers, a few micrometers of vibration amplitude are enough to drive primary spindle endings at the frequency of the vibration.

5.3. THE GAMMA SYSTEM

Primary and secondary spindle endings are unique among proprioceptors in their ability to change their sensitivity

to muscle length and velocity in response to signals from special groups of neurons that form the **gamma system** (γ-system).

Intrafusal muscle fibers receive signals from the efferent axons of neurons of a particular type whose bodies are located in the spinal cord. These neurons belong to the class of **motoneurons** together with spinal neurons that send their signals to power-generating, extrafusal fibers. Motoneurons innervating muscle fibers inside muscle spindles belong to the gamma system and are called γ-**motoneurons.** They are much smaller than the other group of motoneurons (α-**motoneurons**); their axons are of approximately the same length, since their target is located in the same muscles, but they are much thinner and, correspondingly, conduct action potentials at much lower velocities (about 20 m/s).

There are two types of γ-motoneurons (figure 5.5), dynamic and static. Dynamic γ-**axons** innervate dynamic bag muscle fibers and thus affect the sensitivity of primary spindle endings located in these fibers. **Static γ-motoneurons** send their axons to static bag and chain fibers. They can change the sensitivity of both primary and secondary endings.

Figure 5.6 shows how stimulation of dynamic γ-axons can change the response of a primary ending to muscle stretching and shortening. Note the increase in the effects of velocity of the spindle response. Static γ-axons innervate intrafusal fibers containing both primary and secondary sensory endings. So the effect of their stimulation can be seen in the response of both groups of sensory endings to muscle length as an increase in their frequency of firing.

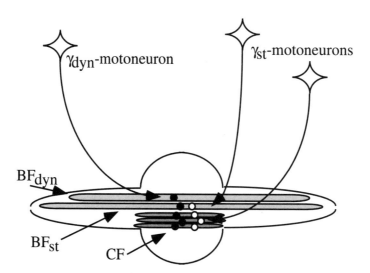

Figure 5.5 There are two types of small motoneurons (γ-motoneurons) innervating intrafusal fibers of muscle spindles. Dynamic γ-motoneurons innervate dynamic bag fibers and change the sensitivity of primary endings. Static γ-motoneurons innervate static bag and chain fibers. They change the sensitivity of both primary and secondary endings.

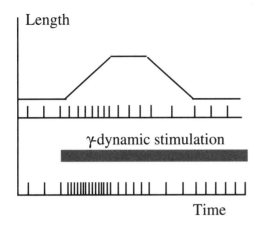

Figure 5.6 The effects of activation of dynamic γ-motoneurons on response of a primary spindle ending to muscle stretch and shortening. In the lower graph, a γ-dynamic stimulation was applied during the same changes in muscle length.

Problem 5.5

How will a secondary ending react to an increase in the activity of dynamic γ-motoneurons innervating the spindle?

Problem 5.6

When we voluntarily contract a muscle, its length decreases. However, the frequency of firing of the spindle endings in the muscle may remain constant. How can this happen?

5.4. GOLGI TENDON ORGANS

Another group of proprioceptors are located close to the junction between tendons and muscle fibers (figure 5.7). These receptors are sensitive to mechanical deformation and are called **Golgi tendon organs.** Note that tendons may be considered elastic structures (springs). This means that mechanical deformation of a tendon increases with muscle force, so Golgi tendon organs appear to be nearly perfect **force sensors.** Golgi tendon organs do not receive any additional innervation (like muscle spindles); they are also not responsive to the rate of force change. Thus their response to muscle force is relatively independent of other factors. The fact that tendons are nonlinear springs makes Golgi tendon organs nonlinear sensors; however, this is unlikely to be a major problem as long as their properties do not change.

Figure 5.8 illustrates a typical response of a Golgi tendon organ to force generated by muscle fibers that

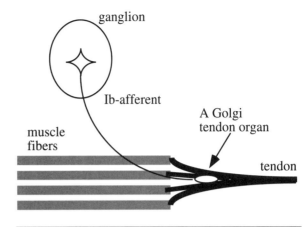

Figure 5.7 Golgi tendon organs are located in series with extrafusal muscle fibers at their junction with the tendon. They are innervated with fast-conducting Ib-group axons of sensory neurons in spinal ganglia.

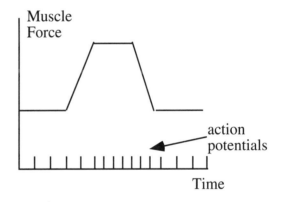

Figure 5.8 A response of a Golgi tendon organ to muscle force. Note that it is similar to the response of secondary spindle endings to muscle length.

---

are in series with the tendon organ. Note, however, that Golgi tendon organs are rather selective; that is, they respond to force generated by "their" muscle fibers. If muscle force is generated by fibers that do not act at the area where a Golgi organ is located, it will not change its firing frequency or even show a drop in activity. This may result from an unloading of a particular "braid" of the tendinous structures where the Golgi organ is located.

Problem 5.7

Imagine that you prevent movement of your right elbow joint and then quickly activate your biceps to a rather large force (isometric conditions). Draw a graph of the change in firing frequency for a primary and secondary muscle spindle and for a Golgi tendon organ.

Problem 5.8

Now do the same for a very fast elbow flexion movement against a constant external force.

Axons originating from Golgi tendon organs are nearly as large as axons of primary spindle endings; their speed of conduction is of the same order of magnitude and may reach about 80 m/s.

5.5. OTHER MUSCLE RECEPTORS

One can find a couple of other types of sensory endings in a muscle. The first is paciniform corpuscles, which are similar in their structure to pacinian corpuscles found in skin (we will consider these later), although smaller. These corpuscles are commonly located at the area of musculotendinous junction and are quite sensitive to high-frequency vibration. Not much is known about their functional significance and central connections.

There are also free sensory endings scattered all around a muscle. They are sensitive to strong mechanical stimuli (such as those occurring during pinching) as well as to certain chemicals. These receptors are likely to play an important role in the sense of pain and in certain reflex responses that we will consider later in this book. They are innervated with small, nonmyelinated axons with a slow conduction speed (on the order of 10 m/s).

5.6. ARTICULAR RECEPTORS

Another group of proprioceptors reside in the joints; these are called **articular receptors.** There are actually several different brands of articular receptors, including sensory endings similar to Golgi tendon organs as well as free nerve endings. They are innervated by axons of variable size, from rather thin ones lacking myelin sheath to large ones, with a diameter of over 10 μm, that are group I fibers and are characterized by fast speeds of conduction (up to 80 m/s).

These receptors were thought for a long time to be perfect angle transducers that inform the central nervous system about the position of the joints. However, a closer inspection of their behavior has revealed that individual articular receptors fire in a rather small range of joint angles (figure 5.9). Moreover, many active receptors are found when joint position is close to one of its physiological extremes, while only a few of them are active in the middle range of joint motion. Thus articular receptors are unlikely to provide reliable information about joint position during natural movements.

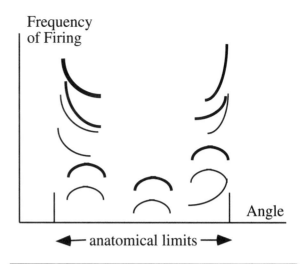

Figure 5.9 Most articular receptors fire in rather narrow ranges of joint angle, mostly close to the anatomical limits. An increase in muscle force leads to an increase in joint capsule tension, and articular receptors increase their response (bold lines).

Articular receptors are also sensitive to changes in joint capsule tension. Typically, a receptor increases the frequency of its firing over the whole range of its activity in response to an increase in joint capsule tension (figure 5.9). Note that joint capsule tension increases with muscle force. All this makes signals from articular receptors even less attractive as a source of information about joint position, because a receptor may demonstrate similar firing frequencies at different positions if muscle forces are different.

5.7. CUTANEOUS RECEPTORS

Human skin houses receptors sensitive to different sensory modalities. Among them are thermoreceptors sensitive to temperature, nociceptors sensitive to potentially damaging stimuli and giving rise to the sense of pain, and mechanoreceptors sensitive to pressure. The last group of receptors play a particularly important role in control of human movements, particularly those involving tactile discrimination (**haptic** perception).

Figure 5.10 shows the major types of cutaneous mechanoreceptors in the glabrous skin of the hand. **Meissner corpuscles** and **Merkel disks** are located most closely to the skin surface, on the border of the epidermis and dermis. Deeper down, in the dermis, are **Ruffini endings,** and even deeper, in subcutaneous tissue, are **pacinian corpuscles.**

Merkel disks respond to vertical pressure on the skin surface but not to lateral displacements. A group of Merkel disks is commonly innervated by one afferent axon. Meissner corpuscles are sensitive to quickly changing pressure on a small area of skin. They quickly adapt and stop responding if the pressure does not change. Each Meissner corpuscle is innervated by two or more axons.

Ruffini endings can be activated from much larger skin areas, from as far as 5 cm away from the location of the ending. They are slowly adapting, and continue firing in response to a stable deformation of the skin. Pacinian corpuscles are the biggest of them all; their size ranges from 1 to 5 mm. Pacinian corpuscles react to very quickly changing mechanical deformation (e.g., vibration).

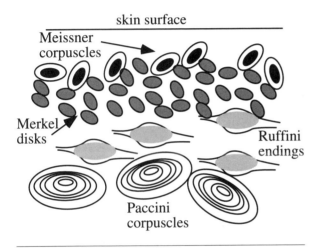

Figure 5.10 Major types of cutaneous and subcutaneous mechanoreceptors in the glabrous skin of the hand.

5.8. WHERE DOES THE INFORMATION GO?

Three major effects of proprioceptor activity are of considerable importance for us at this point.

First, proprioceptors induce changes in muscle activity bypassing human consciousness. Some of these effects are called reflexes, while others are termed triggered reactions or preprogrammed reactions. (We will not get involved now in linguistic debates on the appropriateness of the term "reflex." I will consider this term in more detail in chapter 8. It has been used for "more or less automatic" and "more or less standard" reactions to external stimuli that do not involve conscious participation by the subject. As readers will see in further chapters, reflexes may be not so automatic and not so standard; they may actually occur in different muscles in response to one and the same stimulus. However, they do reflect the stimulus, albeit in a more complex way than was thought in the first half of the 20th century.)

Second, proprioceptors let us know where our arms and legs are as well as how heavy or light, how rough or soft, the objects we handle are.

Third, proprioceptors play a major role in creating an internal system of coordinates that is used by the brain to plan and execute movements.

Signals from proprioceptors travel along afferent axons into the spinal cord (figure 5.11). There they make connections with different kinds of neurons. Primary spindle afferents are the only ones known to make direct connections with spinal motoneurons. The majority of afferent axons make synapses on interneurons that typically are smaller cells processing incoming information and making projections onto other neurons. Careful tracing of spinal projections of different proprioceptors has revealed a rather disturbing picture: different afferents project onto the same interneurons, so that the original information about length, velocity, pressure, force, and joint angles gets totally and seemingly irrecoverably mixed. At first glance, this looks plain stupid, but we will try to understand the logic of this organization later in the book when we consider position sense. Some afferent fibers go as far as the brain without making intermediate connections, which probably makes them the longest neural fibers in the body. After they get into the brain, they apparently participate in such processes as perception of the body, limb position, and movement planning. The time will come for these themes as well.

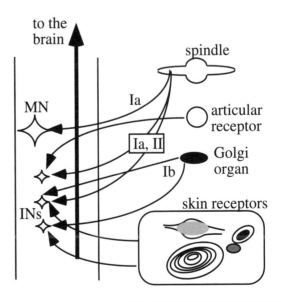

Figure 5.11 Afferent nerves from peripheral receptors enter the spinal cord through the dorsal roots. There they make synapses on interneurons and motoneurons and send signals to the brain. Note that the same interneurons may receive signals from afferents of different modalities.

Chapter 5 in a Nutshell

Receptors are specialized cells or parts of cells that can respond to external stimuli of certain types. Signals from receptors lead to perception of stimuli that is related to the strength of the stimulus by a nonlinear law. Proprioceptors produce information about relative configuration of body segments. Muscle spindles contain sensory endings of two types: those that are sensitive to muscle length and those that are sensitive to both muscle length and velocity. The sensitivity of spindle endings is modulated by a special system of neurons, the fusimotor or gamma system. Golgi tendon organs are sensitive to muscle force. Articular receptors are sensitive to both joint angle (typically, close to the anatomical limits of joint rotation) and joint capsule tension. Skin and subcutaneous receptors measure pressure on the skin. Sensory endings send signals along the peripheral branch of the T-shaped axon to spinal ganglia where bodies of sensory neurons are located. Then, signals travel along the central branch of the T-shaped axon into the central nervous system.

CHAPTER 6

MOTOR UNITS AND ELECTROMYOGRAPHY

Key Terms

motor units   recruitment patterns   electromyography

Henneman principle

6.1. THE NOTION OF MOTOR UNIT

It is time to make a step from the properties of single cells to the next functionally important level of complexity. It would certainly be unwise to expect the central nervous system to control the level of activity of each and every neural and muscular cell separately. Such an approach would impose a computational load beyond imagination. It would be comparable to calculating the trajectory of each individual elementary particle within a baseball in order to assure a desired trajectory of the ball. The central nervous system simplifies the task and decreases the computational load by uniting small elements of the neuromuscular system into functional units that are controlled with just one or two parameters. The smallest functional unit of the neuromotor system is termed **motor unit.**

Figure 6.1 shows a couple of neural cells in the spinal cord innervating a muscle, that is, **α-motoneurons.** Their axons branch at the end and innervate several muscle fibers each. Since each neuron obeys the law of all-or-none, such an arrangement leads to synchronized contraction of all the muscle fibers innervated by one α-motoneuron in response to each action potential delivered by the axon of the motoneuron. So all these muscle fibers also behave according to the law of all-or-none. *The motoneuron and the muscle fibers it innervates are called a motor unit.* Typically, each muscle fiber is innervated by only one axon branch, although during development and during recuperation following nerve injury, muscle fibers may receive inputs from a number of axons. With time, however, "redundant" inputs disappear, and each muscle fiber ends up being innervated by one axon.

Motor units differ in size, which relates to both the size of the motoneuron and the number of muscle fibers innervated by the motoneuron. These two parameters are closely correlated so that large motoneurons (with a large body cell and large axon) innervate more muscle fibers than smaller motoneurons. The number of muscle fibers innervated by a single motoneuron (the **innervation ratio**) varies in a wide range, from under 10 in muscles controlling eye movements to over 1000 in large muscles participating in postural control during standing. With age, the number of motoneurons decreases, and a process of **reinnervation** takes place that leads to an increase in the size of individual motor units and a corresponding increase in the innervation ratio.

Problem 6.1

Can one motor unit produce different levels of muscle force? Why?

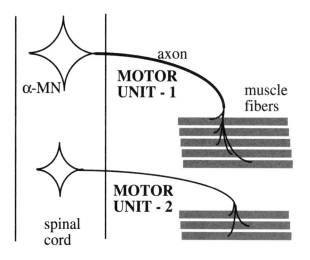

Figure 6.1 Alpha motoneurons in the spinal cord send their axons through the ventral roots. Each axon branches in the target muscle and innervates several muscle fibers. A motoneuron and the muscle fibers it innervates are called **a motor unit.**

Problem 6.2

You want a large motor unit and a small motor unit to contract simultaneously. How would you time commands to the motoneurons?

Up to now I have been discussing the most common muscle fibers that generate action potentials in response to a local membrane depolarization at the neuromuscular synapse, conduct these potentials, and generate twitch contractions in response to each action potential. Another type of muscle fiber is relatively rare and has been seen in muscles involved in eye, throat, and ear movements; these are sometimes called **tonic fibers.** Each tonic fiber is typically innervated at a number of places. It does not generate its own action potential in response to presynaptic inputs but rather spreads local postsynaptic depolarization with local currents. So the response of a tonic fiber to presynaptic stimuli does not obey the all-or-none law and can be graded. However, we will not consider these unusual fibers further, but instead return to the "normal" twitch fibers that are involved in voluntary movements of the human body and limbs.

6.2. FAST AND SLOW MOTOR UNITS

Each muscle consists of a number of motor units. This number ranges from less than a hundred for small muscles controlling eye movements to thousands for large muscles controlling movements of large body segments. Within a muscle, one can see motor units that differ not only in their relative size but also in their contractile properties.

Two basic tests are used to describe the functional properties of motor units. One is **twitch contraction** and the other is **fatigue.** Figure 6.2A shows twitch contractions of three motor units. Note that these motor units generate different levels of peak force and take different times to reach the peak force level. In particular, MU3 takes the longest time to complete its twitch contraction and generates the lowest peak force, while MU1 is the first to reach the peak force level and has the highest peak force. If these motor units are stimulated at a rather high frequency, they produce a **tetanic contraction** (discussed in chapter 4). One can bring about such a contraction by stimulating the axons of these motor units with an external electrical stimulator. If the frequency of stimulation is the same for all three motor units, the peak force will again be the highest for MU1 and the lowest for MU3 (figure 6.2B). If the motor units are stimulated for a rather long time, there will be changes in the level of their contraction force (figure 6.2B) that are related to fatigue. The mechanisms of fatigue will be discussed later. Here it is important to note that the changes in the force level of MU2 and MU3 are small while the force level of MU1 has dropped significantly.

Thus there seem to be three types of motor units. Motor units of the MU1 type are called **fast twitch, fatigable;** motor units of type MU2 are called **fast twitch, fatigue**

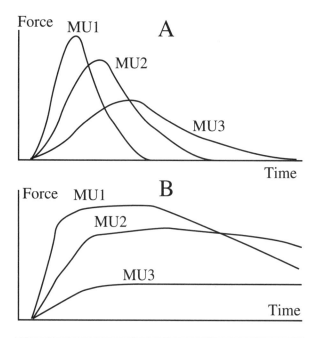

Figure 6.2 Twitch contractions (A) and tetanic contractions (B) of three motor units. Note that the fastest and strongest motor unit (MU_1) shows the largest drop in force with time (fatigue), while the smallest and slowest motor unit (MU_3) does not show fatigue at all.

resistant; and motor units of type MU3 are called **slow twitch, fatigue resistant.** These groups are sometimes referred to as FF, FR, and S motor units. Slow motor units (S) typically have fewer muscle fibers, smaller motoneurons, and thinner axons. Correspondingly, the speed of conduction of action potentials along the axons of slow motor units is the lowest (although it is still rather high, since, as you remember, the axons of α-motoneurons, which are group I neural fibers, are thick and myelinated). The FF motor units are characterized by the highest conduction velocity. The difference in conduction velocity may be more than twofold (from 40 m/s to 100 m/s).

The differences in physical properties of motor units correlate with their different biochemical and morphological characteristics. We will consider three major sources of energy used for muscle contraction. The first is **ATP** contained in myofibrils; the importance of this source may be assessed by the level of activity of the enzyme ATPase participating in metabolizing ATP. The second source is **oxidative metabolism** occurring in mitochondria. Its rate may be assessed by the activity of a couple of enzymes, succinic dehydrogenase and NADH dehydrogenase. The third source is **glycogen,** whose metabolism is anaerobic. Table 6.1 shows three major types of motor units and the relative representation of physiological and biochemical characteristics of their muscle fibers. It shows that S motor units contain mostly slow, oxidative fibers characterized by a high level of mitochondrial oxidative processes and a well-developed blood supply network. Fast motor units use more energy from ATP and glycogen metabolism. The FR motor units have a rich capillary supply comparable to that of S motor units, while FF motor units have a sparse capillary supply.

Most muscles contain a mixture of motor units of different types, although the percentages of slow and fast motor units may differ. Slow muscles (i.e., those with a high percentage of S motor units) are typically

pale (an example is soleus), while fast muscles (i.e., those with a high percentage of FR and FF motor units) are typically red (an example is gastrocnemius). Within a muscle, the central nervous system has come up with a rule that coordinates the order in which different motor units are recruited. This rule is extremely important in itself, but also as a unique example of a **coordinative rule.**

6.3. THE HENNEMAN PRINCIPLE (SIZE PRINCIPLE)

The **Henneman principle** (also known as the size principle) states that *the recruitment of motor units within a muscle proceeds from small motor units to large ones.* That is, if a person contracts a muscle at a low force, nearly all the force will be produced by the slowest motor units (figure 6.3). If the contraction force is increased, larger motoneurons will start to fire, recruiting larger motor units. At the highest levels of muscle contraction (maximal voluntary contraction force), the largest motor units are recruited. Note that derecruitment of motor units with a decline of muscle force follows the inverse order: the largest motor units are the first to be turned off, while the smallest ones are the last to stop firing.

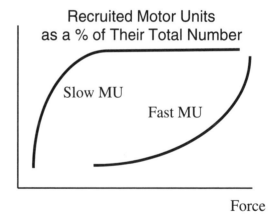

Figure 6.3 Henneman principle. Small motor units recruit first at low muscle forces. An increase in muscle force leads to recruitment of larger motor units.

Note that the contribution of a motor unit to total muscle force depends upon two factors—the **size of the motor unit** and the **frequency** of action potentials that arrive at it. Larger motor units have larger forces generated in response to single action potentials, while all motor units generate more force (up to a limit, of course) when action potentials arrive at a higher frequency. The importance of the frequency of firing for the force contribution of a motor unit gives the central nervous system options for developing a given level of muscle force.

Table 6.1 Properties of Different Motor Units

Type	FF	FR	S
Fiber diameter	Large	Medium	Small
ATPase	High	High	Low
Glycogen	High	High	Low
Succinic dehydrogenase	Low	Medium	High
NADH dehydrogenase	Low	Medium	High

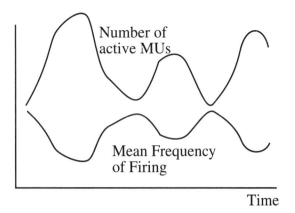

Figure 6.4 Muscle force is kept constant. A change in the number of recruited motor units correlates (negatively!) with their mean frequency of firing.

Figure 6.4 illustrates that the same level of muscle force may result from the recruitment of fewer motor units at higher frequencies or from the recruitment of a larger number of motor units at lower frequencies. *Recruitment and changes in firing frequency are the two major mechanisms of regulating muscle force.*

During sustained contractions, one can commonly see **derecruitment** (turning off) of some motor units accompanied by recruitment of new motor units and/or changes in the firing frequency of already recruited motor units. Thus, the Henneman principle does not define, by itself, which motor units are going to be recruited and at which frequencies for a given level of muscle force. However, it limits the area where the solutions can be searched for to "grammatically correct" or "coordinated" sequences of motor unit recruitment. Thus, the Henneman principle is a **coordinative rule** rather than a prescribing rule.

Problem 6.3

Formulate the size principle for the order of motor unit involvement when the contraction is induced by progressively increasing the strength of electrical stimulation of the muscle nerve.

There are situations in which the Henneman principle does not work perfectly, although these are rare. In particular, if a muscle participates in a task in which it is not the **primary mover,** the order of motor unit recruitment within this muscle may change, leading to a violation of the size principle for certain pairs of motor units: a larger motor unit may be recruited before a smaller one. A reversal of the size principle can also be seen in certain reflex responses (we will consider these later), in particular in responses to cutaneous stimulation.

6.4. FUNCTIONAL ROLE OF DIFFERENT MOTOR UNITS

The functional role of motor units is largely defined by their properties. That is, tasks that require prolonged exertion of muscle force are mostly carried out by slow, fatigue-resistant motor units, while tasks that require a quick but short-lasting increase in muscle force are mostly performed by fast motor units. In particular, many of the postural muscles have a large proportion of S motor units. On the other hand, muscles that participate in quick limb movements such as kicking, hitting, or catching typically have a large proportion of FR and FF motor units. Most muscles, however, have a relatively wide range of motor units of different types.

Problem 6.4

Which motor units would you expect to find in abundance in a marathon runner, in a weight lifter, and in a swimmer?

The rates of sustained firing of motoneurons are commonly rather high (from about 8 Hz to about 35 Hz) so that twitch contractions of individual motor units overlap, leading to a tetanus. The upper limit of the firing rate makes sense because at this rate individual twitch contractions fully fuse, so that an additional increase in firing rate could not lead to an increase in muscle force.

As already mentioned, there are two basic means available to our central nervous system to increase muscle force (figure 6.5). The first is to recruit more motor units, and the second is to increase the firing frequency of already recruited motor units. Both methods are used dur-

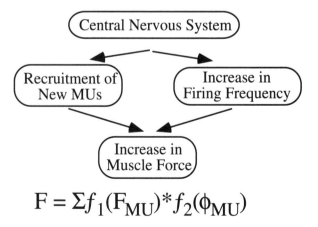

$$F = \Sigma f_1(F_{MU}) * f_2(\phi_{MU})$$

Figure 6.5 To increase muscle force, the central nervous system may recruit new motor units and/or increase the frequency of firing of already recruited motor units. Here, F is force, f is a monotonically increasing function, ϕ is frequency of firing.

ing natural, voluntary movements, although recruitment of new motor units is a more commonly seen phenomenon during voluntary muscle contractions.

During most voluntary movements, individual motoneurons do not demonstrate any substantial level of synchronization. At very high levels of muscle force, however, during fatigue, and in some neurological disorders (such as loss of voluntary muscle force following a spinal cord injury), **synchronization** of motor unit firing becomes a way of achieving higher forces or maintaining a level of force for a considerable period of time. Motor unit synchronization has both positive and negative features. The gain is obvious: synchronized discharges will sum up to higher total muscle force as compared to asynchronous motor unit firing. However, smoothness of the contraction will suffer. There is also a possibility of quicker fatigue.

Problem 6.5

You have invented a way to induce abrupt synchronization of motor units in human muscles. What types of athletes would you recommend this method to, and what types of athletes would you suggest not even try it?

Synchronization of motor units can be measured directly, with the method of cross-correlation, or indirectly, by performing spectral analysis of the "summed" (interferential) electromyogram (EMG). If the activity of a couple of motor units is recorded for a long time, the cross-correlation function will show a peak at a zero delay if the motor units are ideally synchronized.

6.5. ELECTROMYOGRAPHY

There are two basic methods of recording muscle activity: **intramuscular** or **needle electromyography** and **surface** or **interferential electromyography.**

With the first method, a thin needle (with a diameter of less than 1 mm) is inserted into a muscle (figure 6.6). Inside the needle is a very thin wire that is electrically isolated from the needle. The tip of the wire is not isolated. An amplifier picks up the difference of potentials between the tip of the wire and the needle. Since the dimensions of each electrode and the distance between the two electrodes are very small, the electrodes will selectively pick up the signals (action potentials) in closest proximity to their tips. Such electrodes are designed to record the patterns of activity of individual motor units. Note that each motor unit contains many muscle fibers but that they all generate action potentials synchronously, so that the electrode picks up the compound action potential of the whole motor unit. Typically, a

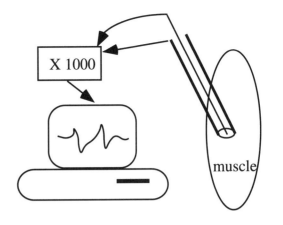

Figure 6.6 Intramuscular EMG uses thin needle electrodes. Inside the needle is a very thin wire that is electrically isolated from the needle. The difference of potentials between the tip of the wire and the tip of the needle is amplified and recorded.

needle electrode is able to record the electrical activity of a few motor units whose muscle fibers happen to be in close proximity to it. However, because each motor unit has a somewhat different number of muscle fibers, and also because the locations of these fibers with respect to the electrode are different, each motor unit will have a different, unique pattern of voltage changes (figure 6.7). These differences make it possible to record several motor units with one electrode and to identify their compound action potentials with a high degree of certainty. Needle electromyography is frequently used in clinical tests.

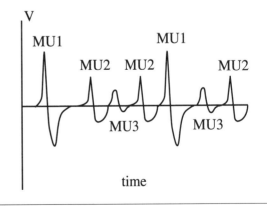

Figure 6.7 A typical record with an intramuscular needle electrode reveals a few motor units with different shapes of the compound potentials, MU_1, MU_2, and MU_3.

Another method is **interferential electromyography,** which is more frequently used in studies of voluntary movements of healthy persons. The main idea of interferential electromyography is to sum up the activity of as many motor units as possible across a muscle.

Typically, two electrodes are taped on the skin over the muscle belly, and the difference of potentials between the electrodes is amplified (figure 6.8). On the one hand, the desire to sum up the activity may suggest using very large electrodes and placing them as far from each other as possible. On the other hand, researchers would probably like to focus on just one muscle and avoid recording the activity of its neighbors. So there is a trade-off that is resolved differently by each experimenter and in each particular case. For example, if one wants to record the activity of a relatively small forearm or facial muscle, it is unwise to use very large electrodes because they will pick up the activity of many other muscles in the neighborhood. Alternatively, if one wants to record the activity of a large postural muscle such as latissimus dorsi or biceps femoris, using large electrodes will probably be appropriate. Typically, electrodes used for surface electromyography vary from 1 mm to 20 mm in diameter, while the distance between the centers of the electrodes varies from 5 mm to 50 mm or even more. The choice of particular electrodes and their placement are part of the art of electromyography.

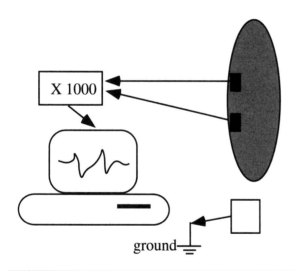

Figure 6.8 Surface EMG uses a pair of electrodes that are placed on a muscle belly. A third electrode (ground) is used to reduce noise.

Note that absolute values of electromyographic signals recorded with surface electrodes are typically on the order of tens to hundreds of microvolts. There are numerous sources of electrical noise that can obscure the biopotentials and make them indistinguishable from the noise. The most frequently encountered sources of noise are the 60 Hz voltage used as the power supply in every laboratory and radio waves that are picked up by a subject's body, which acts like an antenna. Other possible sources include electric motors or strong electrical magnets, even when these are located in an adjacent room. In order to minimize the noise and assure selective recording of biopotentials, the *body surface is usually grounded* with a large "indifferent" electrode.

6.6. FILTERING, RECTIFICATION, AND INTEGRATION

It is impossible to recommend a single method of recording and processing EMGs. There are several standard types of procedures; however, each researcher selects his or her own methods of data processing based on the actual goals of the study and the researcher's own imagination. Three operations are frequently used in processing a surface EMG.

The first is **filtering.** Note that action potentials are very fast events with typical times of potential changes of about a few milliseconds. So a high-pass filter, which cuts off all the frequencies equal to or below 60 Hz, is frequently used. As a result, the 60 Hz noise is reduced, as are possible reactions of the electrodes to purely mechanical factors that are usually much slower than changes in biopotentials. On the other hand, the upper limit of frequency is chosen based on the characteristic times of events that are of interest to the experimenter. If the experimenter is not interested in the microstructure of the electromyographic signals such as shapes of individual action potentials, a low-pass cutoff frequency is commonly on the order of a few hundred Hertz.

The second operation is **rectification.** Basically this consists of turning all the negative values of the difference of potentials into positive values of equal magnitude (figure 6.9). The purpose is to be able to get a quantitative estimate of an electromyographic signal. If an action potential runs along a fiber under a pair of recording electrodes (figure 6.9), the difference of potentials at the electrodes will change gradually, leading to a reversal in its sign. Actually, most biopotentials show a nearly symmetrical picture with respect to zero level. Integrating an unrectified signal over a reasonably long time will yield a very small number (close to zero) because the signal is composed of an approximately equal number of positive and negative values. Integrating a rectified EMG will result in a value reflecting the average magnitude of the activity over the time of integration.

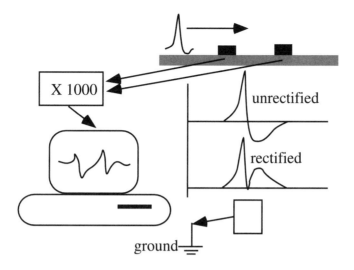

X 1000

unrectified

rectified

ground

Figure 6.9 An action potential runs under a pair of electrodes. The difference of potentials recorded by the electrodes will change its sign (the upper record). Rectification means making all the values of the difference of potentials positive (the lower record).

Problem 6.6

Imagine that you have an EMG record. You can filter it and then rectify it or, alternatively, you can rectify it and then filter. Which method is better? Why?

The third procedure is **integration.** Actually, two types of integration are used for different purposes. If a researcher is interested in the overall shape of the EMG rather than in its microstructure, an EMG "envelope" is calculated. The EMG envelope represents a time function each point of which is the result of integration over small time periods, such as several tens of milliseconds. The other integration procedure is used when an overall measure of the amount of muscle activity over a certain period of time is needed. Integration of a rectified EMG gives a value reflecting total current between the electrodes as well as total resistance. Skin resistance is very hard to control; it can vary in a wide range and may even change during an experiment, for example if the subject sweats. So in order to compare integral electromyographic measures across subjects, one needs to **normalize** the integrals. Normalizing means dividing a measured value by a number that is likely to reflect the differences in the conditions of recording (for example, skin resistance) but not the differences in the signal of interest:

$$E_N = EMG/EMG_{st} \qquad (6.1)$$

where E_N is normalized EMG, EMG is a calculated integral of a signal that you are interested in, and EMG_{st} is a calculated integral over the same time period during a standard task. This procedure is another "piece of art"; it is extremely subjective, and different experimenters use different methods of normalization. Typically, integrated EMGs are normalized with respect to the value recorded when the subject exerts maximal voluntary contraction of the muscle or, alternatively, when the subject exerts a standard level of force.

Problem 6.7

Suggest a way to normalize an EMG during very fast movements and during very small changes in the level of muscle activity.

Figure 6.10 illustrates the effects of different filtering and rectification procedures on an EMG signal recorded from a human biceps muscle. The upper signal is the "raw" (unprocessed) EMG signal amplified and sampled at a high frequency (1000 Hz) by a computer. The next panel shows a rectified signal without any additional filtering. The next two panels show the effects of low-pass filtering (with the "second-order Butterworth filter") at cutoff frequencies of 100 Hz and 20 Hz. The lowest panel shows the same record rectified and processed with a moving-average window of 100 ms to create an EMG envelope signal. Note that filtering can affect the characteristic amplitude of the signal.

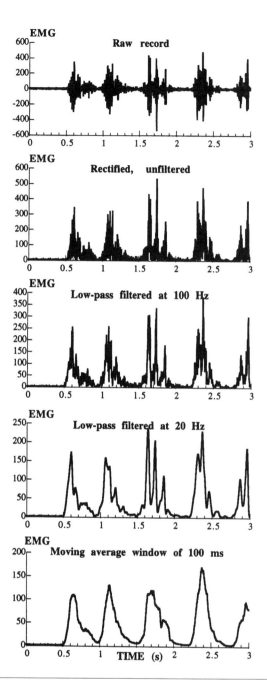

Figure 6.10   The effects of different filtering and rectification procedures on an EMG signal recorded with surface electrodes from a human biceps muscle during a series of brief voluntary contractions. The upper signal is the "raw" (unprocessed) EMG signal sampled at a high frequency (1000 Hz) by the computer. Note the similarities (e.g., burst timing) and differences in the signal under different filtering.

Chapter 6 in a Nutshell

A motor unit consists of a motoneuron and all the muscle fibers innervated by its axon. There are three major types of motor units: slow, fatigue resistant; fast, fatigue resistant; and fast, fatigable. Slow motor units contain neurons with a smaller body, a thinner axon, slower conduction velocity of action potentials, and fewer innervated muscle fibers. During natural muscle contractions, motor units are recruited in a fixed order, from the smallest to the largest (size or Henneman principle). Derecruitment follows the opposite order, from the largest to the smallest. Electromyography is a method for studying muscle activation levels and patterns. It is more an art than a science.

Self-Test Problems

1. You have an atypical neural cell in which the concentration of K^+ ions inside the cell is not 150 mmol/L, but only 50 mmol/L. Everything else is exactly as in "regular" cells. Calculate the equilibrium potential for K^+. How will the equilibrium potential on the membrane and the action potential in this cell differ from those in "regular" neurons?

2. You observe two fibers under changes in temperature. A stimulator is placed at one end of each fiber, and you record the response at the other end. One fiber decreased the speed of transmission of action potentials with a decrease in temperature and eventually stopped transmitting them. The other fiber did not transmit action potentials at higher temperatures, started to transmit them at lower temperatures, and stopped transmitting them at very low temperatures. What can you conclude about these two fibers? Explain the differences in their behavior.

3. You have a neural cell with one excitatory and one inhibitory synapse. At a certain frequency of stimulation of both presynaptic fibers, the neuron does not generate an action potential. You increase the frequency of stimulation of the inhibitory input without changing the frequency of stimulation of the excitatory input. After some time, the neuron starts to generate action potentials. Why? In another experiment, you increase the frequency of stimulation of the excitatory input. The neuron generates several action potentials and then becomes silent. Why?

4. You study the response of a neural cell to a single excitatory input. The cell generates action potentials at a certain frequency. You add an excitatory neurotransmitter to the extracellular space and the cell stops firing. What happened?

5. You induce a twitch contraction of a muscle by a direct electrical stimulus. The external load is zero. Draw time changes in the frequency of firing of a primary spindle ending, of a secondary spindle ending, and of a Golgi tendon organ. Prior to the contraction, each receptor showed steady firing at a constant frequency. Solve the same problem for isometric conditions, that is, when the muscle+tendon complex cannot change its length.

6. A person generates 5% of the maximal voluntary contraction force of a muscle. Then muscle force increases slightly so that only one new motor unit is recruited. What can you say about the properties of this motor unit? The same person generates 95% of the maximal voluntary contraction force. Again, muscle force increases slightly so that only one new motor unit is recruited. What can you say about the properties of this motor unit?

Recommended Additional Readings

Basmajian JV, DeLuca C (1985). *Muscles Alive and Their Functions Revealed by Electromyography.* Baltimore: Williams & Wilkins.

Enoka RM (1994). *Neuromechanical Basis of Kinesiology.* 2nd ed. Champaign, IL: Human Kinetics. Chapters 3, 4.

Granit R (1955). *Receptors and Sensory Perception.* New Haven: Yale University Press.

Hill AV (1938). The heat of shortening and the dynamic constants of muscle. *Proceedings of the Royal Society of London, Series B,* 126: 136-195.

Lieber RL (1992). *Skeletal Muscle Structure and Function.* Baltimore: Williams & Wilkins.

Partridge LD, Partridge LD (1993). *The Nervous System: Its Function and Its Interaction with the World.* Cambridge, MA: MIT Press. Chapters 10, 11, 12, 13, 14.

Popper KR, Eccles JC (1983). *The Self and Its Brain.* London, New York: Routledge & Kegan Paul.

Rothwell JR (1994). *Control of Human Voluntary Movement.* 2nd ed. London: Chapman & Hall. Chapters 2, 3, 4.

WORLD II

CONNECTIONS

CHAPTER 7

EXCITATION AND INHIBITION WITHIN THE SPINAL CORD

Key Terms

anatomy of the spinal cord
excitation

postsynaptic and
    presynaptic inhibition
recurrent inhibition

Renshaw cells
reciprocal inhibition
Ia-interneurons

7.1. THE SPINAL CORD

At this point the reader is ready to make another qualitative step in terms of the complexity of the objects of our study. The story started with the properties of parts of single cells (the membranes, ions, molecules, channels, etc.) and electrical phenomena that form the foundation of information exchange among neural and muscular cells. Then it moved through an overview of the properties and functions of certain individual cells such as muscular cells and receptors. The next step is to consider how various neurons interact with each other within the **spinal cord** and with signals supplied by peripheral receptors. Let us start with relatively automatic reactions to external stimuli that are commonly designated **reflexes.** (A controversy surrounding the term "reflex" has been briefly addressed earlier; this notion will be discussed further in chapter 8). The wiring of the spinal cord is rather complex, and only a tiny fraction of all the connections have been deciphered with any degree of certainty.

The spinal cord has a **laminar structure** (figure 7.1). This word means that it more or less "flows down" from

the brain without abrupt changes in its cross-sectional structure, like crossings-over or other discontinuities. The meaning of "lamina" is very close to that of "layer." If the spinal cord is transected at an intermediate level, a characteristic "butterfly" picture can be seen. The "butterfly" consists of **gray matter,** while the rest of the section is **white matter.** At each level, the same areas (laminae) can be identified in the gray matter. These areas are named after a scientist, Rexed, and are designated by roman numerals from laminae I to laminae X.

It is necessary to introduce a few "geographical" terms that will help in future chapters as well (figure 7.2). **Dorsal** means oriented toward the back of the body; **ventral** means oriented toward the stomach; **rostral** means closer to the head; **caudal** means closer to the tail (or what is left of the tail in humans); **medial** means closer to the center; **lateral** means closer to a side; **proximal** means close to an origin of coordinates (commonly, the trunk); and **distal** means far from the origin of coordinates. Three orthogonal planes are commonly identified with respect to the human body. These are **frontal,** which means a plane parallel to the mirror into which a person looks when combing his or her hair; **sagittal,** which means a

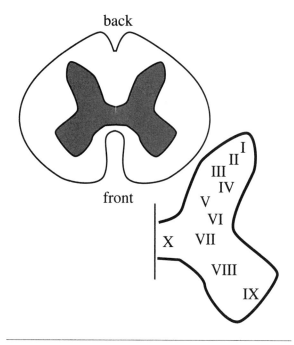

Figure 7.1 The spinal cord has a laminar structure. It "flows" along the body, preserving the general picture of its cross sections (above). At each level, the gray matter forms a characteristic butterfly picture consisting of 10 Rexed's laminae (below).

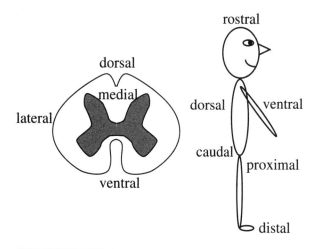

Figure 7.2 These terms will be helpful in future descriptions. The figure of a person is drawn in a sagittal plane.

plane parallel to the plane of arm and leg movements during normal walking; and **coronal,** which means a plane perpendicular to the spine and parallel to the ground if one is standing upright.

The spinal cord is a very important part of the human central nervous system; an injury of the spinal cord may lead to complete and irreversible paralysis. It is protected from possible damaging influences by the spine. The spine consists of vertebrae (bone structures) separated from each other by elastic spinal disks (cartilage struc-

tures). This construction allows the combination of flexibility of the spine, resistance to possible compression forces, and protection of the spinal cord. Each vertebra has two pairs of horns, the **dorsal horns** (closer to the back) and the **ventral horns** (closer to the stomach or chest) (figure 7.3). The dorsal horns serve as input paths for information from peripheral receptors. Remember that bodies of the receptor cells are located in spinal ganglia, just outside the spinal cord. These cells have T-shaped axons whose distal branches go to the sensitive endings, somewhere in the periphery, while the proximal branch enters the spinal cord through the dorsal horns. Axons from numerous peripheral receptors form a dorsal root and come together through the same dorsal horn. The ventral horns serve as output paths of signals to peripheral structures, in particular to muscles (axons of α-motoneurons) and to muscle spindles (axons of γ-motoneurons). Axons of these neurons form **ventral roots.**

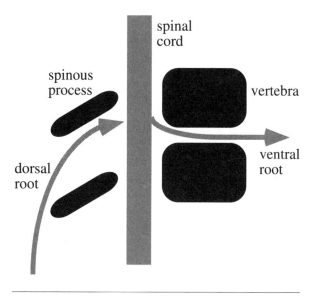

Figure 7.3 Each vertebra has a body and a spinous process. Peripheral information gets into the spinal cord through the dorsal roots, while efferent signals are sent from the spinal cord through the ventral roots.

Spinal vertebrae form four major groups: the **cervical spine** (7 vertebrae), the **thoracic spine** (12 vertebrae), the **lumbar spine** (5 vertebrae), and the **sacrum** (figure 7.4). The vertebrae are numbered through each group starting from the most rostral vertebra. So, starting from the connection between the spine and the skull, the vertebrae are CI to CVII, ThI to ThXII, LI to LV, and the sacrum. The spinal cord is commonly described as consisting of **spinal segments;** this classification refers to the spinal roots that enter the spine and leave it at the level of each vertebra. Each spinal segment receives peripheral information through one pair of dorsal roots and sends command signals through one pair of ventral roots. The segments are also classified into cervical, thoracic, lumbar, and sacral, but this classification does not exactly correspond to the classification of vertebrae. Spinal segments, starting from the brain, go in the order C1 to C8, Th1 to Th12, L1 to L5, and S1 to S5. The size of the spinal segments does not correspond exactly to the size of the vertebrae; thus there is a mismatch between the numbers of segments and numbers of corresponding vertebrae, which increases in the caudal direction. As a result, the spinal cord ends at the level of L1 vertebrae. The caudal part of the spine does not contain spinal cord at all, only the axons forming the dorsal and ventral roots of the lower spinal segments. This part is called **cauda equina** or the horsetail because of its appearance.

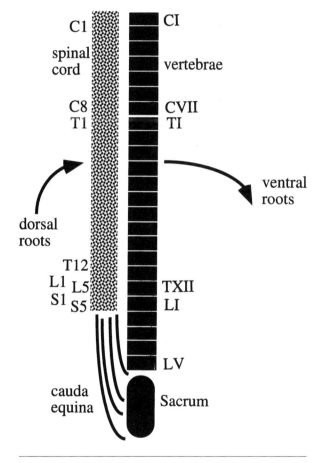

Figure 7.4 Vertebrae are numbered starting from the skull: C_1 to L_5, and then the sacrum. Spinal segments are numbered from C_1 to S_5, but this classification does not exactly correspond to the vertebrae classification. The spinal cord ends at the L_1 vertebra; lower, the roots of the lower segments form the cauda equina.

Each segment of the spinal cord receives peripheral information from a well-defined area of the body and sends command signals to muscles within approximately the same area (figure 7.5). These areas go, like zebra stripes, across the body and down the limbs. It can be said, for example, that the anterior thigh area is **innervated** by segments L2 and L3 while the foot is innervated by segments L5 and S1. The topography of these areas is well known to neurologists, who use it, in particular, to define the level of a spinal cord injury.

Let us get back to the "butterfly" that can be seen on a cross section of the spinal cord at any level. The back parts of the "wings" are the places where dorsal roots enter the spinal cord. The axons forming the dorsal roots spread out and make synapses in various areas of the cross section. The cross section shows areas of different colors commonly designated white matter and gray matter (figure 7.1). The white matter consists mostly of cut axons of descending and ascending pathways, while the gray matter contains cell bodies. The ventral (front) parts of the "wings" are the places where the motoneurons (both α- and γ-) are located and where ventral roots leave the spinal cord. This area will be of particular interest. In this chapter, the discussion will be limited to neurons and events that occur in the ventral areas of the spinal cord. Note, however, that most of the neurons within the spinal cord are not motoneurons but interneurons. These neurons receive information either from afferent fibers or from other neurons within the central nervous system, and generate action potentials that are transduced to other interneurons or to motoneurons.

7.2. EXCITATION WITHIN THE CENTRAL NERVOUS SYSTEM

There are methods that can be used to trace the path of a given axon, or, more frequently, of a group of axons from cells of one type located in one area. These methods involve injection of certain chemicals into the cell bodies or into neural fibers. The chemicals are transported, mostly by simple diffusion, along all the neural cell branches, including the axon and the dendrites. Then a histochemical analysis can be performed that shows the areas where the chemical is present. Certainly such experiments are performed on anesthetized animals. A common substance used for tracing neural pathways is horseradish peroxidase. Specifically it allows one to trace the patterns of termination of various afferent fibers as well as of the axons of neurons within the central nervous system.

Tracing excitatory neural pathways has shown that within the central nervous system, *virtually every neuron is connected to every other neuron* through a certain number of synapses. So if an excitation emerges somewhere, theoretically it has a chance to spread to each and every neural cell and consequently to induce contractions of each and every muscle of the body. It is important to consider that all the synapses made by afferent fibers on neurons within the central nervous system are

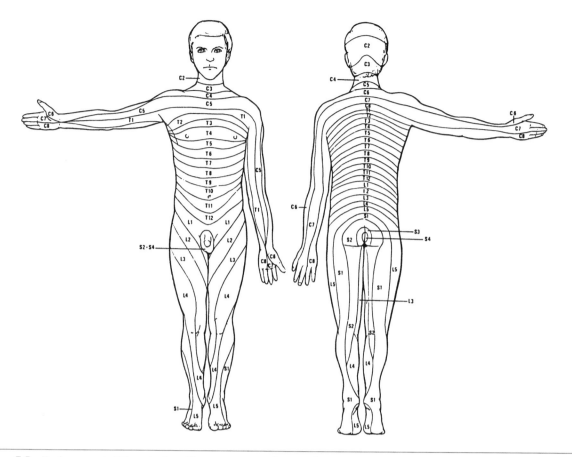

Figure 7.5   Each segment of the spinal cord innervates a certain area of the body. These areas divide the body surface into zebra-like stripes.
Reproduced by permission of Appleton & Lange from "Anatomy of the Somatic Sensory System" by J.H. Martin and T.M. Jessell published in "Principles of Neural Science," third edition, edited by E.R. Kandel, J.H. Schwartz, and T.M. Jessell, Elsevier: New York.

excitatory. This means that the human central nervous system is always under the influence of an inflow of excitatory stimuli that may lead to undesirable motor effects unless balanced by inhibitory stimuli. In some pathological conditions, something like this actually may happen, when pinching an arm may lead to a spasm of virtually all the body muscles. It is obvious that the central nervous system needs strong and reliable mechanisms to prevent uncontrolled spread of excitation. One may even go a step further and make the statement that the essence of information transmission within the central nervous system is in cutting off undesirable routes. Consider the following analogy: in order to control the flow of a river, you need to build dams to prevent the water from flowing astray.

Thus we have come to the conclusion that the central nervous system needs means to make excitatory synapses ineffective. There are two basic mechanisms of inhibition within the central nervous system, termed **postsynaptic inhibition** and **presynaptic inhibition.** The first of these makes a neuron less sensitive (or insensitive) to any excitatory signal that may arrive. The second one is more subtle and selective; it makes certain inputs (cer-

tain synapses) into the neuron less effective without affecting other inputs.

7.3. POSTSYNAPTIC INHIBITION

First, think back to chapter 3 and recollect that a synapse consists of a presynaptic membrane, a synaptic cleft, and a postsynaptic membrane (figure 7.6). So the term postsynaptic inhibition means that the inhibition occurs on the postsynaptic membrane. The mechanism of postsynaptic inhibition is rather straightforward. Excitatory synapses lead to a depolarization of the postsynaptic membrane, that is, to a decrease in the absolute value of its negative resting potential (an EPSP). If the combined action of a number of excitatory synapses reaches the threshold, the postsynaptic neuron generates an action potential.

Synapses between neurons within the central nervous system may be either excitatory or inhibitory. Inhibitory synapses use special mediators that lead to an increase in the absolute value of the membrane resting potential, that is, to membrane hyperpolarization (figure 7.7). Thus,

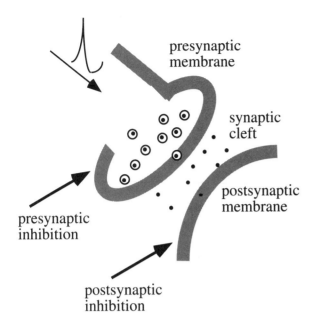

presynaptic
membrane

synaptic
cleft

postsynaptic
membrane

presynaptic
inhibition

postsynaptic
inhibition

Figure 7.6 A synapse consists of a presynaptic membrane, a synaptic cleft, and a postsynaptic membrane. Inhibition of synaptic transmission means a decrease in the efficacy of the synapse and may occur as a result of events on the presynaptic or the postsynaptic membrane.

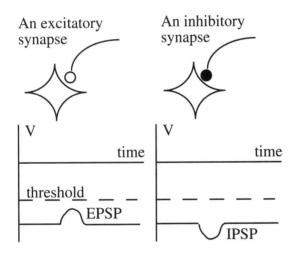

An excitatory
synapse

An inhibitory
synapse

V

time

threshold

EPSP

V

time

IPSP

Figure 7.7 An excitatory synapse leads to a depolarization of the postsynaptic membrane (EPSP), i.e., bringing it closer to the threshold, while an inhibitory synapse leads to a hyperpolarization (IPSP) of the postsynaptic membrane.

inhibitory postsynaptic potentials (IPSPs) bring the membrane potential further away from its threshold and make the membrane less likely to generate an action potential in response to excitatory stimuli. Note that IPSPs have properties similar to those of EPSPs, such as temporal and spatial summation. So a large number of inhibitory synapses may cancel out potential excitatory effects of a

comparably large number of comparably effective excitatory synapses.

Problem 7.1

Can you use an inhibitory neuron to increase the excitability of another neuron?

Consider two examples of postsynaptic inhibition within the spinal cord that are particularly important for the control of voluntary muscle contractions.

7.4. RENSHAW CELLS

Motoneurons (and some interneurons) are organized in pools, that is, in groups with a similar function. In particular, all the α-motoneurons innervating a single muscle are called a **motoneuronal pool.** Figure 7.8 shows schematically a few motoneurons (α and γ) innervating the same muscle. The axons of α-motoneurons travel to the muscle and induce contraction of its fibers, while the axons of γ-motoneurons innervate intrafusal muscular fibers and change the sensitivity of spindle sensory endings to muscle length and velocity. The axons of α-motoneurons, however, branch very closely to the cell body, within the ventral horns, and make excitatory synapses on special interneurons that are called **Renshaw cells.**

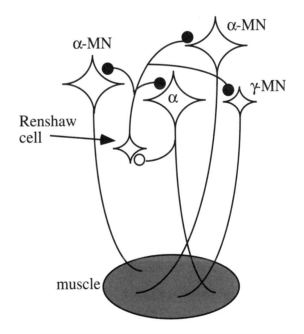

α-MN

α-MN

γ-MN

α

Renshaw
cell

muscle

Figure 7.8 Axons of α-motoneurons branch very close to the cell body and make excitatory synapses on Renshaw cells, which in turn make inhibitory synapses on α-motoneurons of the same pool as well as on γ-motoneurons sending their axons to spindles in the same muscle.

The axons of the Renshaw cells go back to the bodies of α-motoneurons as well as to the bodies of γ-motoneurons and form inhibitory synapses. Note that inhibition by Renshaw cells spreads over all the motoneurons of the pool.

This scheme may look strange: the output of α-motoneurons excites cells that inhibit the same α-motoneurons! However, it makes a lot of sense as a mechanism limiting the level of activity of a pool of motoneurons. Such schemes are called **negative feedback.** There are quite a few examples of negative feedback in the mechanisms of control of voluntary movements. It seems that the central nervous system does not like any changes and that if a change occurs, there is always a mechanism available to scale it down. Negative feedback mechanisms allow the central nervous system to minimize the effects of external perturbations as well as to keep down our reactions to such perturbations.

Problem 7.2

A muscle is actively contracting against a constant load. What effects do you expect from the action of Renshaw cells upon γ-motoneurons?

Renshaw cells also receive descending inputs, that is, signals from the brain. These signals may be considered as means to control the effectiveness (gain) of the negative feedback. For example, if the brain "wants" to achieve a high level of muscle contraction force in the shortest possible time, it makes sense to turn the Renshaw cells off. On the other hand, if the task is to have precise control over the output to a muscle, Renshaw cells must be activated to counteract any accidental changes in the level of activity of α-motoneurons.

7.5. Ia-INTERNEURONS

Another important group of inhibitory interneurons receive signals from Ia-spindle afferents (figure 7.9). Note that these signals are always excitatory. These interneurons (**Ia-interneurons**) send their axons to α-motoneurons controlling an antagonist muscle, that is, a muscle whose contraction opposes the action of a muscle from where the Ia-afferents originate. Such neuronal projections are called **heterogenic,** while projections from afferents within a muscle to motoneurons controlling the same muscle are called **autogenic.** Ia-interneurons make inhibitory synapses on the mem-

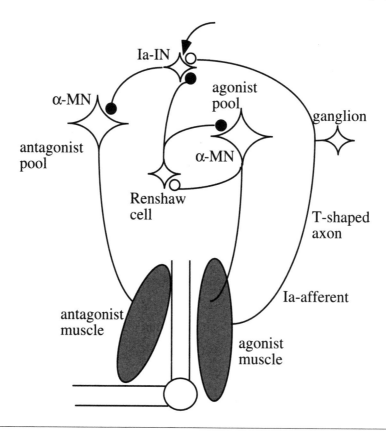

Figure 7.9   Ia-interneurons (Ia-IN) receive excitatory inputs from Ia-afferents and make inhibitory synapses on motoneurons innervating the antagonist muscle. Ia-INs are inhibited by Renshaw cells and also receive descending inputs.

brane of the α-motoneurons that belong to the antagonist pool.

This arrangement is another example of negative feedback (figure 7.10). Imagine that a muscle is being stretched. Typically this occurs because the antagonist muscle is shortening as a result of its active contraction. The spindle endings of the stretched muscle will become more active and will excite Ia-interneurons. These interneurons will inhibit the antagonist α-motoneurons, thus bringing down the level of contraction of the antagonist muscle. Thus, the action of Ia-interneurons will counteract an increase in the level of activity of the antagonist α-motoneurons.

Ia-interneurons are inhibited by Renshaw cells as shown in figure 7.10. Again, this is a mechanism of negative feedback. Imagine that α-motoneurons increase their level of activity. This would bring about an active contraction of a muscle controlled by the α-motoneurons and a corresponding joint motion. The Renshaw cells inhibit the Ia-interneurons and thus decrease their inhibitory effects on antagonist α-motoneurons. Such an action is called **disinhibition** and is equivalent to additional excitation of antagonist α-motoneurons. An increase in the activity of the antagonist muscle will apparently counteract the joint motion that would otherwise occur.

Problem 7.3

You stimulate a pool of Ia-interneurons. How will muscle force change for an agonist and for an antagonist? What kind of change do you expect to see in the firing rate of Renshaw cells?

7.6. PRESYNAPTIC INHIBITION

Note that both Renshaw cells and Ia-interneurons decrease the potential response of their target neurons to all possible excitatory stimuli. The second major type of inhibition within the central nervous system is more selective. Its purpose is to decrease the effectiveness of just one type (or a few types) of inputs to a neuron without affecting other inputs. Let us once again take a look at a typical inhibitory synapse (figure 7.11). Apparently, any action on the postsynaptic membrane will affect the effectiveness of other synapses because of the passive spread of membrane potential changes. So in order to shut down only one synapse, the system needs to act at a presynaptic level.

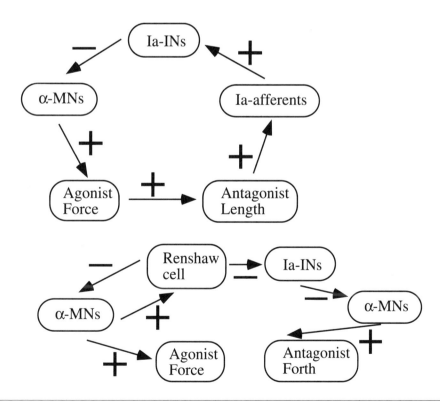

Figure 7.10 Feedback loops involving Ia-interneurons and Renshaw cells. Pluses mean that an increase in the input leads to an increase in the output; minuses mean that an increase in the input leads to a decrease in the output.

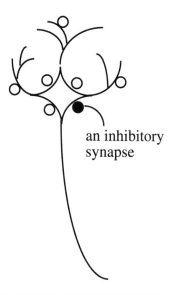

an inhibitory
synapse

mediator. The GABA induces a long-lasting depolarization of the presynaptic membrane. This certainly does not prevent the action potential from getting to the synapse. However, the amount of the excitatory mediator released in response to an action potential very strongly depends upon the peak-to-peak amplitude of the action potential. Depolarization of the presynaptic membrane leads to a decrease in the peak-to-peak amplitude of the action potential and, as a result, to a substantial decrease in the amount of mediator released into the synaptic cleft. Consequently, depolarization of the postsynaptic membrane decreases and may become unable to bring the membrane potential to its threshold. Thus, an additional excitatory synapse becomes an effective tool of inducing selective inhibitory effects!

Figure 7.11 A postsynaptic inhibitory synapse hyperpolarizes the postsynaptic membrane and decreases its responsiveness to all the excitatory synapses (open circles).

Problem 7.4

Is postsynaptic inhibition equally effective in decreasing the response of the cell to all the presynaptic excitatory synapses?

Problem 7.5

What will happen if an inhibitory synapse is acting at a presynaptic membrane close to the synaptic cleft?

Problem 7.6

What will happen if a presynaptic inhibitory mechanism is acting on a postsynaptic inhibitory synapse? What will happen if a presynaptic inhibitory mechanism is acting on another presynaptic inhibitory synapse?

This is achieved in a paradoxical way. An **excitatory** synapse acts at the presynaptic axonal membrane near the synaptic cleft (figure 7.12). It uses GABA as a

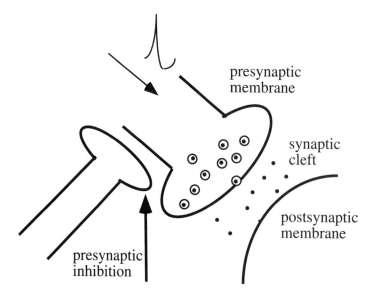

presynaptic
membrane

synaptic
cleft

postsynaptic
membrane

presynaptic
inhibition

Figure 7.12 Presynaptic inhibition acts selectively on certain synapses. It involves an excitatory synapse acting on the presynaptic membrane, inducing its steady subthreshold depolarization and thus decreasing the amount of mediator released in response to a single presynaptic action potential.

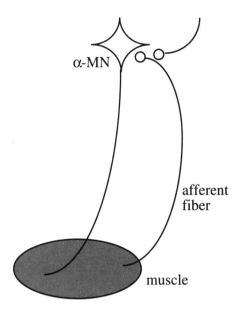

Figure 7.13 presents an example of the action of presynaptic inhibition. In this figure, an excitatory synapse is acting at the presynaptic afferent (sensory) fiber close to its synapse at an α-motoneuron. The activity of the presynaptic synapse can lead to a decrease in the reflex response to the afferent fiber activity, while the activity of the motoneuron can be unchanged or even increased. Such examples will be discussed in the next chapter.

Figure 7.13 An example of the action of presynaptic inhibition. In this figure, an excitatory synapse is acting at a presynaptic afferent (sensory) fiber close to its synapse at the target α-motoneuron.

Chapter 7 in a Nutshell

The spinal cord is protected by the spine; it has a laminar structure and is divided into segments that innervate certain areas of the body. The spinal cord contains numerous motoneurons, interneurons, and conduction pathways that carry both descending and ascending information. Afferent information enters the spinal cord through the dorsal roots, while efferent nerves that carry motor signals exit through the ventral roots. Inhibition within the central nervous system is vital for its proper functioning. Postsynaptic inhibition hyperpolarizes the postsynaptic membrane and makes the neuron less sensitive to all excitatory inputs. Presynaptic inhibition works through depolarization of presynaptic fibers and selectively decreases the effectiveness of only some of the inputs. Renshaw cells are interneurons that are excited by axons of α-motoneurons and inhibit motoneurons of the same pool (recurrent inhibition). Ia-interneurons are excited by Ia-afferents from primary spindle sensory endings; they inhibit α-motoneurons of the antagonist pool (reciprocal inhibition).

CHAPTER 8

MONOSYNAPTIC REFLEXES

Key Terms

general scheme of a reflex

reflex arc

latency

H-reflex

M-response

T-reflex

effects of voluntary muscle activation

F-wave

8.1. REFLEXES

The noun "reflex" means something that reflects or is a consequence of another something. Correspondingly, a muscle reflex is a muscle contraction induced by an external stimulus. However, many actions induced by external stimuli are not considered reflexes. For example, if a driver sees a red light, he or she presses the brake pedal. Is this a reflex? Most people would probably argue that if the driver presses the pedal automatically, "without thinking," this is a reflex (remember, there are drivers with "good reflexes" and those with "bad reflexes"). If the same driver saw the light from far away and then decided to brake, this is probably not a reflex but a voluntary action. This example shows that it is very hard to distinguish formally a reflex from a nonreflex. For our purposes, I am going to accept the following definition of muscle reflex, and stick to it, even when it apparently fails: a reflex is a muscle contraction induced by an external stimulus that cannot be changed by "pure thinking," that is, by a volitional act that is not accompanied by another muscle contraction.

This definition is not perfect, but at least it provides a starting point.

Many reflexes have been studied in animal preparations, that is, in animals whose central nervous system has been experimentally damaged. Such procedures frequently induce surgical separation of the spinal cord from the brain. In this case, the animal is referred to as **spinalized** or as a **spinal preparation.** If one assumes that everything volitional comes from the brain, all muscle reactions to external stimuli in a spinalized animal are apparently reflexes, because signals from the brain cannot reach the spinal cord.

In the beginning of the century, muscle reflexes were considered as building blocks for voluntary movements. This view was based on a very impressive series of experiments on spinalized animals performed by Sherrington and his school. Later, the growing awareness of the complexity and variability of voluntary movements, and of their relative independence of transient changes in the external conditions of movement execution (external force field), led to another extreme in which muscle reflexes were considered relatively insignificant mechanisms that play an important role only when a movement gets off its planned track. Recently, muscle reflexes have been once again brought into the center of attention by hypotheses of motor control that consider voluntary movements to be consequences of central modulation of parameters of certain reflexes.

8.2. REFLEX ARC

A central notion related to all muscle reflexes is that of the **reflex arc** (figure 8.1). The reflex arc consists of an

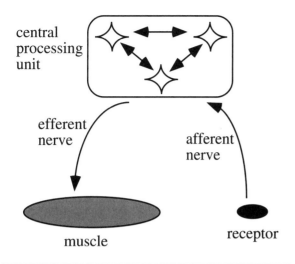

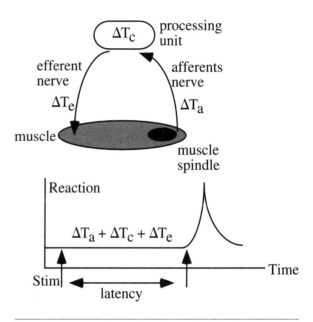

Figure 8.1 Reflex arc consists of a sensory element (receptor), an afferent (sensory) nerve, a central processing unit, an efferent (command) nerve, and an effector (e.g., a muscle).

afferent neuron that senses an external stimulus, a **central processing unit,** and an **efferent neuron** that induces a muscle contraction. The central processing unit may be very simple, consisting of just one synapse, or very complex, involving numerous synapses and integration of information from different sources. The simplest reflexes involve only one central synapse (we do not count the neuromuscular synapse that is apparently involved in any muscular contraction). These reflexes are called **monosynaptic** (figure 8.2). Reflexes that involve many synapses are called **polysynaptic.** Reflexes that involve two to three synapses are called **oligosynaptic.**

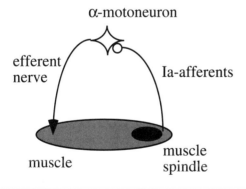

Figure 8.2 A monosynaptic reflex has only one synapse in its reflex arc. This synapse is between an afferent fiber and an α-motoneuron.

Each reflex involves a time delay between a stimulus and a reaction. This time delay is called **reflex latency** (figure 8.3). It consists of three components: time of af-

ferent conduction, central delay, and time of efferent conduction. Conduction time apparently depends on the speed of action potential propagation along the involved neural fibers and the length of the fibers. Central delay depends mostly on the number of synapses involved in processing the afferent volley and generating an efferent command. The simplest monosynaptic reflexes have a central delay of about 0.5 ms. An increase in the number of synapses leads to a proportional increase in the central delay.

Figure 8.3 The delay between a stimulus and a reflex reaction is called **reflex latency.** It consists of an afferent conduction time (ΔT_a), a central delay (ΔT_c), and an efferent conduction time (ΔT_e).

Problem 8.1

What is missing in the suggested definition of reflex latency?

I will start with the simplest monosynaptic reflexes and consider two versions of the same reflex, one certainly known to everybody: this reflex can be induced by a tendon tap and induces a joint jerk (e.g., a knee jerk).

8.3. H-REFLEXES, T-REFLEXES, AND M-RESPONSE

Monosynaptic reflexes are the only ones whose afferent source and reflex pathway are relatively well defined. They originate from primary spindle endings and make only one intraspinal excitatory connection (synapse) with α-motoneurons of the muscle that houses the spindle or, sometimes, its agonist, that is, a muscle causing joint movement in the same direction.

Let us imagine that an experimenter places a pair of stimulating electrodes close to a muscle nerve (figure 8.4). Note that **afferent fibers** (axons of muscle receptors) and **efferent fibers** (axons of motoneurons) travel between the spinal cord and the muscle together, that is, within one nerve. Nerves contain numerous efferent fibers, that is, axons of α-motoneurons, as well as numerous afferent fibers, that is, peripheral branches of the axons of sensory neurons. So when the experimenter stimulates the nerve with a short pulse of electrical current, both afferent and efferent fibers "feel" the same stimulus.

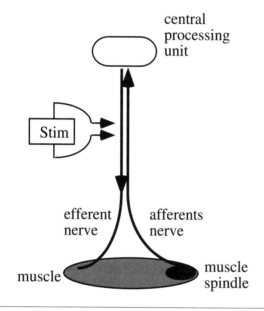

Figure 8.4   A scheme of experiments with an electrical stimulation of a muscle nerve. Note that the stimulus is applied to both afferent and efferent fibers.

Let the experimenter apply a short rectangular pulse of stimulation (its duration is typically about 0.5 to 1 ms) and slowly increase its amplitude. Each stimulus will induce a depolarization of the membrane of all the axons within the nerve. The magnitude of the depolarization in individual fibers will depend on two factors. The first is the location of the fiber with respect to the stimulating electrodes. In general, fibers closer to the electrodes will show higher depolarization. Second, the magnitude of depolarization will depend on the properties of individual fibers. In particular, thick fibers show higher depolarization than thin fibers. If one assumes that individual axons within the nerve are mixed randomly, the first, "geographical," factor will

not play a major role. The second factor is very important in defining the pattern of muscle reaction to the stimulation.

The biggest fibers within a muscle nerve are Ia-afferents that originate from muscle spindles. The axons of the α-motoneurons are just a little bit smaller. So when the experimenter starts to increase the strength of the stimulation, the first fibers to react will be Ia-afferents. These fibers travel from muscle spindles into the spinal cord and make monosynaptic connection with α-motoneurons innervating the muscle that houses the spindles (figure 8.2). Thus, a burst of activity in Ia-afferents may be expected to induce a **monosynaptic reflex.** When this reflex is induced by electrical stimulation of the muscle nerve, it is called an **H-reflex** (named after a famous German scientist, P. Hoffman). H-reflexes are commonly studied in the calf muscles (triceps surae) in response to electrical stimulation of n. tibialis (a nerve that innervates the calf muscles). The latency of the H-reflex in triceps surae is about 30 to 35 ms, depending mostly on the length of the subject's leg.

If the experimenter continues to increase the amplitude of the stimulation (figure 8.5), the amplitude of the H-reflex will increase because more and more Ia-afferents will be excited by the stimulus and consequently more and more α-motoneurons will be activated. At some point, the stimulus will also be able to induce action potentials in the axons of α-motoneurons.

Problem 8.2

In which direction will the action potential travel if the axon of an α-motoneuron is excited by an external electrical stimulus?

Since the place of stimulation is rather close to the muscle, action potential in the axons of α-motoneurons will take a short time to get to the muscle and induce its contraction. This contraction in triceps surae occurs at a delay of about 8 ms and is called an **M-response** (the *M* stands for "muscle"). Sometimes it is called a **direct contraction** in contrast to a **reflex contraction,** which is mediated by Ia-afferents.

If the experimenter continues to increase the strength of the stimulation, the amplitude of the M-response will start to increase because the membranes of more and more axons of α-motoneurons will be depolarized to the threshold. The amplitude of the H-reflex may continue to increase for a short while and then will start to decrease. This nonmonotonic behavior of the H-reflex with an increase in the strength of electrical stimulation is due to the physiological mechanism of the H-reflex. Note that when the axon of an α-motoneuron is excited by an external stimulus it generates an action potential, and the

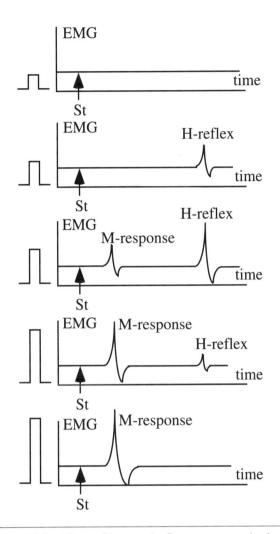

Figure 8.5 Afferent fibers are the first to react to a slowly increasing electrical stimulus. They induce a reflex muscle contraction (H-reflex). Later, efferent fibers become excited and induce a direct muscle contraction (M-response). Further increase in the strength of the stimulation leads to an increase in the M-response and suppression of the H-reflex.

action potential travels along the fiber **in both directions**—that is, to the muscle (this is called **orthodromic conduction**) and to the spinal cord (this is called **antidromic conduction**). The action potential that travels to the muscle will induce its contraction (the M-wave). The other action potential will travel to the spinal cord, to the motoneuron body, and two things may happen. The action potential may either disappear or induce an orthodromic action potential (we will discuss the latter case further on).

Problem 8.3

What may happen with a motoneuron if an antidromic action potential arrives to the axon hillock?

Problem 8.4

What will happen if two action potentials (one orthodromic and one antidromic) are moving toward each other and meet at a certain point on the axon?

Consider now what happens when an action potential comes along a Ia-afferent to an α-motoneuron (figure 8.6). Normally, this action potential would have induced a depolarization of the motoneuronal axon hillock over the threshold, and the motoneuron would have fired and induced a muscle contraction. However, an action potential is already traveling antidromically along the same axon. Note that the velocity of action potential in Ia-afferents is a little higher than that in the axons of α-motoneurons. However, the path for an action potential in a Ia-afferent fiber is slightly longer and involves a 0.5 ms synaptic delay. So it may be expected that these two signals will arrive at the target α-motoneuron virtually simultaneously. In this case, they will extinguish each other because of the **refractory period** of the membrane. For an analogy, imagine that there is fire in a dry, open field. The best way to stop the fire is to start another fire that will spread toward the first one. When the two fires meet, there is no fuel to enable the fire to move in either direction, and it will extinguish itself. You may view a neural fiber as a "fire conductor" that needs time to become able to conduct another "fire."

Thus, an increase in the strength of the stimulation leads to more and more axons of α-motoneurons directly

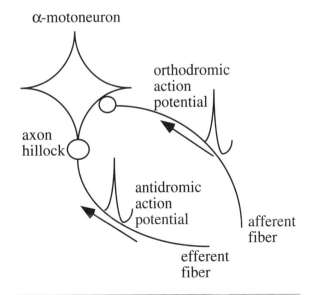

Figure 8.6 When an afferent fiber delivers a presynaptic action potential to an α-motoneuron whose action hillock has just responded to an antidromic efferent action potential, the motoneuron is unable to generate another efferent action potential because of the refractory period.

responding to the stimulation, conducting action potentials both ortho- and antidromically, and consequently making more and more motoneurons unable to respond to action potentials that are conducted by Ia-afferents. Eventually, all the efferent axons will be stimulated directly and the H-reflex will disappear, while the M-response will achieve its peak.

If two or more electrical stimuli are applied to a muscle nerve at one or more relatively short delays, the direct muscle response and the reflex response demonstrate dramatically different behaviors. M-responses in response to successive stimuli will be very similar to each other (unless you get to *very* high frequencies). The H-reflex in response to the second stimulus will be smaller; if there is a third stimulus, the reflex may even be smaller, and may eventually disappear (figure 8.7). The difference in the behaviors of M-response and H-reflex is attributable to the properties of the synapse that is part of the H-reflex arc. Remember that the refractory period for a typical membrane is due to the inactivation of sodium channels and is rather short, so that a relatively short time is required to restore the membrane's sensitivity and ability to conduct action potentials.

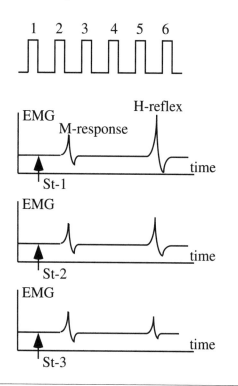

Figure 8.7 Successive stimuli at a high frequency (above) induce similar M-responses but progressively smaller H-reflexes. Time scales are certainly different in the lower graphs as compared to the upper panel.

Problem 8.5

What is the frequency of stimulation at which you may expect to see the M-response become smaller?

Synapses, on the other hand, need more time to restore the original amount of the mediator in synaptic vesicles. So synaptic transmission shows signs of attenuation even at time delays of about 1 s.

A monosynaptic reflex, similarly to the H-reflex, may be induced by a more physiological stimulus, that is, by a quick muscle stretch (figure 8.8). Primary endings of muscle spindles are very sensitive to muscle length and velocity, so a quick muscle stretch will lead to their synchronized firing. This volley of action potentials will travel along the Ia-afferents to the spinal cord and induce a reflex response of α-motoneurons leading to a twitch contraction of the muscle. This reflex is called a **T-reflex** (or tendon reflex). Muscle stretch may be induced by a tendon tap leading to the well-known knee jerk or ankle jerk. Note that a quick muscle stretch does not induce direct excitation of the axons of α-motoneurons, so there is no antidromic conduction. As a result, an increase in the amplitude and/or velocity of the stretch will lead to a monotonic increase in the amplitude of the T-reflex until it reaches its peak value.

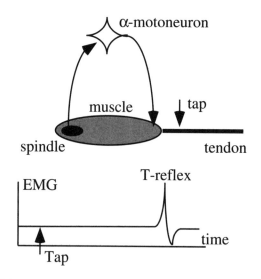

Figure 8.8 A tendon tap excites spindle endings and may induce a monosynaptic reflex contraction (T-reflex). Its reflex pathway is the same as for the H-reflex.

8.4. THE EFFECTS OF VOLUNTARY MUSCLE ACTIVATION ON MONOSYNAPTIC REFLEXES

Monosynaptic reflexes are very poorly controlled by the subject's will, although prolonged training of monkeys has been shown to lead to their ability to modulate the amplitude of a monosynaptic reflex. Human subjects can modulate amplitude of monosynaptic reflexes indirectly by activating certain muscle groups. Voluntary muscle activation leads to a postsynaptic excitation of agonist motoneuronal pools and to a postsynaptic inhibition of antagonist motoneuronal pools. For example, a voluntary activation of the calf muscle group increases the H-reflex in response to electrical nerve stimulation (figure 8.9). This increase in the H-reflex amplitude results from a general increase in the excitability of the motoneuronal pool. A voluntary command leads to a sub-threshold membrane depolarization of many of the motoneurons in the pool. As a result, more neurons are able to generate action potentials in response to a standard afferent discharge induced by an electrical stimulus.

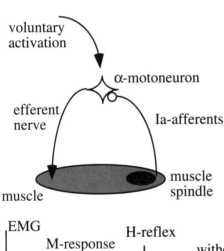

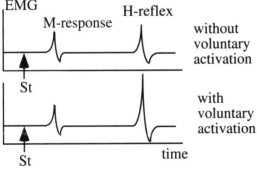

Figure 8.9 Voluntary muscle activation increases the amplitude of the H-reflex in the activated muscle through an excitation of the motoneuronal pool.

On the other hand, voluntary activation of an antagonist muscle decreases the amplitude of a monosynaptic reflex (e.g., an H-reflex in the calf muscle group will decrease if you activate the tibialis muscle). This effect is assumed to result from the action of Ia-inhibitory interneurons that are excited by the descending voluntary command to the antagonist muscle and induce postsynaptic inhibition of the motoneuronal pool that is being activated by Ia-afferents responding to the electrical stimulus.

In addition, activation of distant, large muscle groups can lead to a modulation of the H-reflex in the calf muscles. This can be achieved, for example, with a procedure called the Jendrassik maneuver. To perform this maneuver one clenches the hands in front of the chest and tries to separate them by a strong contraction of the shoulder and back muscles. After several seconds, there will be a change (usually, an increase) in the amplitude of the H-reflexes in the calf muscles. The mechanism of this effect is not known.

8.5. F-WAVE

The H-reflex can be readily seen only in some muscles. This may be due to a number of factors, in particular to differing density and effectiveness of monosynaptic connections of Ia-afferents on α-motoneurons, as well as to differing relations between the diameters of Ia-afferents and efferent axons.

Problem 8.6

How can a synapse on an α-motoneuron be more or less effective than another synapse?

Some muscles demonstrate a response to an electrical stimulation of the muscle nerve at a latency similar to that of the H-reflex. However, this response does not become smaller with an increase in the stimulation amplitude, and does not suffer from an increase in the stimulation frequency as the H-reflex does. This response is termed the F-wave. The described properties of the F-wave suggest that no synaptic transmission is involved. The F-wave results from antidromic conduction along the axons of α-motoneurons. However, because of the peculiarities of the time course of membrane depolarization at the neuron body, the membrane at the axon hillock gets out of its refractory period in time to respond to its continuing

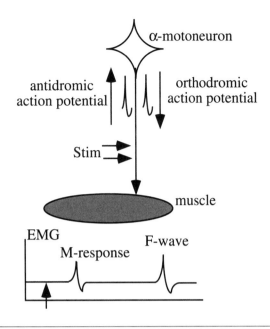

Figure 8.10 An antidromic action potential in an efferent fiber, induced by an electrical stimulus, can induce an orthodromic action potential leading to a muscle contraction called F-wave.

depolarization. In a sense, this is a unique case, in which an antidromic action potential comes to a neuron and gives rise to another, orthodromic action potential (figure 8.10).

Accurate measurement can show that the latency of the F-wave is just a little smaller than the H-reflex latency. To be exact, the difference is about 0.5 ms, corresponding to the typical synaptic delay, because the H-reflex arc involves a synapse while the F-wave arc does not.

Chapter 8 in a Nutshell

"Reflex" is a loosely defined notion meaning an involuntary motor reaction to an external stimulus. The simplest reflex consists of a receptor, an afferent nerve, at least one synapse on a central neuron, an efferent nerve, and an effector. Monosynaptic reflexes contain only one central synapse; they always induce excitatory effects on α-motoneurons. They can be induced by an abrupt change in the activity of primary muscle spindle afferents, as during a tendon tap (T-reflex), or in response to an electrical stimulation of a muscle nerve (H-reflex). In the latter case, motor axons are also stimulated, leading to a direct muscle response (M-response). Voluntary activation of a muscle leads to an increase in its monosynaptic reflexes. In some muscles an F-wave can be observed; this is a direct response of α-motoneurons to an antidromic volley traveling up their axons that has been induced by an electrical stimulus.

CHAPTER 9

OLIGOSYNAPTIC AND POLYSYNAPTIC REFLEXES

Key Terms

oligosynaptic reflexes

polysynaptic reflexes

pasic vs. tonic reflexes

flexor reflex

tonic stretch reflex

tonic vibration reflex

inter-joint and inter-limb reflexes

9.1. OLIGOSYNAPTIC REFLEXES

Monosynaptic reflexes are the simplest among the variety of muscle reflexes acting in the human body. Their functional importance, however, is questionable. Because they induce brisk, short-lasting contractions and are poorly controlled voluntarily, they are unlikely candidates as important parts of the mechanism of voluntary muscle control.

Oligosynaptic reflexes are assumed to involve, by definition, a "small" number of synapses, but more than one. Typically, oligosynaptic reflexes are assumed to involve two or three synapses. One of the best-known inhibitory oligosynaptic connections is from the primary endings of muscle spindles to α-motoneurons of the antagonist muscle, mediated by one interneuron, a Ia-interneuron (figure 9.1). The latency of inhibitory muscle reactions mediated by these connections is very close to the latency of monosynaptic reflexes induced by the same stimulus in a muscle housing the spindles. The difference is due to the additional synapse, which adds 0.5 ms to total transmission time.

Another important group of oligosynaptic reflexes originate from Golgi tendon organs, whose axons be-

long to the group of **Ib-afferents** (figure 9.2). The action of Ib-afferents looks the exact opposite of that of Ia-afferents. That is, Ib-afferents from a group of Golgi tendon organs induce a disynaptic inhibition of the homonymous α-motoneurons (i.e., those controlling the muscle whose tendon contains the Golgi tendon organs) and a disynaptic or trisynaptic excitation of the antagonist α-motoneurons. Note that both excitatory and inhibitory pathways from Ib-afferents involve at least one interneuron that belongs to the group of **Ib-interneurons.** The action of Ib-afferents is another example of negative feedback: if a muscle develops active force, its Golgi tendon organs become active and inhibit the motoneurons of this muscle while exciting the motoneurons of its antagonist.

On the basis of a recent series of studies in cats, American neurophysiologist T.R. Nichols has suggested that reflex effects from Golgi tendon organs can play a major role in muscle coordination across joints of a limb. This suggestion was based on observations of different force-related reflex effects in single-joint and multi-joint muscles that are commonly considered agonists (in particular, different heads of the triceps surae muscle).

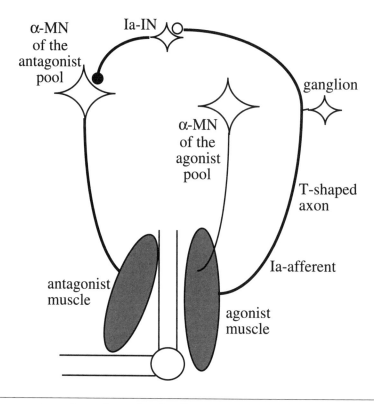

Figure 9.1 Ia-interneurons receive excitatory inputs from Ia-afferents and make inhibitory synapses on α-motoneurons innervating the antagonist muscle. Thus, they have an oligosynaptic (disynaptic) inhibitory reflex effect.

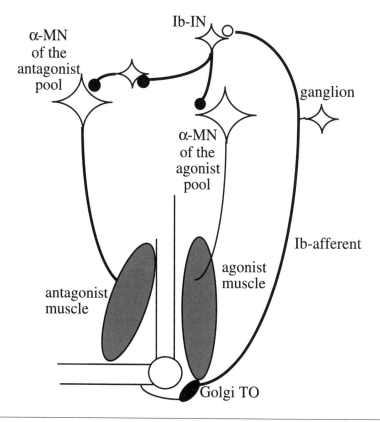

Figure 9.2 Golgi tendon organs send their axons (Ib-afferents) to Ib-interneurons, which exert an inhibitory action on the agonist α-motoneurons and disinhibit (excite) antagonist α-motoneurons.

Problem 9.1

What kind of reflex effects can be expected from the action of Ib-afferents during a fast flexion movement against a constant external load?

Problem 9.2

What can be expected from the action of Ib-afferents during a fast development of extension force against a stop?

Many of the properties of oligosynaptic reflexes are similar to those of monosynaptic reflexes, with the only exception that they have a slightly longer reflex delay. However, the presence of at least one additional synapse changes the properties of the reflex arc, in particular its reaction to a high-frequency stimulation. Usually when more synapses are involved in the transmission of a stimulus to α-motoneurons, a more pronounced suppression of reflex effects is observed with an increase in the stimulation rate.

Since in everyday movements there are not too many twitch-like contractions (humans would probably like to avoid them!), monosynaptic and oligosynaptic reflexes are likely to represent rather artificial phenomena that might be helpful during research and clinical studies but are rarely observed in "normal" life. This statement certainly does not mean that the **mechanisms** underlying these reflexes are not functioning or are insignificant for everyday motor control. The point is that in daily life, people make smooth movements, and most of the peripheral stimuli induce muscle stretches that do not induce strong synchronized afferent discharges that would give rise to monosynaptic reflexes resembling those studied in laboratories.

9.2. POLYSYNAPTIC REFLEXES

Most of the muscle reflexes are considered to be polysynaptic, that is, to involve "many" (more than three) synapses in the reflex arc. These reflexes are generally characterized by noticeably longer latencies and more complex behavior than monosynaptic or oligosynaptic reflexes. Since they involve more interneurons in their reflex arc, they can potentially provide more information about other levels of the neural hierarchy that are beyond the reach of the simpler reflexes.

Neurophysiological phenomena, including the reflexes, are commonly classified into two groups: **phasic** and **tonic. Tonic** typically means steady state, showing little change over time, while **phasic** means time-varying. This classification is far from clear and straight-

forward; depending on the time scale (e.g., a typical time of observation), one and the same phenomenon can be qualified as tonic or as phasic. Complex processes can have both tonic and phasic components.

Phasic reflexes emerge in response to a *change* in the level of a specific to the receptor stimulus. They usually represent a burst (or a short-lasting depression) of muscle activity leading to a twitchy movement or a series of twitchy movements. Note that all the monosynaptic reflexes are phasic.

Tonic reflexes emerge in response to the level of a stimulus itself. They lead to sustained muscle contractions and/or relatively smooth movements. These reflexes are always polysynaptic. One should take into account that a **succession** of stimuli inducing monosynaptic reflexes can lead to a smooth, tonic muscle contraction due to a superposition of successive twitch contractions. Thus we need to clearly distinguish tonic reflexes from tonic muscle contractions.

For example, activity of length-sensitive spindle endings can lead to both types of reflexes (figure 9.3). If a muscle is quickly stretched, monosynaptic and polysynaptic reflexes can be observed in response to the **process of stretch.** If the muscle stays in a new, stretched state, the phasic reflexes quickly disappear. However, if the muscle was active before the stretch, it is possible to record tonic changes in the muscle activity at any time after the stretch is completed and the muscle is at a new steady state. This mechanism is frequently termed **tonic stretch reflex** in contrast to the **phasic stretch reflex,** which is another term for the T-reflex.

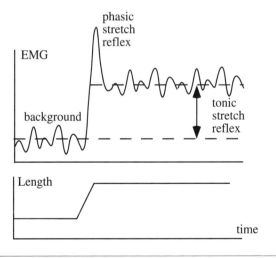

Figure 9.3 Tonic and phasic components of the muscle reflex to stretch.

The phasic-tonic dichotomy is rather conventional and is based on quantitative rather than qualitative differences in the mechanisms. For example, monosynaptic reflexes are mediated by monosynaptic connections of

Ia-afferents with α-motoneurons. Spindle Ia-afferents are sensitive to both muscle length and the rate of its change. Their monosynaptic projections certainly function during slow stretches or maintenance of a constant muscle length, but do not evoke monosynaptic reflexes. Therefore, monosynaptic connections of Ia-afferents can and are likely to play a role in apparently tonic reflexes. When the rate of muscle stretch reaches a threshold, monosynaptic reflexes emerge; when it is lower than this threshold, only tonic reflexes are observed.

There is a big difference between monosynaptic and polysynaptic reflexes. For the former, the afferent source and the reflex arc are known with a degree of certainty. For the latter, next to nothing is known about the exact neural mechanism leading to reflex muscle contractions. So polysynaptic reflexes are usually considered **functional notions.** Figure 9.4 illustrates a typical scheme for a polysynaptic reflex. A stimulus is applied, leading to activation of a number of receptors (commonly of different modalities). The stimulus leads to a change in the level of activation of a muscle. The muscle may be located in close proximity to the stimulus or be rather far away, even on a different limb. As a result, polysynaptic reflexes are described as **input-output relations** between a stimulus and its mechanical or electromyographic consequence.

9.3. FLEXOR REFLEX

The **flexor reflex,** as its name suggests, represents a reflex contraction of flexor muscles in response to a stimulus. There are many proprioceptors contributing to the flexor reflex; they are frequently united into one group and are called the **flexor reflex afferents.** This group involves, among others, secondary endings of muscle spindles (group II afferents); free endings scattered all over muscles and innervated by thin, slowly conducting axons of groups III and IV; some cutaneous receptors; and nociceptors (receptors of painful stimuli). The flexor reflex may be induced by a painful stimulus to the skin or by electrical stimulation of a cutaneous nerve, for example the sural nerve (figure 9.5). It has a relatively long latency (typically about 70 ms), which is due both to the slow conduction of most of the afferent fibers and to long central delays. An appropriate stimulus induces a quick but sustained contraction of all the major flexor muscles of the limb to which the stimulus is applied. These reflexes look somewhat different in babies and are sometimes changed in certain pathologies, such as spinal cord injury, brain trauma, and multiple sclerosis.

9.4. TONIC STRETCH REFLEX

I have already identified the **tonic stretch reflex** as a sustained muscle contraction in response to a slow

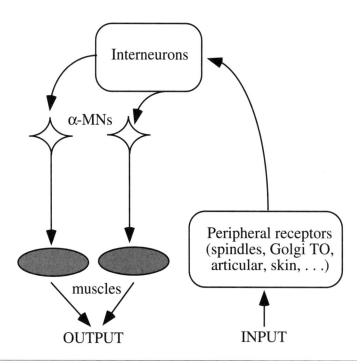

Figure 9.4 A functional scheme of a polysynaptic reflex. Commonly these reflexes receive contribution from receptors of different modalities, and their central pathways are unknown.

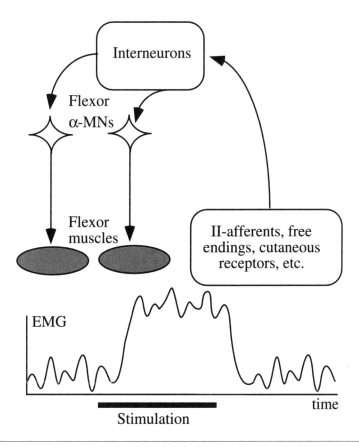

Figure 9.5 Flexor reflex is induced by a group of afferents called flexor reflex afferents. These include secondary endings of muscle spindles, free nerve endings, some cutaneous receptors, and some others. Flexor reflex leads to an activation of flexor muscles within the limb. Below: A typical reflex reaction in a flexor muscle of a hindlimb (e.g., tibialis anterior) to an electrical stimulation of n. suralis.

stretch or maintenance of the muscle at a new, longer length. In a sense, the tonic stretch reflex is a mechanism providing for a very important feature of our muscles: their **springlike behavior.** This reflex was first described by a great British physiologist, Sir Charles Sherrington, and has been studied by many since his time.

Let us consider what will happen if an intact muscle (i.e., a muscle with all its neural connections in place) is slowly stretched by an external force (figure 9.6). First, the muscle will resist stretching because of its **passive elastic properties** (remember that the muscle has parallel and series elastic elements). Then, at a certain length, the increased activity of muscle spindles will bring about an **autogenic recruitment** of a few motoneurons whose activation will lead to active force development by the muscle, also opposing the stretch. The muscle length at which the recruitment begins is termed the **threshold of the tonic stretch reflex.** If one continues to stretch the muscle, more and more motoneurons will be recruited, leading to an increase

in muscle force. Eventually, such an experiment will yield a **tonic stretch reflex characteristic** (a force-length characteristic). The slope of the characteristic may be considered muscle stiffness; actually, it is better to use a different term, **apparent stiffness,** because muscle and its reflexes cannot be considered a single, ideal spring. Note that this apparent stiffness has two components. The first component is purely peripheral and is independent of any reflex effects. The second component has a reflex nature. Note also that the slope of the curve changes with muscle length. This means that *the muscle behaves like a nonlinear spring.*

Actually, the term "tonic stretch reflex" is somewhat misleading, because this reflex has a velocity-dependent component due to the velocity sensitivity of the primary endings in muscle spindles. This means that if a muscle is stretched at a certain velocity and moves through a certain value of muscle length, its force of contraction will be higher than if the same length is maintained constant.

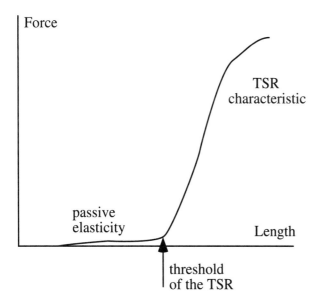

Figure 9.6 A muscle is slowly stretched by an external force. First, it resists the stretching only due to its passive elasticity. Then, at a certain threshold, recruitment of α-motoneurons begins, leading to an active force development (tonic stretch reflex). The whole curve is called a tonic stretch reflex characteristic.

Problem 9.3

What will happen with muscle force when the muscle passes through a certain length during its shortening, as compared to the force developed at the same length in static conditions?

9.5. TONIC VIBRATION REFLEX

High-frequency, low-amplitude **muscle vibration** is a very potent stimulus for spindle sensory endings. For example, in humans, vibration of a muscle at a frequency of about 100 Hz and an amplitude of about 1 mm may be strong enough to "drive" virtually all the primary endings of all the spindles within the muscle. **Driving** means inducing an action potential in response to every cycle of vibration. Secondary muscle endings are also rather sensitive to vibration, as are numerous skin and subcutaneous receptors. In fact, skin vibration is sometimes used to test individual skin sensitivity.

Problem 9.4

If all the Ia-afferents are driven by vibration, why don't they induce monosynaptic reflexes in response to each vibration cycle?

Vibration typically induces a tonic contraction of the muscle to which it is applied. This contraction is termed **tonic vibration reflex.** (Think about what a strange word combination this is: "tonic" means steady state, while "vibration" implies high-frequency oscillations. These two words become compatible, however, when a high-frequency stimulus leads to a relatively slowly changing muscle contraction.) The contraction starts a few seconds after the beginning of the vibration (figure 9.7), increases gradually, and stays at a relatively constant level until the vibrator is turned off. Then the contraction gradually subsides over a few seconds. The EMG

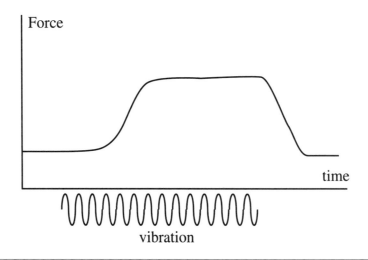

Figure 9.7 High-frequency muscle vibration leads to a slow reflex increase in muscle force (tonic vibration reflex). It starts at a delay and lasts for some time after the stimulus is turned off.

of a muscle during the tonic vibration reflex looks very similar to EMGs during voluntary muscle contractions. However, deeper analysis shows a large number of motor units firing synchronously with vibration cycles (which is not surprising because Ia-afferents are being driven by the vibration), while the voluntary EMG is rather asynchronous.

An analysis of the excitatory postsynaptic potentials during muscle vibration in animal experiments revealed that two types of EPSPs exist during vibration: those that are synchronized with the vibration, and a slow depolarization that is not synchronized with the vibration. The slow depolarization was attributed to the action of a polysynaptic pathway from the Ia-afferents (with a possible contribution of other muscle afferents), while the synchronized EPSPs were attributed to the action of monosynaptic or polysynaptic connections among Ia-afferents and α-motoneurons.

Muscle vibration is accompanied by four rather unusual phenomena. The first is the ability of subjects to suppress the tonic vibration reflex voluntarily, that is, by "pure thinking." Sometimes the desire to suppress the reflex is so strong that subjects need to be taught how not to suppress it. This fact makes the tonic vibration reflex a "nonreflex" according to our earlier definition. However, I warned earlier that the definition was going to fail; here is just one example.

The second phenomenon is suppression of monosynaptic reflexes on the background of vibration (figure 9.8), sometimes leading to their total elimination. These effects look rather paradoxical, since a tonic voluntary contraction of a muscle is typically associated with a process of postsynaptic excitation, leading to an increase in H-reflexes observed in the same muscle (this point was discussed in chapter 8). Thus, a voluntary muscle contraction mimicking a tonic vibration reflex leads to an increase in the amplitude of H-reflexes.

Problem 9.5

Suggest an explanation for the suppression of H-reflexes during a tonic vibration reflex.

The suppression of monosynaptic reflexes by vibration has been demonstrated to be presynaptic. That is, the complex afferent inflow induced by vibration leads to selective presynaptic effects on the terminals of Ia-afferents at their synapses with α-motoneurons. Other synapses do not suffer. As a result, the polysynaptic pathways induce a tonic muscle contraction (tonic vibration reflex), while the monosynaptic pathways become relatively ineffective.

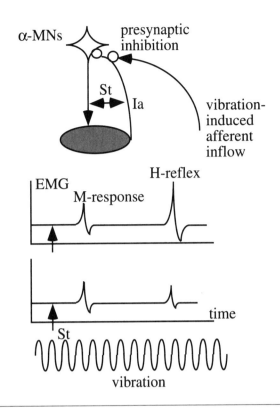

Figure 9.8 Tonic vibration reflex is accompanied by a suppression of monosynaptic reflexes in the same muscle (e.g., of the H-reflex). This suppression is of a presynaptic origin (upper drawing).

The third unusual effect of muscle vibration is its ability to induce reflex contractions of muscles that are not subjected to vibration. In particular, if vibration is applied to a muscle, reflex contractions may be observed in the muscle or its agonists, or in the antagonist muscles, or even in muscles acting at different joints of the limb. Which muscle will be activated depends on a number of factors including, in particular, the configuration of the limb (joint angles), its orientation with respect to the field of gravity, the presence of support under the foot, and other factors (figure 9.9). These patterns suggest that vibration involves rather "high" (intersegmental) mechanisms that may also be used during such common activities as standing and walking.

The fourth effect is kinesthetic illusions, and we will consider these later on.

9.6. INTERACTION AMONG REFLEX PATHWAYS

In the previous sections, the reflex effects of certain afferents such as Ia- and Ib-afferents were considered as

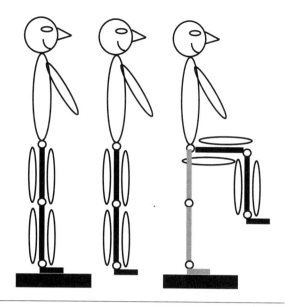

Figure 9.9 Muscle vibration can induce reflex contractions of different muscles of the same limb (shown by black). Note that these muscles are the same as would be active during locomotion when the postures shown are passed through. The vibration is applied to the Achilles and the patellar tendons.

separate phenomena, out of context. But what happens if all the afferents are acting simultaneously, as occurs in everyday life? Actually, the exact answer is unknown. However, a series of experiments by an outstanding Swedish research group headed by A. Lundberg and E. Jankowska has demonstrated that most interneurons, including the Ia-interneurons and Ib-interneurons previously mentioned, receive information that is very mixed (figure 9.10). That is, if the level of firing of a Ib-afferent is kept constant, the output of Ib-interneurons may change depending on the level of firing of Ia-afferents. The neural wiring of the spinal cord creates the impression of a total mess rather than of a well-designed set of feedback circuits, each having its own function.

These findings should not be a cause for desperation, however. They demonstrate the limits of the classical neurophysiological approach, which is good for testing certain neural circuits but is probably too simplistic for analysis of the functioning of the central nervous system as a whole. This is another illustration of the limitations of the reductionist approach in studies of the functions of the human body.

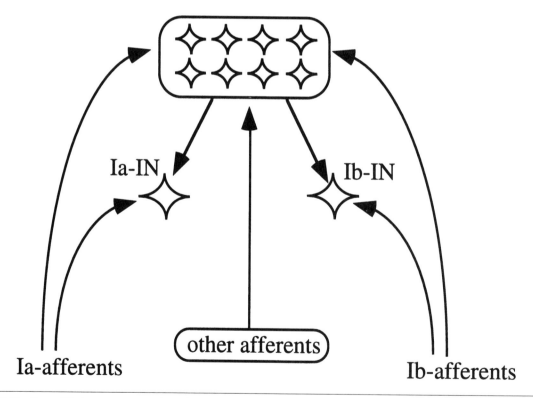

Figure 9.10 Ia- and Ib-interneurons receive mixed information from afferents originating from different receptors.

9.7. INTERJOINT AND INTERLIMB REFLEXES

In the previous section we encountered examples of interjoint reflexes in which vibration of a muscle could induce a tonic reflex contraction of another muscle within the same limb, acting at a different joint. Actually, the flexor reflex also induces muscle contractions of virtually all the flexor muscles of a limb and may be considered an interjoint or a whole-limb reflex.

Interlimb reflexes are commonly observed in animal preparations, that is, in animals whose neural axis has been cut, separating the "upper" brain structures from the rest of the central nervous system. In such animals, many spinal reflexes become released from the suppressing descending influence. In particular, electrical stimulation of a skin nerve, or a pinprick, will induce a "normal" flexor response in the limb to which the stimulus is applied and an extensor reflex in the contralateral limb. This reaction is termed "crossed extensor reflex" (figure 9.11).

Some of the more complex polysynaptic receptors involving the vestibular, ocular, and postural systems will be discussed later.

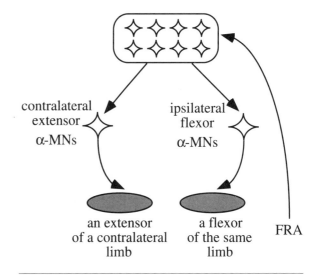

Figure 9.11 A stimulation of the flexor reflex afferents (FRA) in one limb induces a reflex response in flexor muscles of this limb, and a crossed extensor reflex in extensor muscles of the contralateral limb.

Chapter 9 in a Nutshell

Oligosynaptic reflexes contain a few central synapses, while polysynaptic reflexes contain many central synapses. Reflexes of these two groups can have excitatory or inhibitory effects. Phasic stimuli or responses are those that change quickly; tonic stimuli or responses are those that are steady state. Muscle spindles and Golgi tendon organs are sources of oligosynaptic reflexes that can be viewed as negative feedback loops. Reflexes can involve muscles of a whole limb, as in the flexor reflex, which is induced by the activity of a variety of receptors with relatively thin axons. The tonic stretch reflex is an increase in the activity of motoneurons innervating a muscle that is being stretched by an external force. The tonic vibration reflex is a steady increase in the level of activation of a muscle that is being vibrated at high frequency and low amplitude. It is accompanied by suppression of monosynaptic reflexes induced by an increase in the presynaptic inhibition.

CHAPTER 10

VOLUNTARY CONTROL OF A SINGLE MUSCLE

Key Terms

elements of control theory

feedforward and feedback control

servo-hypothesis

alpha-gamma coactivation

equilibrium-point hypothesis

role of reflexes in muscle control

Now it is time to take another step and, following Sherrington's tradition, to discuss how the described neurophysiological subsystems (reflexes) can be used in the control of voluntary movements. Let me start from the most simple case, control of a single muscle. Even for a single muscle, there is evidence for numerous reflex mechanisms originating from different types of peripheral receptors and mixed at the level of interneurons. All these mechanisms are likely to be mediated by *thousands of neurons,* even for the simplest voluntary movement. It is certainly unrealistic to try to trace each and every reflex pathway and describe its functioning during voluntary muscle activation. However, we can consider a different question: *Is it possible to describe the action of all the variety of muscle reflexes with just a few parameters?* In order to do so, we need to move from consideration of individual reflex pathways to a new level of complexity that will be characterized by a new set of functionally significant variables—just as we did when we proceeded from the physiology of membranes and ions to the physiology of cell interactions (reflexes).

10.1. FEEDFORWARD AND FEEDBACK CONTROL

Moving into the area of control requires the introduction of a few basic notions from this area. Consider figure 10.1. A command signal comes from a hypothetical central controller and, after some processing, produces a certain output. Variables used by the controller to formulate command signals are addressed as **independently controlled variables.** The word "independently" means that these variables may be supplied by the controller without regard to possible changes in the output or in any other external factor. This does not mean that the controller cannot change an independently controlled variable based on peripheral information. What is important is that it has a choice of reacting or not reacting to this information.

If the controller supplies the signal (a variable or a few variables) independently of the output, this type of control is termed **feedforward.** A typical example of feedforward control is kicking a soccer ball. The brain sends commands to the muscle during the kick that have

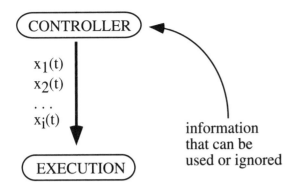

Figure 10.1 A scheme of feedforward control. The controller uses independently controlled variables [$x_1(t)$; ... $x_i(t)$] to formulate command signals to the "lower" (executive) structures.

been generated before the kick and certainly before the outcome of the kick becomes known.

If a controller changes command signals on the basis of their outcome, this type of control is termed **feedback** (figure 10.2). An important component of a feedback control system is a **comparator,** that is, a unit that compares current output of the system with a desired output and changes command signals based on the discrepancy between the actual and desired effects. For example, when you drive a car at a certain constant speed, you use visual information from the speedometer or from the moving environment to change the force with which you are pressing on the gas or brake pedal. This type of control allows you to maintain a preferred speed when the road

goes uphill or downhill, when the wind changes, or when you see a police car.

A **negative feedback loop** acts to subtract from a control variable (x) an amount (Δx) proportional to a deviation in a peripheral variable (Δy), typically leading to a decrease in the original deviation (figure 10.2A). Such a system tends to maintain a certain value (or a certain time function) of the output variable. **Positive feedback** acts to add to a control variable an amount proportional to a deviation in a peripheral variable, typically leading to an increase in the original deviation (figure 10.2B). Positive feedback systems tend to amplify any deviation of the peripheral variable and commonly get out of control, leading to a qualitative change in the behavior of the system (cf. action potential generation as described in chapter 2).

Two important parameters characterize feedback loops, **gain** and **delay.** Gain can be defined as a ratio of a change in a control variable to a change in a peripheral variable ($\Delta x/\Delta y$). Delay can be measured in time units, for example in seconds or milliseconds, or in relative timing units, for example in a percentage of a time interval typical of the process. Both positive and negative feedback loops achieve their functional purpose of amplifying or decreasing error only if their gain is high enough and their delay is within certain limits. Large delays can, however, lead to unexpected circumstances. For example, figure 10.3 shows what can happen if a steady output signal is perturbed by a function sin(t), and a negative feedback loop is acting with the gain of 0.9 and time delay (Δt) of either 0 or half the period of the perturbing function (π). In the first case, there is a nearly

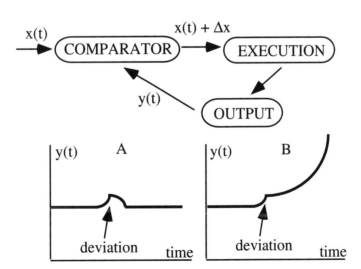

Figure 10.2 Feedback control changes command signals based on their outcome. This is done by a unit termed the comparator. Negative feedback (A) changes the output of the comparator to bring down any possible deviations of the output, while positive feedback (B) amplifies any deviations of the output.

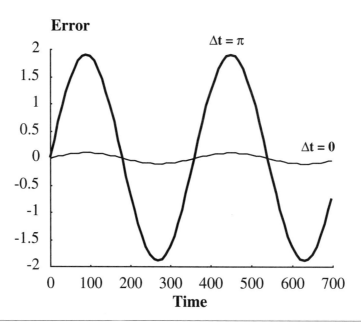

Figure 10.3 Large delays in a feedback loop can lead to unexpected consequences. For example, in this figure a perturbing signal (a sine function with a peak value of 1) is acting on the output of a system that includes a negative feedback with the gain of 0.9. If the time delay in the feedback loop is zero, the error is nearly ideally compensated (thin line); if the time delay is π, the error is actually amplified (bold line).

perfect compensation of the perturbing function. In the second case, the "error" is actually amplified although a negative feedback loop is acting. Thus, while talking about negative or positive feedback loops, one needs to distinguish between actual structural components of the system and their overall functional effects.

Time delay is an important drawback of feedback control. Therefore, if speed is vital, feedforward control may become preferred, whereas if accuracy is more important, feedback control has an advantage.

Problem 10.1

Suggest examples of negative and positive feedback from the material we have already considered in this book and from everyday life.

10.2. SERVO CONTROL

Feedback and feedforward types of control are frequently combined into schemes of differing complexity that have an ability to generate command signals in a feedforward manner and to correct the signals—if their effect is different from some desired outcome—using feedback. When a cat chases a mouse, it uses a combination of feedforward and feedback control. On the one hand, it tries to predict what the mouse will do and to intercept it (feedforward control); on the other hand, it uses visual information and corrects its movements based on actual

movements of the mouse (feedback control). Schemes combining feedforward and feedback control frequently consist of a few **control circuits** (figure 10.4). Among various types of control circuits, let us single out the so-called **servo mechanism,** which is sometimes simply called the **servo.**

In figure 10.4, a signal is sent by a central controller in a feedforward manner to a servo loop. The signal encodes a desired value of an output parameter that needs to be kept constant. The servo loop is taking care of keeping this value constant with the help of a feedback mechanism. A sensor is used to measure current values of the parameter and to supply these measurements to the comparator. The comparator compares the measured value to the specified one and changes its output (Δx) on the basis of the **error,** that is, the difference between the prescribed and actual values. Note that the presence of errors is a necessary component of the functioning of a servo. Good servos allow only very small errors to emerge and correct them promptly. In other words, they have high gains and small time delays, while bad servos may have considerable delays in their corrective actions so that errors may be rather large.

A thermostat is a typical example of a servo controller (figure 10.5). It keeps room temperature constant by using a comparator that compares actual room temperature to its preset value. If the temperature differs from the preset value by a large enough margin, a heater or air conditioner is turned on. Note that the input into this servo is specified by setting the dial of the thermostat.

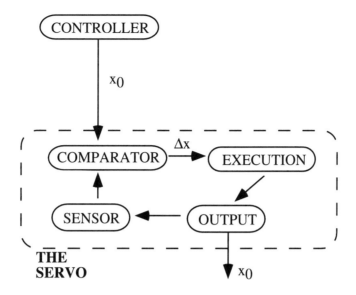

Figure 10.4 This circuit combines feedforward and feedback mechanisms of control. The feedback loop (the servo) keeps constant a value of a variable specified by the controller despite possible changes in the external conditions that may "try" to change this variable.

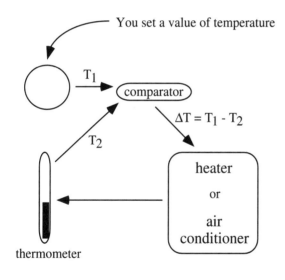

Figure 10.5 A scheme of a simple thermostat that keeps room temperature constant.

Problem 10.2

Suggest an area of sport in which having a servo mechanism would be vital for good performance. Suggest another area in which such a mechanism would be disastrous.

I have already mentioned an important characteristic of any servo (or any feedback system), namely its **time delay.** Apparently, the bigger the delay is, the bigger the errors that are likely to accumulate before a corrective action of the servo takes place. In electrical systems, the errors may be very small. However, in the human body, the speed of information transmission is limited by the speed of action potential propagation. Thus, delays of several tens and up to a hundred milliseconds are common. These delays are comparable to the movement time of the fastest voluntary movements; thus, even the best servos within our body are likely to function suboptimally.

The servo is an **autonomic** element of a control system. This means that setting a desired value of an output parameter makes a servo mechanism do its job independently of other factors as long as the specified value remains constant. Using servos apparently simplifies control within a complex system because part of the responsibility may be delegated to the "lower" servos, and the "smart controller" may ignore the details and concentrate on specifying more general and important variables.

10.3. THE SERVO HYPOTHESIS

Early in the 1950s, R.A. Merton suggested a principle that was the first **control hypothesis** in the area of human movement studies. This hypothesis, called the **servo hypothesis,** was the first to formulate the problems of generation of voluntary movements in terms of **control** using information about the neurophysiological mechanisms of muscle reflexes. Merton suggested that the control of muscle spindles with the gamma system was part of a servo mechanism controlling muscle length.

The main idea of the servo hypothesis is illustrated in figure 10.6 and involves the following steps:

1. A descending signal comes to γ-motoneurons and thus changes the sensitivity of the sensory endings in muscle spindles to muscle length. The effects of an increased γ-activity are similar to the effects of an increase in muscle length (both lead to an increase in the spindle afferent activity level), while a decrease in γ-activity is similar to the effects of a decrease in muscle length. So, we may say that the descending signal in figure 10.6 simulates a new value of muscle length.

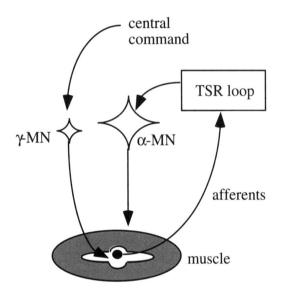

Figure 10.6 The servo hypothesis of Merton considers the feedback loop muscle length—muscle spindle—tonic stretch reflex (TSR)—activity of α-motoneurons—changes in muscle force—movement—changes in muscle length a perfect servo. Descending signals specify a level of activity of γ-motoneurons, thus setting a value of muscle length.

2. The activity of the spindle endings changes and, via the mechanism of the **tonic stretch reflex,** leads to a change in the level of activity of α-motoneurons innervating the muscle. Actually, the original version of Merton's hypothesis was based on monosynaptic action of Ia-muscle afferents on homonymous α-motoneurons. However, later, the mechanism underlying the servo action was reconsidered on the basis of the tonic stretch reflex.

3. The level of muscle contraction changes, leading to movement, that is, to a change in muscle length (we will assume that there are no changes in the external load, i.e., **isotonic conditions**). Note that an increase in spindle activity will lead to an additional muscle contraction, leading to muscle shortening, which will lead to a decrease in the spindle activity. So the tonic stretch reflex mechanism acts as a negative feedback system.

4. The movement will continue until muscle length comes to a new value at which the activity of muscle spindles leads to a muscle contraction exactly balancing the external load, that is, to a new **equilibrium state.**

If the descending command remains constant, the mechanism of the tonic stretch reflex is assumed to assure constant muscle length despite possible changes in external load, that is, to work as a **perfect servo.** For example, if the load increases, this increase leads to an increase in muscle length, which in turn leads to an increase in the activity of α-motoneurons and an increase in muscle contraction force. According to Merton's servo hypothesis, the increase in muscle force will exactly balance the external load change so that muscle length will not change.

Figure 10.7 illustrates the servo hypothesis with the help of force-length muscle characteristics. The central command specifies the location of a characteristic corresponding to a certain value of muscle length. In order for the servo mechanism to assure perfect compensation of possible changes in external load, the characteristic must be vertical; then muscle length will not depend on muscle (and external) force. Voluntary movements are performed by shifting the characteristics along the x-axis, so that the independently controlled variable may be associated with the signal to γ-motoneurons (γ1, γ2, γ3 in figure 10.7).

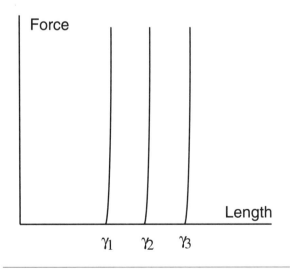

Figure 10.7 The servo hypothesis of Merton may be illustrated with vertical force-length curves whose position along the abscissa axis is defined by the descending signal (γ1, γ2 γ3). Note that even a large change in the external force is assumed to be perfectly compensated by the tonic stretch reflex mechanism; i.e., this mechanism has a very high (infinite) gain.

Problem 10.3

What will happen, according to the servo hypothesis, if you try to activate a muscle in isometric conditions, or in isotonic conditions, or against an elastic load?

10.4. ALPHA-GAMMA COACTIVATION

Note that the servo model predicts that voluntary movements are initiated by a change in the activity of γ-motoneurons while changes in the activity of α-motoneurons follow at a delay that is characteristic of the tonic stretch reflex arc. The development of new methods, in particular direct recordings from human peripheral nerves pioneered by the Swedish scientist A. Vallbo, allowed direct assessment of the relative timing of changes in the activity of α- and γ-motoneurons during voluntary muscle contractions. These observations showed that during virtually all voluntary movements, changes in the activity of α- and γ-motoneurons happen simultaneously. This phenomenon is termed **α-γ coactivation.**

In mid-1960s, researchers were very reluctant to abandon the servo hypothesis and suggested that the servo mechanism worked as suggested by Merton while voluntary movements were initiated by a combination of a feedforward command signal (to α-motoneurons) and a signal to the length-controlling servo (to γ-motoneurons).

Problem 10.4

What will happen with the activity of spindle afferents in a flexor muscle during a voluntary increase in flexion force against a stop?

Problem 10.5

What will happen during a fast flexion movement against a constant external load?

This is a very elegant model, indeed! Note, however, that it still implies a very high (actually an infinite) **gain** in the tonic stretch reflex loop, so that any change in the external load (which may be rather large) is readily balanced by a change in muscle force while the change in muscle length is assumed to be extremely small (in fact, zero). Unfortunately for the servo hypothesis, later measurements of the gain in the tonic stretch reflex arc demonstrated relatively low values, so the mechanism of this reflex cannot be considered a perfect servo. Thus eventually the servo hypothesis was replaced by new models.

10.5. VOLUNTARY ACTIVATION OF MUSCLES

Presently, two views exist on the nature of voluntary muscle activation. According to the first view, central commands directly specify the levels of activity of α-motoneuronal pools and therefore the levels of muscle activation. Reflex mechanisms are assumed to play a minor role, mostly in cases of unexpected changes in the external forces (perturbations). This view, however, is incompatible with some observations. For example, ask a person to activate a muscle to a high level against a large load and not to change the level of muscle activation (figure 10.8). Now, unexpectedly and quickly remove the load. A fast movement will occur. If you record an EMG of the muscle, you will see that immediately after the unloading there is a period of virtually total silence in the muscle activity. This effect is called the **unloading reflex.** Note that an unloading leads to a quick shortening of the muscle (a decrease in its length at a high negative velocity) so that the sensory endings in the muscle spindles become silent, and their reflex effects on the homonymous α-motoneurons disappear. So the unloading reflex may be considered an inverse of the stretch reflex. The disappearance of the muscle activity during the unloading reflex shows that the reflex effects may be strong enough to eliminate 100% of voluntary muscle activation and certainly cannot be considered "minor additions." Thus, the alternative view looks much more attractive.

10.6. EQUILIBRIUM-POINT HYPOTHESIS

According to the second view, central commands use the mechanisms of muscle reflexes to induce changes in the levels of muscle activity and specify parameters of these reflexes. This view is compatible with all the observations on the reflex effects on voluntary muscle activation. On the other hand, it does not go to an extreme implying an infinite gain in any of the reflex arcs and thus avoids the problems of the servo hypothesis. This view emerged as a formal language for describing a body of experimental data on observations of single-muscle force-length characteristic curves in animals and single-joint torque-angle characteristic curves in human subjects. Animal experiments were performed on cats with a lesion of the central nervous system such that the cats lacked the ability to make voluntary movements. Then an electrical stimulator was placed on the "stump" of the residual part of the brain. This stimulator simulated different descending commands.

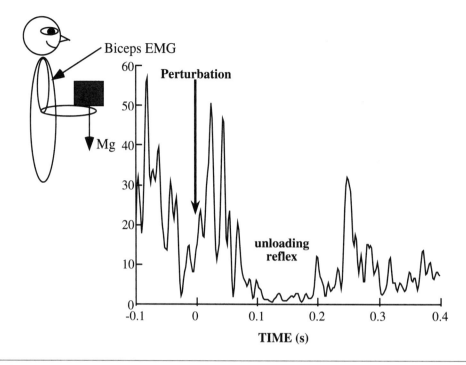

Figure 10.8   The subject is holding a position in the elbow by activating the biceps. The load is suddenly removed. Biceps EMG shows a period of nearly complete silence (the unloading reflex) even if the subject tries to keep the biceps activity constant. This illustrates that muscle EMG is not an independently controlled variable.

At a "fixed" descending command and a constant external load, the muscle-load system will be in an equilibrium at a certain length. The combination of muscle length and force at the equilibrium is called the equilibrium point (figure 10.9). This is a central notion within the hypothesis that is known as the **equilibrium-point hypothesis.** A change in the external load leads to a change in muscle length that induces changes in the level of muscle activation via the tonic stretch reflex arc. Thus, a constant descending command does not mean a constant level of muscle activation. Changed muscle activation leads to a parallel change in muscle length and force until a new equilibrium point is achieved. For a fixed descending command, all the equilibrium points form a curve on the force-length plane that is termed an **invariant characteristic** (IC).

If the "central command" in an animal experiment is changed by using a different level of electrical stimulation, a new invariant characteristic emerges that is shifted with respect to the first one (figure 10.10). Now a variable can be introduced that encodes the location of an invariant characteristic, for example, the point at which activation of α-motoneurons occurs (the **threshold of the tonic stretch reflex**). This variable is an **independently controlled variable** as defined earlier, because changes in the external load are able only to move the equilibrium point along the invariant characteristic.

Within this scheme, movements may occur because of changes in the external load, as in figure 10.9, or may be induced by central shifts of the invariant characteris-

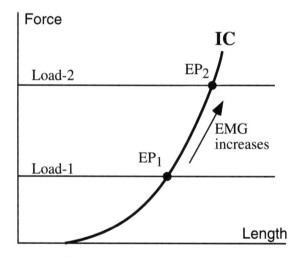

Figure 10.9   According to the equilibrium-point hypothesis, muscle reflexes specify a relation between muscle force and muscle length—an invariant characteristic (IC). The system muscle+load is in an equilibrium when muscle force is equal to the external force (load). This point is termed the equilibrium point (EP). If the external load changes, both muscle force and length will change corresponding to a new EP (EP$_2$). Note that muscle activity (EMG) changes along the IC.

tic, as in figure 10.10. Note that a shift of the invariant characteristic may have different peripheral effects depending on the external load. In figure 10.10, a standard shift of the invariant characteristic may lead to a change in muscle length (cf. EP$_0$ and EP$_1$, isotonic conditions),

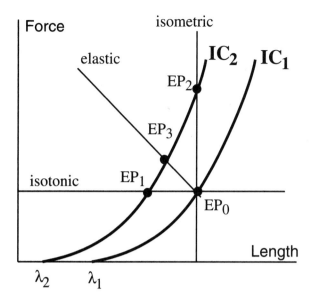

Figure 10.10 Central command specifies the location of an IC for the muscle. This can be described as a shift in the threshold of the tonic stretch reflex (λ). Depending on the external load, a shift in λ can lead to a change in muscle length (isotonic conditions, EP_1), or in muscle force (isometric conditions, EP_2), or in both (elastic load, EP_3). Note that EMG changes will depend on both central λ changes and the external load.

or in muscle force (cf. EP_0 and EP_2, isometric conditions), or in both (cf. EP_0 and EP_3, if the load is elastic).

Problem 10.6

How can you change the velocity of a voluntary movement according to the equilibrium-point hypothesis?

As far as the neurophysiological mechanisms are concerned, the equilibrium-point hypothesis assumes that the tonic stretch reflex, providing for the invariant characteristics, incorporates all the reflex loops that can be influenced by levels of activity or excitability of

γ-motoneurons, α-motoneurons, and interneurons. It does not single out one anatomical structure as the "most important." Moreover, the feedback loops from receptors other than muscle receptors (e.g., skin and subcutaneous receptors) can also play an important role in defining the shape of the invariant characteristics. Thus, it is assumed that central commands for voluntary movements involve a balanced combination of signals to all types of spinal neurons (figure 10.11). Actual levels of muscle activation (EMGs), muscle forces, and movements occur as consequences of these central commands.

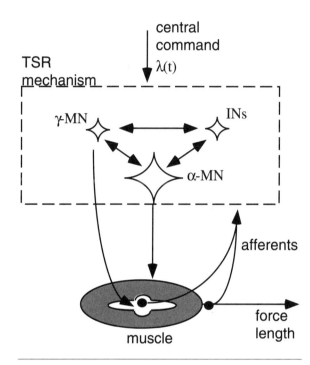

Figure 10.11 According to the equilibrium-point hypothesis, central command represents a balanced combination of descending signals to all groups of spinal neurons including α-MNs, γ-MNs, and interneurons (INs). The tonic stretch reflex is assumed to incorporate all the reflex effects from all the peripheral receptors. Changes in muscle length (movement), muscle force, and levels of muscle activation emerge with equally important contributions from the central command and signals from peripheral receptors.

Chapter 10 in a Nutshell

Control signals can be generated in a feedforward fashion or based on feedback signals. Positive feedback tends to amplify the error, while negative feedback tends to eliminate errors; however, the exact effects depend on gains and time delays of feedback loops. The servo is a particular form of feedback loop that keeps output at a preset value. Merton's theory considers muscle spindles the sensor in the perfect servo controlling muscle length; the theory has been proven to be wrong. Voluntary activation of a muscle is accompanied by simultaneous activation of the α- and γ-motoneurons. The equilibrium-point hypothesis considers control of voluntary movements as a process of central modulation of the threshold of the tonic stretch reflex for the participating muscles. The tonic stretch reflex and peripheral muscle/tendon elasticity provide for springlike muscle behavior. Reflex effects play an important role in defining levels of muscle activation.

CHAPTER 11

PATTERNS OF SINGLE-JOINT MOVEMENTS

Key Terms

multi-joint and single-joint movements

performance and task parameters

isotonic movements

isometric contractions

tri-phasic EMG pattern

kinematic profiles

dual-strategy hypothesis

11.1. ISOTONIC MOVEMENTS AND ISOMETRIC CONTRACTIONS

Our everyday movements usually involve many joints and are performed in conditions of changing external forces. Even if a person tries to do "the same thing" a few times, for example to pick a cup of tea from the table, individual movements will be slightly different during different attempts (figure 11.1). This phenomenon is termed **motor variability,** which is always present even in the best-trained subjects. Moreover, all people are unique and are characterized by different dimensions of body segments, different experiences, and different abilities to learn new motor tasks. A scientific study, however, implies the possibility of reproducing an experiment in another laboratory and with another subject, and getting similar data.

In order to solve at least one part of this problem, experimenters frequently try to reduce the number of parameters describing a motor task and also the variables available to the subject in performing the task. This is commonly done by confining the movements to a single joint, one axis of rotation, and, frequently, a constant

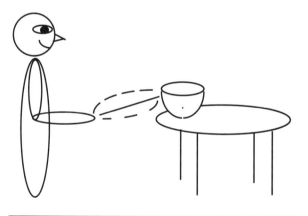

Figure 11.1 If a person is trying to perform "the same" movement several times, e.g., to pick up a cup of tea, the trajectories of all the joints and of the hand will be different in different attempts.

external load. Movements against an apparently constant external load are termed **isotonic.** Isotonic conditions are usually achieved by restricting movements to a horizontal plane in which there are no apparent changes in the force of gravity.

Problem 11.1

What will happen with the activity of Golgi tendon organs during a fast isotonic movement?

Another favorite among experimenters' regime of muscle work is termed **isometric contraction.** The word "isometric" implies the lack of changes in muscle length, which can never be secured even in animal experiments. Any active contraction of muscle fibers leads to a decrease in their length. Even if this decrease is relatively small, it can be realized at high velocities and can lead to changes in the activity of length- and velocity-sensitive muscle receptors (spindle endings). In human studies, tendons and soft tissues surrounding the joints and muscles lead to inevitable changes in muscle fiber length when the muscle activation level changes.

Problem 11.2

What will happen with the level of activity of muscle spindles (primary and secondary endings) during an isometric muscle contraction?

Unfortunately for the experimenters, most of the commonly studied joints of human limbs (e.g., shoulder, elbow, wrist, and ankle) have more than one axis of rotation (so-called kinematic **degree of freedom**) and are controlled by more than two muscles, some of which are biarticular, meaning that their contractions directly induce changes in joint torque and/or movements in two adjacent joints. In addition, a movement in a joint may lead to a change in the relation between muscle force and joint torque; thus, different active muscle forces may be required to balance a constant external load. So we are coming to the conclusion that single-joint movements against a constant external load (isotonic) as well as without changes in muscle length (isometric) do not exist.

Even if single-joint movements and contractions existed and were obtainable in experimental conditions, we might question their relation to "real-life" movements and to problems of motor control of voluntary movements in general. However, experimenters stubbornly continue to study these fictitious phenomena. They have good reasons to do so.

First, the progress of science proceeds from simple to complex, and studies at a certain advanced level usually require understanding of the lower functional levels.

Second, although results of single-joint studies cannot be directly generalized to multi-joint movements, they provide theoretical frameworks and experimental approaches that can be helpful for understanding general principles of motor control irrespective of the number of joints and muscles involved.

Third, investigations of single-joint movements have proven useful in clinical studies. In some patients, voluntary motor control is restricted to single muscles or single joints; therefore, understanding basic principles of control of such movements is likely to be useful.

And fourth, experimental studies require reproducible conditions in the performance of experiments and necessitate taking into account all the important factors likely to influence a subject's performance. Even for human single-joint movements, it is, strictly speaking, virtually impossible to take into account all the factors. For multi-joint movements, the situation is likely to be even more complicated, since joint interaction forces come into play, biarticular muscles are likely to start playing an important role, the force of gravity changes its direction with respect to individual joints for most of the movements, and the number of involved variables increases dramatically. Therefore, the chances of performing poorly controlled experiments increase for multi-joint movement studies.

So, let us consider experimental situations in which subjects are asked to perform single-joint isotonic movements or isometric contractions. Assume that these regimes of muscle work exist, keeping in mind that the assumption is likely to be false.

11.2. PERFORMANCE AND TASK PARAMETERS

In most motor control experiments, relations between **task parameters** (what is required from the subject) and **performance parameters** (what the subject is doing) are studied. For single-joint movement studies, task parameters may include movement amplitude, movement time (or speed), external load, accuracy requirements, and other specific instructions to the subjects (e.g., "Make a smooth movement," "Avoid oscillation at the end of the movement," "Do not correct the final position if you miss the target"). Performance parameters include kinematic variables (joint position, speed, and acceleration), kinetic variables (joint torque and its derivatives), EMGs, accuracy indexes (e.g., variability of the final position or the percentage of trials hitting the target), and other recorded or calculated indexes.

Why do experimenters care about relations among performance and task parameters or variables? This is an example of a typical "black box" approach in which input-output relations are studied in a complex system in order to check hypotheses on the internal structure and/or principles of functioning of the "black box." It is expected that any new hypothesis is able to generate both previously unobserved, experimentally testable **predictions** about the relations between task and performance parameters and previously observed relations among the parameters that can be called **"postdictions."** An absolute prerequisite for any new hypothesis that it must be experimentally disprovable. This means that a hypothetical experiment studying relations among task and performance parameters or variables should be able to generate results incompatible with the hypothesis, so that the hypothesis can be rejected and replaced with an alternative one. Therefore, studies of relations among these two groups of parameters or variables are crucial for the development of the field of motor control.

For example, predictions can be generated based on a given hypothesis, and experimental questions can be formulated such as "What happens with peak velocity with an increase in inertial load?" or "How does integrated EMG change with an increase in movement amplitude?" Note that performance parameters are characterized by normal **variability,** that is, changes that occur during repeated attempts at the same task. Because of normal variability, one cannot expect absolutely identical signals even when the subject is seemingly performing the same movement in the same conditions. Thus any experiment is this area necessitates collecting several trials and using appropriate statistical approaches.

Problem 11.3

You want to show that there are no changes in a performance parameter with a change in a task parameter. How can you do this?

A favorite index in motor control studies is movement time, although it seems that it would be hard to find a less reliable measure. Look at figure 11.2, which shows typical kinematic traces for a fast elbow flexion. The beginning of the movement is relatively easy to define, although even here one can pick a moment at the beginning of the biceps EMG burst or a deviation of one of the kinematic traces above a certain threshold (cf. T_{acc}, T_{vel}, and T_{ang}). This choice may considerably affect the measured value. As far as the moment of movement termination is concerned, the problem becomes much worse, since fast movements are frequently accompanied by oscillations at the final position. One can pick the time when a position trace first hits the target, or when a velocity trace crosses zero, or when an acceleration trace crosses zero for the second time, or some other measure. Each index has its own pluses and minuses and can be used as "movement time." Actual choice of a particular criterion is made by each researcher on the basis of his or her theory and the particular research questions asked in the study.

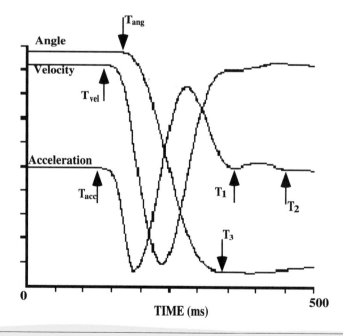

Figure 11.2   A typical kinematic pattern of a single-joint movement (six elbow flexions over 54° were averaged). The beginning of the movement will be defined differently based on the first visible change in the acceleration (T_{acc}), velocity (T_{vel}), or angle (T_{ang}). It is even harder to define the end of the movement. One can use an instant when the acceleration reverses its direction (T_1), or when it comes to zero (T_2), or when the joint signal first hits the target (T_3), or some velocity-based criterion. Note that the figure shows a relatively smooth movement without major oscillations at the end, which can only complicate the problem. Reprinted, by permission, from M.L. Latash, 1993, *Control of Human Movement* (Champaign, IL: Human Kinetics), 109.

11.3. ELECTROMYOGRAPHIC PATTERNS DURING SINGLE-JOINT ISOTONIC MOVEMENTS

Before proceeding any further, two basic notions of **agonist** and **antagonist** need to be introduced. The word "agonist" (or agonist muscle) will be used for a muscle whose activation accelerates the limb or increases joint torque in a required direction. A muscle whose activation brakes the movement or resists joint torque developed by the agonist will be termed an antagonist (or antagonist muscle). These notions are as good or as bad as those relating to isotonic movements and isometric contractions, but they help to describe the major findings in this area.

Problem 11.4

Can one and the same muscle be both an agonist and an antagonist for the same movement (or contraction)?

Recording muscle activity during fast isotonic single-joint movements reveals a typical EMG pattern usually termed the **triphasic pattern** (figure 11.3). The beginning of the agonist EMG burst is usually the first detectable event accompanying fast voluntary movement. It precedes the first detectable kinematic changes by several tens of milliseconds. The initial agonist burst is accompanied by a relatively low **coactivation** of the antagonist muscle and is followed by an antagonist EMG burst during which the agonist is relatively quiet. The antagonist burst can be followed by a second burst in the agonist. At the final position, there is usually a visible increase in both agonist and antagonist tonic muscle activity. The triphasic pattern is obvious during very fast movements. A decrease in movement speed leads to less pronounced EMG bursts, and eventually, slow movements are accompanied by a sustained agonist activity with a low activation of the antagonist.

Changes in other task parameters lead to a variety of reproducible changes in the triphasic pattern. Typically, subjects are asked to make movements "as fast as possible," or "at different speeds," or to be "both fast and accurate." Then the movement amplitude, load, target size, or more than one of these parameters are changed. As a result, regularities can be seen in certain parameters describing the triphasic pattern. These parameters may include the duration of the EMG bursts, the integrals of the bursts, the delay between two successive bursts, the level of muscle coactivation at the end of the movement, etc.

1. An increase in the velocity of movements over a constant amplitude against a constant load (figure 11.4) leads to an increase in the rate of EMG rise, peak value

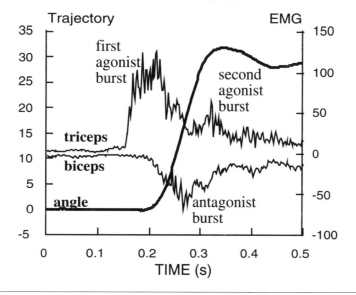

ELBOW EXTENSION

Figure 11.3 The triphasic EMG pattern begins with a burst of activity in the agonist muscle (triceps), followed by an antagonist burst (biceps; its EMG is inverted for better visualization), which sometimes is followed by a second agonist burst. Note that the first agonist burst starts several tens of milliseconds prior to joint trajectory.

Adapted, by permission of Cambridge University Press, from M.L. Latash and J.G. Anson, 1996, "What are normal movements in atypical populations," *Behavioral and Brain Science,* 19: 57. © 1996 Cambridge University Press.

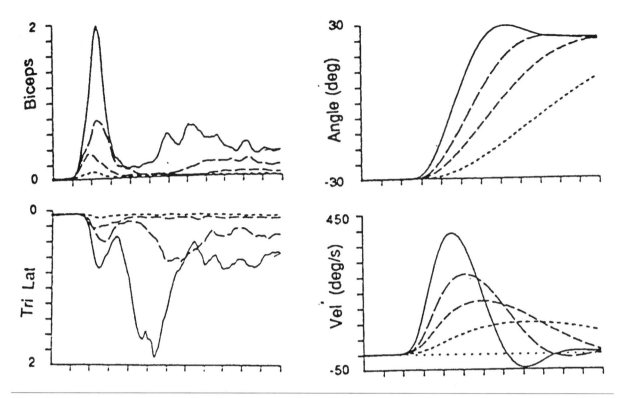

Figure 11.4 Typical changes in the triphasic EMG pattern during movements over a constant amplitude, against a constant external load, but at different speeds.

Adapted, by permission, from D.M. Corcos, G.L. Gottlieb, and G.C. Agarwal, 1989, "Organizing principles for single-joint movements: II. A speed-sensitive strategy," *Journal of Neurophysiology,* 62: 358-367. © 1989 The American Physiological Society.

and area of the first agonist burst (biceps curve during elbow flexions illustrated in figure 11.4), a decrease in the delay before the antagonist burst, and an increase in the antagonist burst amplitude and area. Duration of the first agonist EMG burst is sometimes reported to increase and sometimes to stay constant. These differences are likely to reflect different methods used for assessing burst duration rather than any fundamental differences in EMG patterns. The level of final coactivation of agonist and antagonist muscles increases with movement velocity.

2. An increase in movement amplitude without changes in external load or instructions concerning movement velocity (e.g., "as fast as possible" or "at a constant speed") leads to relatively uniform rates of agonist EMG rise, a higher and longer first EMG burst with a corresponding increase in its area (biceps curve in figure 11.5), longer delays before the antagonist burst, and inconsistent changes in the antagonist burst amplitude and duration. An increase in movement amplitude for relatively small movements leads to an increase in the antagonist burst, while further increase may lead to a decrease in the antagonist activity.

3. An increase in inertial load without changes in movement amplitude or instructions concerning movement velocity (e.g., "as fast as possible," figure 11.6)

leads to a higher and longer agonist EMG activity (although without changes in the rate of the EMG rise), a longer delay before the antagonist burst, and no apparent changes in the antagonist burst characteristics. Final coactivation of agonist and antagonist muscles increases with inertial load.

Variations in more than one of the three major task parameters (amplitude, velocity, and load) lead to combined effects on the EMG bursts, as seen, for example, in experiments in which subjects are required to perform movements of different amplitudes within the same movement time.

Problem 11.5

What will happen with the first agonist burst and the antagonist burst if the subject is performing movements of different amplitudes within the same movement time?

Problem 11.6

What kind of an EMG pattern do you expect to see if a subject is doing a fast isotonic movement to a target and quickly back to the initial position?

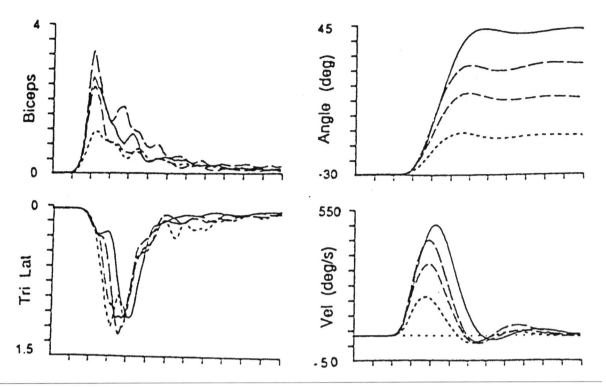

Figure 11.5   Typical changes in the triphasic EMG pattern during movements over different amplitudes, against a constant external load, and under an instruction to move "as fast as possible."

Adapted, by permission, from G.L. Gottlieb, D.M. Corcos, and G.C. Agarwal, 1989, "Organizing principles for single-joint movements: I. A speed-sensitive strategy," *Journal of Neurophysiology,* 62: 342-357. © 1989 The American Physiological Society.

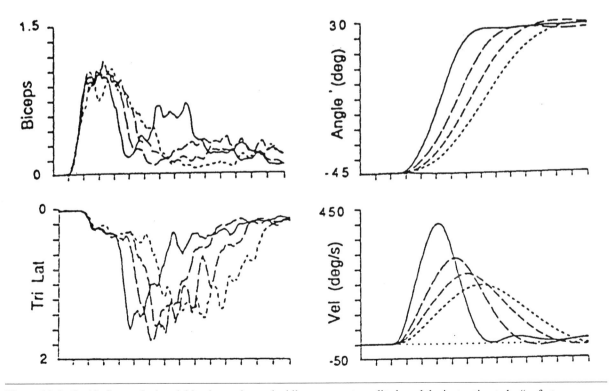

Figure 11.6   In this figure, the inertial load was changed while movement amplitude and the instruction to be "as fast as possible" were preserved.

Adapted, by permission, from G.L. Gottlieb, D.M. Corcos, and G.C. Agarwal, 1989, "Organizing principles for single-joint movements: I. A speed-sensitive strategy," *Journal of Neurophysiology,* 62: 342-357. © 1989 The American Physiological Society.

11.4. ELECTROMYOGRAPHIC PATTERNS DURING SINGLE-JOINT ISOMETRIC CONTRACTIONS

Two types of isometric contractions have usually been studied: step and pulse contractions. Step contractions require the subject to increase joint torque up to a certain level, while pulse contractions require also returning quickly to the initial level of joint torque (commonly, relaxation). Other instructions have been used to specify time of the torque increase, accuracy constraints, and the like—similarly to what is done with single-joint isotonic movements. Fast isometric contractions are accompanied by triphasic EMG patterns similar to those observed during fast isotonic movements. However, the second delayed agonist burst is more frequently absent. Bursts of the EMG activity become smaller and more poorly defined with a decrease in the rate of torque increase, and slow increases in joint torque are accompanied by a tonic increase in the agonist EMG and a smaller increase in the antagonist EMG.

Similar measures have been used for relating parameters of isometric contractions and isotonic movements to changes in the EMG patterns. Let me describe them, starting from the step experiments.

1. An increase in the rate of torque rise keeping the final torque level constant leads to an increase in the rate of EMG rise, peak value and area of the first agonist burst (see biceps in figure 11.7), no apparent changes in the delay before the antagonist burst, and an increase in the antagonist burst amplitude and area. There are no obvious changes in the duration of either burst or the level of final coactivation of agonist and antagonist muscles with the rate of torque rise.

2. An increase in the final torque level without changes in instructions concerning the rate of torque rise (e.g., "as fast as possible," figure 11.8) leads to relatively uniform rates of agonist EMG rise, higher agonist and antagonist burst amplitudes, higher integrated EMG activity for both muscles, higher final levels of both agonist and antagonist EMGs, and inconsistent changes in the duration of both bursts.

During pulse contractions, EMG patterns become more "phasic," with better-defined bursts, a better-pronounced second agonist burst, and a lower level of muscle co-contraction at the final state. In this case, an increase in pulse torque amplitude without changes in the rate of torque increase leads to a longer first agonist burst, a delay in the antagonist burst, and inconsistent changes in the antagonist burst amplitude and area (figure 11.9). An increase in the rate of torque rise without

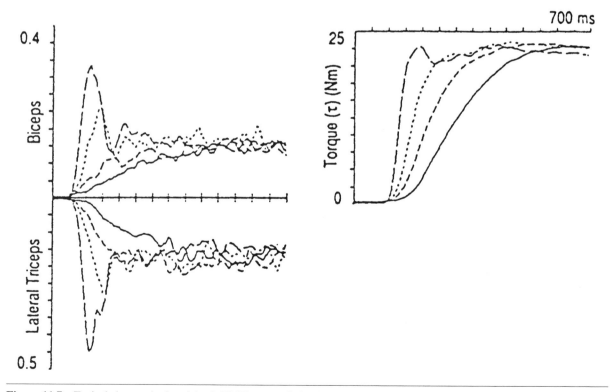

Figure 11.7 Typical changes in the triphasic EMG pattern during isometric contractions with different rates of torque rise. Adapted, by permission, from D.M. Corcos, G.L. Gottlieb, G.C. Agarwal, and B.P. Flaherty, 1990, "Organizing principles for single-joint movements: IV. Implications for isometric contractions," *Journal of Neurophysiology,* 64: 1033-1042. © 1990 The American Physiological Society.

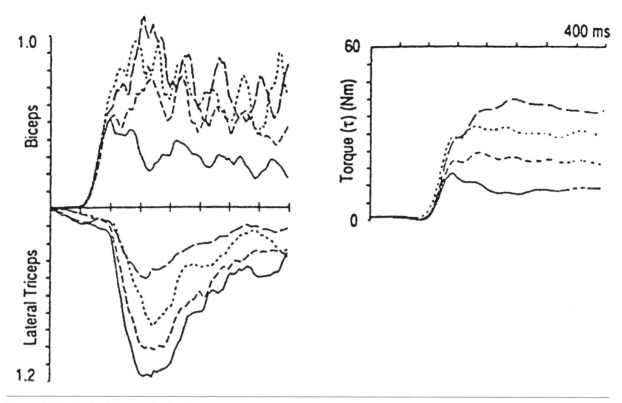

Figure 11.8 Typical changes in the triphasic EMG pattern during isometric contractions with the same rates of torque rise but to different target values of torque.

Adapted, by permission, from D.M. Corcos, G.L. Gottlieb, G.C. Agarwal, and B.P. Flaherty, 1990, "Organizing principles for single-joint movements: IV. Implications for isometric contractions," *Journal of Neurophysiology,* 64: 1033-1042. © 1990 The American Physiological Society.

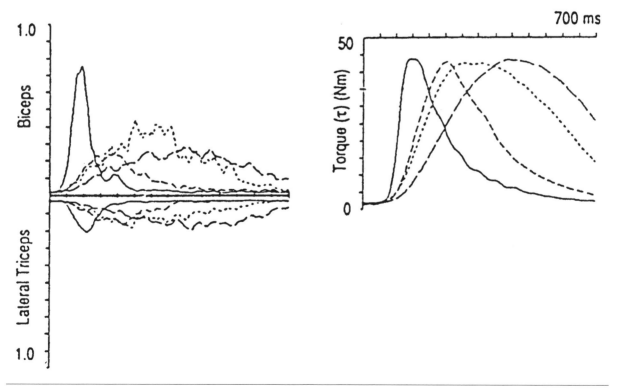

Figure 11.9 A typical EMG pattern during an isometric pulse contraction.

Adapted, by permission, from D.M. Corcos, G.L. Gottlieb, G.C. Agarwal, and B.P. Flaherty, 1990, "Organizing principles for single-joint movements: IV. Implications for isometric contractions," *Journal of Neurophysiology,* 64: 1033-1042. © 1990 The American Physiological Society.

changes in pulse amplitude leads to faster-rising first agonist and antagonist EMG bursts.

11.5. THE DUAL-STRATEGY HYPOTHESIS

Changes in the EMG patterns during simple movements have been used as the basis for a number of hypotheses on control of such movements. Some of these hypotheses assume that EMGs are reliable indexes of control signals within the central nervous system, reflecting processes of voluntary motor control. An alternative group of hypotheses are based on an assumption that EMGs are generated with equally important contributions from central control signals and from the activity in peripheral reflex loops. Analysis of EMG patterns is an important tool for both groups of hypotheses. One of the most fully developed hypotheses within the first group is the **dual-strategy hypothesis.**

The variety of findings in single-joint experiments creates an impression of total chaos. An attempt to introduce an order (a classification) into this array of data was undertaken in the form of the dual-strategy hypothesis. The basic idea of the hypothesis is rather simple: you can perform movements "at the same speed" or "at different speeds." Movements performed "at the same speed" are assumed to be controlled using a **speed-insensitive strategy,** while movements performed "at different speeds" are assumed to be controlled using a **speed-sensitive strategy.** Note, however, that actual movement speed is a time function that depends, in particular, on external loading conditions. So the dual-strategy hypothesis implies not the actual movement speed (or its measure, such as average speed or peak speed), but an internal variable that is used by the brain to vary movement speed. For example, if a subject is asked to perform movements "as fast as possible," he or she is probably using the highest available value of this "internal speed" variable. Actual speed, however, may be very different if, for example, movements are made against different inertial loads (see figure 11.6).

This hypothesis was based originally on an idea that we control movements by sending commands to the α-motoneuronal pools of the agonist and antagonist muscles that define the EMG patterns of these muscles. Unfortunately for this version of the hypothesis, the α-motoneuronal pools receive not only descending signals from the brain but also signals from peripheral receptors that induce reflex changes in their activity. These changes will certainly be reflected in the EMG patterns. The activity of the peripheral receptors depends on actual changes in muscle length, joint angles, and tendon forces. Imagine

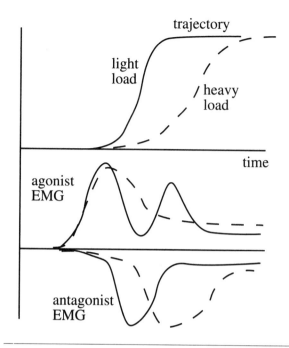

Figure 11.10 Schematic illustration of kinematic and EMG patterns for two movements, both performed over the same amplitude and under the same instruction to be "as fast as possible." The inertial load was, however, four times as high during the second movement. Note the difference in movement kinematics, which will apparently be reflected in different reflex effects on both agonist and antagonist α-motoneurons.

that you use the same signals from the brain to control a couple of movements (figure 11.10). During the second movement, the inertial load is increased fourfold. Apparently, movement speed will drop. This will be reflected in changes in the activity of virtually all the peripheral receptors. As a result, the reflex effects of the receptors on the α-motoneurons will change, leading to a change in the EMG patterns. This example illustrates that EMG patterns are not reliable indexes of central control signals.

Problem 11.7

Can you consider EMG patterns during isometric contractions as pure reflections of hypothetical central commands? Why?

The dual-strategy hypothesis was rather successful in describing the regularities in the first agonist EMG burst during single-joint movements. This is not surprising, because during fast movements the first agonist burst is commonly about 100 ms long, so that there is no time for the reflexes to exert significant effects on it. The problems of the dual-strategy hypothesis became obvious when the same approach was used for delayed events, like the antagonist burst, or for muscle contractions with significantly different kinematics, for example, in comparisons of isotonic movements and isometric contractions. However, the basic idea of classifying hypothetical motor commands into two categories may be applied without assuming an exclusive central control over the activity of α-motoneurons (and EMGs). It helps to introduce order into a large number of experimental findings performed in different laboratories.

Chapter 11 in a Nutshell

Investigation of relations among task and performance parameters or variables is a common method of studying a complex system. Fast single-joint movements are typically accompanied by a triphasic EMG pattern seen in the agonist-antagonist muscle pair—a nearly symmetrical bell-shaped velocity and a double-peaked acceleration. There is a set of reproducible relations among task parameters and parameters of the triphasic pattern. Such relations have been extensively studied in isotonic and isometric loading conditions. The dual-strategy hypothesis introduces a classification of all movements into two groups, with and without explicit or implicit control over movement time. The original version implies independent central control over the total presynaptic input into motoneuronal pools; thus it does not take into account the reflex effects on EMG patterns.

CHAPTER 12

PREPROGRAMMED REACTIONS

Key Terms

corrective reactions to
perturbations

nature of pre-programmed
reactions

postural corrections

corrective stumbling
reaction

Human voluntary movements are typically performed not in a Motor Control Laboratory but in the real world full of unexpected changes in sensory information, force fields, targets, and so on. As a result, people are never able to predict ideally the external force field (among other unpredictable things) and its possible changes. When a command is issued whose purpose is to assure a certain movement or a certain posture, at the time the command in being realized by muscles, the external conditions will have changed somewhat and the planned movement or posture will be **perturbed** by these changes. Posture and movement must be in some sense stable to such everyday perturbations, and human bodies are equipped with a variety of mechanisms designed to assure such stability. Each of these mechanisms has its own functional purpose.

Some of these mechanisms have already been described briefly in previous chapters, for example, muscle and tendon elasticity (chapter 4) and muscle reflexes (chapter 9) that generate changes in muscle force against the perturbing force. In this chapter we will look at another very important group of muscle reactions to perturbations that come at a relatively short delay (although

the delay is longer than that for monosynaptic reflexes) and provide context-specific corrections of movement or posture in cases of unexpected external perturbations.

12.1. PREPROGRAMMED REACTIONS

There is one more group of semiautomatic reactions to muscle length changes (or, sometimes, to other stimuli) that may be tentatively termed "reflexes." In fact, there is a whole group of terms used for these reactions: **long-latency reflexes, preprogrammed reactions, functional stretch reflex, M_2-M_3,** and **triggered reactions.** The variety of terms reflects different understandings of the nature and functional significance of these reactions. For the sake of convenience, we will call them preprogrammed reactions.

In the most common procedure for eliciting a preprogrammed reaction, a subject maintains a constant position in a joint against an external load, provided, for example, by a motor, with steady contraction of a muscle. The subject is given the instruction, "Return to the starting position as fast as possible in cases of external perturbations." Unexpected rapid load changes by the motor give rise to a sequence of EMG events in the muscle (figure 12.1). The first one corresponds, according to its latency, to monosynaptic transmission and probably represents the phasic stretch reflex, just like the one observed during a tendon tap (T-reflex). After that, two peaks (sometimes poorly differentiated) appear at an intermediate latency. The first peak is commonly designated M_2 and the second one is designated M_3, and after that there is a voluntary reaction. The latency of the intermediate reactions is typically in the range from 50 to 100 ms. The bottom panel of the figure shows an actual EMG record of the activity of a human biceps muscle in response to its loading with clear M_2-M_3 peaks.

In the past it was hypothesized that preprogrammed reactions represented a **transcortical reflex** (i.e., a reflex whose loop involves neurons in the brain cortex;

see chapter 13), and this idea is still very much alive. However, these reactions (or other reactions that are very similar to M_2-M_3) were observed in decerebrated and even spinalized animals, that is, animals without a cortex.

Problem 12.1

The difference between the latencies of the monosynaptic response and those of M_2 is the same in arm muscles and leg muscles. What does this finding tell us about the possible transcortical nature of M_2?

Preprogrammed reactions differ significantly from other reflexes in that they strongly depend on the instruction to the subject. For example, if you repeat the experiment described earlier but give the subject the

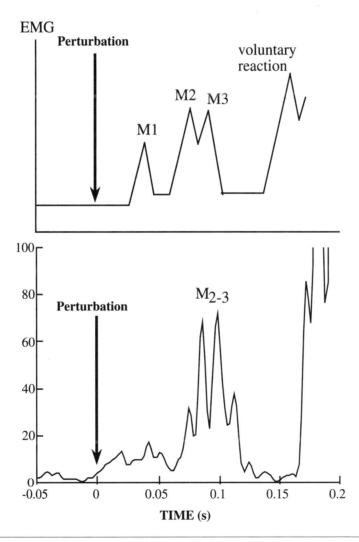

Figure 12.1 An unexpected perturbation of a joint gives rise to a sequence of EMG events in a stretched muscle. The first one comes at a short latency (under 40 ms; M_1); then there are two peaks (M_2 and M_3) that come at a latency of between 50 and 100 ms. M_2 and M_3 are considered preprogrammed reactions. Later, a voluntary reaction comes. The bottom panel shows an actual recording of the reaction of a human biceps muscle to an unexpected loading (perturbation).

instruction, "Do not resist external perturbations; let the motor move your arm," the amplitude of the preprogrammed reactions will decrease significantly, and the reactions may even disappear (figure 12.2).

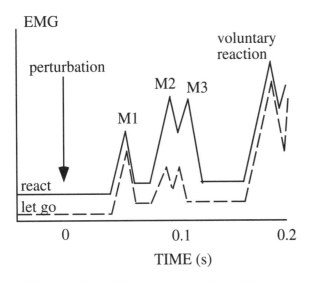

Figure 12.2 Preprogrammed reactions demonstrate a strong dependence on the instruction. If the subject is instructed to resist perturbations, the preprogrammed reactions are large (solid lines); if the subject is asked to let the limb move, the preprogrammed reactions are much smaller (dashed lines). Note that the M_1 reaction is the same.

12.2. PREPROGRAMMED REACTION IS NOT A STRETCH REFLEX

Several experimental findings prevent one from considering preprogrammed reactions as a kind of stretch reflex because they do not demonstrate an unambiguous dependence between the response and changes in muscle length. Depending on the instruction to the subject, preprogrammed reactions can be observed not only in stretched muscles but also in a muscle shortened because of the perturbation or even in a muscle whose length is not changed by the perturbation at all. In addition, the amplitude of the preprogrammed responses does not correlate with the amplitude of the applied perturbation if the latter cannot be predicted by the subject. Thus, the compensation of the perturbation by preprogrammed reactions can vary in different trials from 0% to 100% or even to overcompensation.

The fact that these responses are independent of the perturbation magnitude suggests that the perturbation represents a nongraded signal for the response generation, a trigger, and that the response magnitude is defined prior to the stimulus on the basis of other factors.

Then, certainly, these reactions can be called **triggered** or **preprogrammed.**

Consider the following scheme for the generation of preprogrammed reactions (figure 12.3). The instruction to keep a joint position against a load requires the subject to generate a voluntary command to muscles controlling this joint. If the subject knows that a perturbation can occur, a corrective command can be prepared in advance and is ready to be triggered by an appropriate peripheral signal. Note that this scheme implies preparation of a preprogrammed reaction by some "higher" cen-

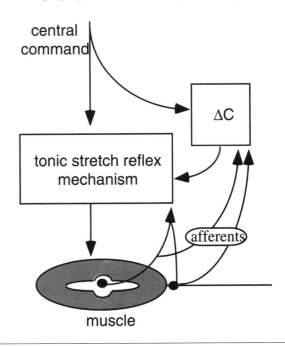

Figure 12.3 A subject is holding a position in a joint against a load with a central command to a muscle. If the subject knows that a perturbation can occur, he/she can prepare an addition to the central command that would compensate for the predicted perturbation. The preprogrammed command (ΔC) is triggered by peripheral signals generated by the perturbation and attenuates the mechanical effects of the perturbation.

ter, for example the cortex, while the loop of the reaction may not involve the "higher" centers.

Let us now try to define what an "appropriate peripheral signal" is.

12.3. IN SEARCH OF THE AFFERENT SOURCE OF PREPROGRAMMED REACTIONS

Consideration of the preprogrammed reactions as triggered responses to a signal provided by the perturbation suggests that the search for the "afferent source" of these responses is likely to provide unreliable results. In fact, if the perturbation provides only a triggering signal, the source of this signal is not really significant (figure 12.4). It must be sufficient to provide necessary information about occurrence of the perturbation. In this context, signals for preprogrammed reactions can be provided by virtually any group of peripheral receptors that deliver information on changes in load, position, pressure on the skin, and, in certain experimental situations, also by visual, auditory, and vestibular receptors.

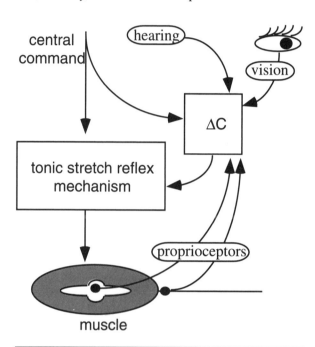

Figure 12.4 Actual source of the triggering signal for a preprogrammed reaction is not important as long as the signal carries sufficient information. It can be provided by proprioceptors, by a flash of light, by a loud tone, etc.

That's why experiments with selective blocking of the transmission along certain afferent systems did not provide conclusive information on the role of these afferents in the generation of preprogrammed responses. The preprogrammed responses disappear after total deafferentation of the limb, that is, when the central nervous system does not receive any signals about the perturbation.

An elegant example of preprogrammed reactions can be observed in experiments with the **grasp reflex.** A subject is given an instruction to position his or her thumb and index finger just near a glass, positioned on a table in front of the subject, "as if going to grasp it." Although no command to grasp occurs, the instruction clearly implies preprogramming of a grasping movement by the subject. This movement is actually observed, at a latency that is characteristic for the preprogrammed response, when the subject's arm is unexpectedly lifted so that the glass remains below the hand.

Note that in this case the perturbation has nothing to do with the length of the muscles directly involved in the grasping task.

Problem 12.2

What would you expect to happen if, in the previous example, the glass suddenly started to fall?

Imagine now that these experiments are performed with anesthesia of various arm segments. If the hand is anesthetized, the reaction is still there. Then the experimenter anesthetizes the forearm; the reaction does not disappear. Only after the whole arm is anesthetized up to the shoulder are the preprogrammed reactions eliminated. These observations may lead to the conclusion that the afferent source of the observed reaction is in the proximal segments of the limb. In fact, information from these segments has proven to be **sufficient** as a signal for the preprogrammed reaction, but it has not proven to be **necessary.** It is quite probable that in a naive subject the same response could have been observed to an unexpected loud sound.

12.4. PREPROGRAMMED REACTIONS DURING MOVEMENT PERTURBATIONS

Up to now we have considered preprogrammed reactions that occur when the posture of a limb is perturbed. Similar reactions, at similar latencies, can be seen when a perturbation occurs unexpectedly in the course of a movement.

For example, imagine that a subject is performing a fast elbow flexion against a constant external load from a certain initial to a certain final position. An unperturbed movement will be accompanied by a typical **triphasic EMG pattern,** as described earlier (figure 12.5). Unexpected changes in the load can be introduced in different ways, depending on the equipment; for example, an electrical motor can be programmed to generate force simulating an increase or decrease in the inertial load. If the load unexpectedly increases, an increase in the activity of the elbow flexors and a decrease in the activity of the elbow extensors will be seen at a latency of about 70 ms. Alternatively, if the load unexpectedly decreases, a decrease in the activity of the elbow flexors and an increase in the activity of the elbow extensors will be seen at a similar latency. As typically happens with preprogrammed reactions, these adjustments will not be able to fully compensate for the effects of the perturbation and will be followed by later, voluntary corrections that are not shown in figure 12.5.

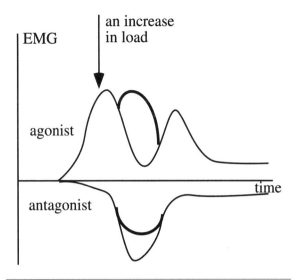

Figure 12.5 If a perturbation occurs during a fast voluntary movement, EMG changes are seen at a latency characteristic of preprogrammed reactions. Generally, they involve an increase in the activity of a muscle that acts against the perturbation, and a decrease in the activity of a muscle that is assisted by the perturbation (bold lines).

Problem 12.3

You are carrying a bundle of firewood with extended arms. Suddenly it drops. What kinds of reactions can you expect in your biceps and triceps?

Let us formulate the following important hypothesis: The analysis of preprogrammed responses to perturbations applied during a number of motor tasks suggests that *the execution of any motor task is associated with preprogramming of fast compensatory reactions to conceivable external perturbations.*

This suggestion is mainly based on common sense, since execution of familiar movements in everyday life is inevitably connected with certain unpredictable but frequently encountered changes in the external conditions of movement execution. These changes include, in particular, rapid changes in the external load or obstacles on the movement trajectory. Therefore, one may assume that any motor task is always associated with preprogrammed compensations triggered in response to unexpected loadings or unloadings of effectors. The magnitude of a preprogrammed reaction can be generated based on the previous experience of the subject.

12.5. BASIC FEATURES OF PREPROGRAMMED REACTIONS

1. It has already been noted that these reactions depend significantly on the instruction to the subject (on what is perceived as major task components). Namely, the responses take place when the subject is instructed, "Compensate as fast as possible," and are small or absent when the instruction is, "Do not pay attention. . . ." This property of pre-programmed reactions is obvious since the subject is free to preprogram or not to preprogram.

2. Emergence of preprogrammed reactions in a muscle shortened by perturbation is also quite understandable, since the subject can preprogram any combination of command functions to any muscle or muscle group (depending on the instruction given or the intention) independently of the influence of a future perturbation on muscle length.

3. Since amplitude of preprogrammed movements should be defined prior to the perturbation, random changes in the perturbation amplitude cannot lead to any correlation of the preprogrammed response amplitude with that of the perturbation. Reproduction of the same perturbation amplitude in a series of trials should lead to an improvement in the compensation due to the preprogrammed responses (such effects were observed experimentally).

Problem 12.4

You measure an integral of a preprogrammed EMG reaction in response to a sequence of perturbations in the same direction but of different magnitude. Do you expect this integral to correlate with any characteristic of your perturbations?

---

4. As discussed earlier, high-frequency muscle vibration leads to a pronounced suppression of the muscle monosynaptic reflexes. However, the preprogrammed responses remain unchanged on the background of the vibration (figure 12.6).

Vibration-induced changes in muscle afferent activity may not be directly related to preprogramming, and thus they influence only the amplitude of a signal for preprogrammed response playback. On the other hand, the amplitude of the preprogrammed response does not depend upon the magnitude of the triggering signal giving rise to the response, which explains the lack of vibration influence upon preprogrammed reactions. Note that muscle vibration suppresses monosynaptic reactions through the mechanism of presynaptic inhibition, which is a selective inhibition mechanism. Apparently it acts on the terminals of Ia-afferents on α-motoneurons but not on the terminals of interneurons that participate in the hypothetical loop bringing about preprogrammed reactions.

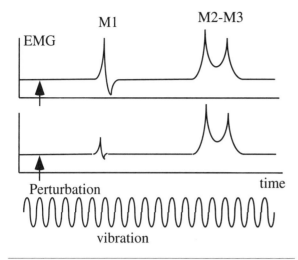

Figure 12.6 Muscle vibration has different effects on different components of the responses to an external perturbation. The early response (M_1) is suppressed just as the H-reflex is, while the preprogrammed response (M_2-M_3) is unchanged.

12.6. PREPROGRAMMED CORRECTIONS OF VERTICAL POSTURE

Unexpected perturbations of **vertical posture** bring about compensatory reactions at latencies resembling those of preprogrammed reactions in limb muscles, that is, intermediate between the phasic stretch reflex and voluntary reactions. These reactions have been observed during maintenance of the vertical posture and during walking. Perturbations of vertical posture not only come from the environment but are frequently generated by a person's own movements. As the reader will see in the chapter on postural control, fast arm movements create large reactive torques acting on the trunk that effectively perturb vertical posture.

Note that maintenance of vertical posture is probably the most common motor task and is a part of many voluntary movements. Therefore, it is reasonable to assume that the mechanism of control of vertical posture is very well "defended" against possible unexpected changes in external conditions. This means, specifically, that various preprogrammed corrections of vertical posture are ready to be initiated in response to certain triggering signals without any special instructions. The complicated problem of maintaining vertical posture in the field of gravity requires relatively complex corrective reactions involving activation of different muscle groups of the legs and the trunk.

Changes in the activity of postural muscles have been seen in response to perturbations applied to various parts of the body of a standing person. These **corrective postural reactions** are specific to the mechanical effects of the perturbation on body equilibrium but not to the exact

point of application of the perturbation. They may occur, in particular, in muscles whose length is not directly affected by the perturbation. According to our general view, these reactions represent preprogrammed motor commands realized when peripheral signals provide information about a perturbation *independently of the afferent source.*

Sometimes people use arm muscles for additional support during standing. In this case, corrective postural reactions can be seen in these muscles in addition to reactions in postural muscles of the legs and trunk. For example, imagine a subject who stands grasping an object for additional support. When the object is fixed to the floor, in other words, provides reliable support, a certain pattern of preprogrammed reactions can be seen in the shoulder muscles. However, if the object has low inertia, the responses can invert and emerge in antagonistic muscle groups, and the overall pattern of the movement resembles that observed in a person holding a cup of tea in his or her hand in response to a postural perturbation.

Let us consider another example. A person is standing on a platform holding in front of him or her a cup filled with play dough (figure 12.7). The platform starts to move. There will be changes in the person's posture, including the posture of the arm holding the cup. If an experimenter records the activity of muscles that maintain the vertical posture of the body and the posture of the arm, there will be changes in the levels of muscle activation. Some of these changes will happen at latencies

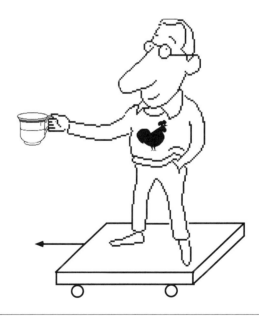

Figure 12.7 Preprogrammed postural corrections to a perturbation created by platform movement are context dependent. They will be different when the cup is filled with play dough than when it is filled with hot tea.
Reprinted, by permission, from M.L. Latash, 1996, The Bernstein problem: How does the central nervous system make its choices? In *Dexterity and Its Development*, edited by M.L. Latash and M.T. Turvey (Mahwah, NJ: Erlbaum), 279.

typical for preprogrammed reactions. Now, let the experimenter repeat the same experiment but put into the cup not play dough, but hot tea. The platform starts to move in exactly the same fashion. Imagine that all the forces, all the initial postures, and all the other conditions are the same (this is impossible to assure, by the way). Preprogrammed changes in the person's posture and his or her arm movements will be quite different. This difference is due to the difference in the person's intentions. In the first case, the major task was not to fall down, while there were no major restrictions on arm movements. In the second case, not spilling the tea becomes comparable in its importance to not falling down. So, human intentions contribute to the patterns of preprogrammed reactions even when the "physics" of the postural task remains the same.

Problem 12.5

You are picking up a small object that turns out to be very heavy (unexpectedly for you). What kinds of reactions do you expect to see?

12.7. CORRECTIVE STUMBLING REACTION

Locomotion is another very commonly used movement in everyday animal and human activity. Therefore it is conceivable that *the mechanism of locomotor movement generation is always in a preprogrammed state.*

A particular pattern of long-latency reflex responses has been observed during cat (and human) locomotion associated with overcoming an unexpected obstacle— the **corrective stumbling reaction.** This pattern could be observed in cats during weak mechanical stimulation of skin areas of the paw or leg (even with an air puff) or during short electrical stimulation of skin nerves.

The application of any of these stimuli during the swing phase gave rise to a flexor reaction with the hindlimb transferring over a hypothetical obstacle (figure 12.8). The same stimulation applied during the stance phase could give rise to an extensor reaction. The coordinated, functionally appropriate pattern of this reaction

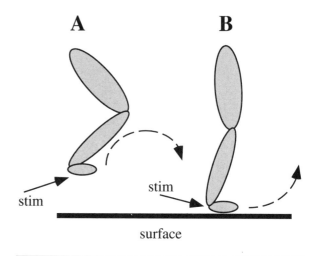

Figure 12.8 A mechanical or electrical stimulation of the paw during locomotion induces different reactions in the swing and the stance phases. In the swing phase (A), there is a flexor reaction, so that the leg "steps over" a fictitious obstacle. In the stance phase, there is an extensor reaction leading to shortening of the stance phase for this limb.

and its relative independence of the stimulus suggest that it is in fact a preprogrammed response of a mechanism responsible in everyday life for the compensatory reactions during real stumbling.

Problem 12.6

Can you define the afferent source of the corrective stumbling reaction with the method of successive limb denervation, that is, eliminating afferent inputs from areas of the leg?

One can present an example of a very complex but obviously preprogrammed reaction. Imagine an officer giving commands to soldiers: "Lie down," "stand up," "lie down," "stand up," . . . "lie down," "stand up," "stand up!" It is obvious that some of the participants in this experiment would lie down in response to the last command. After numerous repetitions of the presented sequence, the motor reactions become preprogrammed, and the voice of the officer plays the role of a triggering signal.

Chapter 12 in a Nutshell

A group of reactions to external stimuli (commonly, to mechanical perturbations) that come at a latency longer than typical reflex latencies and shorter than voluntary reaction time are called preprogrammed reactions, triggered reactions, or long-latency responses. These responses can be modulated by prior instruction. They produce quick, crude corrective actions counteracting the mechanical effects of the original perturbation. They can be seen in muscles whose length is increased, decreased, or not changed by the perturbation. The exact sensory source of preprogrammed reactions is not important as long as it is sufficient to provide information about a perturbation. Preprogrammed responses are important components of all everyday activities, particularly of postural control and locomotion.

Self-Test Problems

1. You placed an electrode close to a group of identical fibers in a dorsal root of the spinal cord. When you stimulate the fibers, in response to a single impulse you get a transient increase in the activity of a flexor muscle and a decrease in the activity of an extensor muscle at the same joint. When you flex the joint with an external force, you see an increase in the activity of these fibers. When you stimulate γ-motoneurons innervating the extensor muscle, there are no changes in the activity of these fibers. Where do these fibers originate?

2. A subject is performing a series of very fast elbow flexions over 40° against a constant external load. Movement time is 200 ms. Unexpectedly, in one trial, the movement is completely blocked. Draw time patterns of the biceps and triceps EMGs based on central programming of EMG patterns and on equilibrium-point control ideas.

3. You placed an electrode close to a group of identical fibers in a dorsal root of the spinal cord. When you stimulate the fibers, in response to a single impulse you get a transient increase in the activity of a flexor muscle and a decrease in the activity of an extensor muscle at the same joint. When you extend the joint with an external force, you see an increase in the activity of these fibers. When you stimulate dynamic γ-motoneurons innervating both flexor and extensor muscle, there are no changes in the activity of these fibers. Where do these fibers originate?

4. A subject is performing a series of very fast elbow flexions over 40° against a constant external load. Movement time is 200 ms. Unexpectedly, in one trial, an opposing force blocks the movement before it can start and releases it after 100 ms. Draw EMG and kinematic (trajectory and velocity) patterns of an unperturbed trial and of the blocked trial. Use different graphs for the agonist and antagonist EMG and for each kinematic variable.

5. You record H-reflexes in a soleus muscle of a subject. Under a certain additional external stimulus, the amplitude of the H-reflexes decreases by 50%. What can you say about changes in the level of excitability of the α-motoneuronal pool controlling the muscle? In another experiment, your subject takes a pill, and both H-reflex and M-response drop by 50%. What can you say about the central and peripheral effects of the pill?

6. A subject is holding a position in a joint against a constant external load. The instruction is "Try your best to keep this position in cases of possible peturbations." Unexpectedly the external load increases and moves the joint. Describe all the mechanisms that help the subject to follow the instruction.

Recommended Additional Readings

Evarts EV, Granit R (1976). Relations of reflexes and intended movements. *Progress in Brain Research* 44: 1-14.

Feldman AG, Levin MF (1995). The origin and use of positional frames of reference in motor control. *Behavioral and Brain Sciences* 18: 723-804.

Gottlieb GL, Corcos DM, Agarwal GC (1989). Strategies for the control of voluntary movements with one mechanical degree of freedom. *Behavioral and Brain Sciences* 12: 189-250.

Houk JC (1979). Regulation of stiffness by skeletomotor reflexes. *Annual Reviews in Physiology* 41: 99-114.

Latash ML (1993). *Control of Human Movement.* Champaign, IL: Human Kinetics. Chapters 1, 3, 4.

McInryte J, Bizzi E (1993). Servo hypotheses for the biological control of movement. *Journal of Motor Behavior* 25: 193-202.

Nichols TR (1994). A biomechanical perspective on spinal mechanisms of coordinated muscular action: An architecture principle. *Acta Anatomica* 151: 1-13.

Prochazka A (1996). Proprioceptive feedback and movement regulation. In: Rowell L, Sheperd JT (Eds.), *Handbook of Physiology.* Section 12, *Exercise: Regulation and Integration of Multiple Systems,* pp. 89-127. New York: American Physiological Society.

Rothwell JR (1994). *Control of Human Voluntary Movement.* 2nd ed. London: Chapman & Hall. Chapters 5, 6.

Stein RB (1974). Peripheral control of movement. *Physiological Reviews* 54: 215-243.

WORLD III

STRUCTURES

CHAPTER 13

METHODS OF BRAIN STUDY AND ELEMENTS OF THE BRAIN ANATOMY

Key Terms

methods of brain study	PET	**Elements of functional anatomy of the medulla and the brain**
EEG	MRI	
CT		

The human **brain** contains at least a hundred billion neurons. Each neuron represents a complex structure that is theoretically capable of processing incoming information in many ways, receives inputs from many other neurons, and has numerous output connections (synapses). The efficacy of each synapse can be modified by numerous factors including the activity of the neighboring neurons. This is probably enough to persuade the reader that trying to compile a full description of brain activity that would account for the activity of each individual neuron would be unrealistic and a waste of time. However, this is not the purpose of the neuroscientists who study brain structures and their connections. Modeling the activity of the central nervous system within the complex system approach can easily lead to models and hypotheses that belong to science fiction rather than to science. Researchers should not forget that the object of interest is not a black box but an actual structure that imposes limitations on the otherwise unlimited imagination of theoreticians. The ultimate test for any hypothesis will always be its ability to map on the substrate and to reproduce its behavior in a variety of activities. Therefore, anatomical, morphological, and neurophysiologi-

cal studies of the brain provide crucially important information for the understanding of brain functioning. Furthermore, these studies have extreme importance for clinicians who deal with patients experiencing various types of brain trauma (for example, stroke) or dysfunction.

A lot of behavioral, neurophysiological, and pathological information has been collected that allows us to make certain inferences about the functioning of the brain and its major structures. Before considering elements of this huge database, let us look at the major methods that have been used to accumulate all this information.

13.1. SINGLE-NEURON RECORDING

Single-neuron recording techniques are similar to intramuscular electromyography, which we discussed earlier. It is based on inserting a **needle with a thin wire** (or a number of thin wires) into a neural structure. Typically the difference of potentials between the wire and the needle or between different pairs of wires is recorded. This method may be highly selective, allowing registration of the activity of even the smallest single neurons. It has provided a wealth of information about the organization and function of various brain and spinal structures. However, it apparently requires direct access to the neural structure, and its use is restricted to animal studies and certain neurosurgical procedures that allow or even require the insertion of needles into the brain for testing purposes.

In animal experiments, however, this method has been used both for acute recording of the activity of the brain and for chronic recording. In the latter case, a number of needle electrodes are implanted into the brain and connected to a "crown" that is mounted on the top of the head of the animal and does not interfere with its daily activities. When the experimenter wants to record the activity of the neurons, a connector is placed on the crown and the recording is performed. This technique allows recording of neurons from the same area of the brain for weeks or even months.

13.2. ELECTROENCEPHALOGRAPHY

Electroencephalography (EEG) is a method of studying the collective electrical behavior of large groups of neurons. It is similar to surface electromyography in using macroelectrodes located on the surface of the body. The EEG electrodes are placed on the skull over certain areas of the brain, commonly over the four major **cortical lobes:** frontal, parietal, occipital, and temporal (figure 13.1). An indifferent electrode is commonly placed on an ear.

Electroencephalography reflects the flow of currents through the extracellular space. These currents may be considered either as an **epiphenomenon,** that is, as a reflection of functionally important processes that in itself does not have any functional significance, or as an important component of brain functioning. Note that information transmission within the brain is based on electrical processes (such as action potentials and synaptic currents). Thus, we can expect synchronized, rather large changes in the external electromagnetic field, reflected by EEG, to be able to affect the processes of generation of action potentials in individual neurons. If so, EEG becomes a product of the neuronal activity that is also an important factor in determining this activity.

The EEG may look like a random signal, or it may demonstrate relatively regular oscillations at certain frequencies. Typical EEG frequencies range from 1 to 30 Hz, while its amplitude on the surface of the skull is of the order of several tens of microvolts. EEG waves are classified into four major groups depending on their frequency (figure 13.2). These are **beta waves** (from 13 to 25 Hz), **alpha waves** (from 8 to 13 Hz), **theta waves** (from 4 to 8 Hz), and **delta waves** (from 0.5 to 4 Hz). The low-frequency waves (delta and theta) have the largest amplitude and are commonly seen during certain

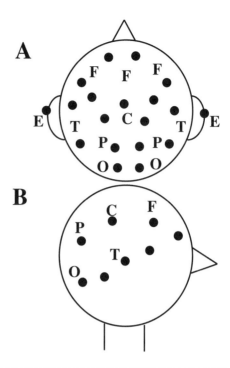

Figure 13.1   Typical placement of EEG electrodes. A: at the top of the head; B: at the side of the head; C: central; F: frontal; O: occipital; P: parietal; T: temporal; E: ear.

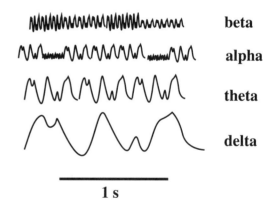

Figure 13.2   Typical EEG waves include beta waves (13-25 Hz), alpha waves (8-13 Hz), theta waves (4-8 Hz), and delta waves (0.5-4 Hz).

phases of sleep. Alpha waves are associated with a state of relaxed wakefulness, although their representation varies widely among different persons. Beta waves dominate during episodes of intense mental activity.

Problem 13.1

Characteristic times of action potential generation are about 10 ms corresponding to a frequency of about 100 Hz. How can neuronal activity give rise to slow waves observed in EEG?

The general pattern of EEG changes dramatically in certain pathological cases such as epileptic seizures. During a seizure, synchronized, large-amplitude oscillations are seen in the signals from all electrodes.

13.3. EVOKED POTENTIALS

A sensory stimulus may give rise to a synchronized volley of action potentials generated by peripheral receptors of the corresponding modality that send their axons to the central nervous system. These action potentials eventually reach brain structures and induce changes in the EEG signal. Commonly, these changes are rather small (of the order of a few microvolts or even fractions of a microvolt) and cannot be clearly seen on the noisy background of the EEG signal in the absence of the sensory stimulus. However, the noisy background is not synchronized with the stimulus, while the induced EEG changes are. Therefore, averaging a number of responses to standard stimuli increases the signal-to-noise ratio and allows visualization of the EEG reaction to the sensory stimulus (figure 13.3). Such reactions are called **evoked potentials.** Depending on the strength and modality of the stimulus, detecting evoked potentials may require the averaging of a few responses or, sometimes, of a few hundred or thousand responses.

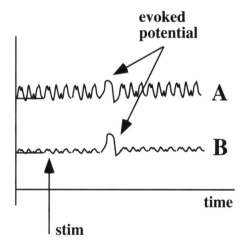

Figure 13.3 Evoked brain potentials to a peripheral stimuli (e.g., to an electrical stimulus) are frequently obscured by the background activity (A). However, averaging a large number of trials may reveal an evoked potential (B).

Note that one sensory stimulus may induce a series of peaks within an evoked potential (or a series of evoked potentials) with different time delays depending on the exact path of the induced volley of action potentials, the conduction speed, the number of synapses, etc. This makes evoked potentials a powerful tool for neurophysiological and clinical research, because changes in the

relative amplitude of different peaks may provide information on the efficacy of corresponding transmission paths.

Evoked potentials can be seen not only in EEG but also in the activity of the spinal cord with surface electrodes placed on the back. They may be induced, for example, by peripheral stimuli to a sensory nerve, in particular in conditions that are commonly used for H-reflex studies. The amplitude of spinal evoked potentials is also very small and is obscured by the resting activity of the large back muscles. Thus, recording these potentials requires averaging several hundred individual responses. This method may provide potentially valuable information about the damage to spinal conduction systems following spinal cord injury (figure 13.4).

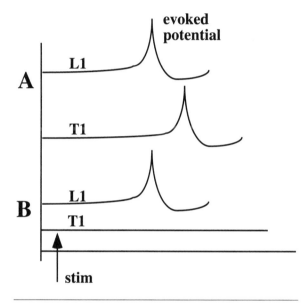

Figure 13.4 Evoked potentials of the spinal cord can be recorded from the back in response to an electrical stimulation of a peripheral nerve. In A, stimulation of the tibial nerve leads to evoked potentials over both L1 and T1 vertebrae, while in B, there is a potential over L1 but not over T1. Probably transmission along the spinal cord is damaged in B.

Problem 13.2

You see a brain evoked potential induced by a stimulus applied to a leg nerve, but no spinal potential. What is your conclusion?

Problem 13.3

You observe a brain evoked potential induced by a stimulus applied to a leg nerve, but no muscle response when you stimulate the corresponding cortical motor area. What is your conclusion?

13.4. RADIOGRAPHY

Using **x-rays** allows the creation of visual images of structures with different abilities to absorb x-rays (gamma rays). Thus, radiography is very effective in **imaging bones,** particularly the cranium. However, it cannot detect gray or white matter or reveal differences between the two. Another major limitation of conventional radiography is in that it creates a two-dimensional image of an object while we are certainly interested in its three-dimensional structure. The major advantage of radiography is its very high spatial resolution, which may be as high as a few percent of a millimeter.

There are variations of conventional radiography that make it more useful for brain imaging. The first is **pneumoencephalography,** which is based on the ability of air to be virtually transparent to radiation. So if one removes a small amount of the cerebrospinal fluid and replaces it with air, the air bubble will eventually reach the brain ventricles and allow one to observe changes in the ventricular system. This method is painful, however, and may be dangerous, so it is not normally used today.

There is another, much more widely used variation on conventional radiography, called **angiography.** During angiography, a gamma ray-opaque substance (a contrast) is injected into the circulatory system. As a result, it is possible to detect changes in the structure of **blood vessels,** in particular those in the brain. This method is invasive but is also more precise than magnetic resonance angiography, which is a noninvasive version of angiography. Angiography is effective in determining vascular malformations, aneurysms, and strokes.

13.5. COMPUTERIZED TOMOGRAPHY

Computerized tomography (CT) is based on radiography and involves the use of a *series of narrow beams of radiation* (figure 13.5). The source of x-rays is placed at one side of the skull while x-ray detectors are placed at the opposite side. Then both the source and the detectors of the x-rays are rotated in steps, and at each step a series of x-ray transmissions is recorded. Thus for each small area of the brain a large number of measurements are taken. Eventually, areas with relatively small differences in radiodensity can be seen as different shades of gray ranging from black to white. More specifically, this method allows visualization of gray and white matter, although the resolution is somewhat lower than that of conventional radiography. Note that CT creates a two-dimensional image of a two-dimensional thin slice of the tissues, while conventional radiography creates a two-dimensional image of a three-dimensional object.

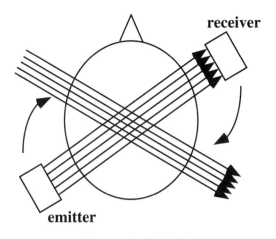

Figure 13.5   Computer tomography involves making a series of x-ray images while rotating the emitter and the receiver of the x-rays.

Computerized tomography can be combined with angiography (injecting an x-ray-opaque substance into the circulatory system), increasing the accuracy of both methods with respect to blood vessels in the brain.

13.6. POSITRON EMISSION TOMOGRAPHY

Positron emission tomography (PET) is somewhat similar to computerized tomography in that it is based on an analysis of x-rays in different directions (figure 13.6). However, the source of the x-rays is not an external emitter but a **radioactive isotope** that is injected into the circulatory system. For example, an analogue of glucose can be labeled with a radioactive ion. Then it is metabolized by neurons, and one of the products of metabolism accumulates in the cells. Consequently, the amount of radiation emitted by the cells is proportional to the number of metabolized glucose-like molecules, that is, to the general level of the cell activity. Recently, many inferences about specific functions of certain brain structures have been made based on this technique. However, one needs to be cautious in jumping to such conclusions, because they are similar to the conclusion that the most important political decisions are made in stadiums where many people shout together.

Problem 13.4

What can you conclude from observing an increase in the general level of cell activity in a certain brain area during a certain action?

Positron emission tomography is based on substituting, for an atom that has a low molecular weight, another

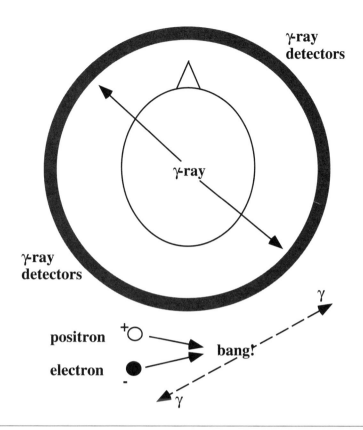

Figure 13.6 Positron emission tomography uses radioactive isotopes of low-molecular-weight elements that emit positrons. Positrons collide with electrons and emit x-rays (gamma rays), which are detected by an array of gamma-ray detectors surrounding the head.

radioactive atom that decays, emitting a **positron.** A typical example is substituting fluorine [^{18}F] for carbon, nitrogen, or oxygen. The emitted positron quickly meets an electron (there are many of those anywhere) and is annihilated, producing a pair of gamma quants. The **gamma rays** are detected with an array of detectors surrounding the head. Then the same method as in CT is used to create a two-dimensional image of a thin slice of the brain. The resolution of this method is of the order of 1 mm.

13.7. MAGNETIC RESONANCE IMAGING

Still another version of CT is **magnetic resonance imaging** (MRI). It is based on differences in the properties of different atomic nuclei and is very efficient in visualizing structures with different chemical compositions. For example, MRI is superior to any other noninvasive method in differentiating between white matter and gray matter. It can also be used to visualize the motion of water molecules and thus to make images of blood vessels, presenting a noninvasive version of angiography.

Magnetic resonance imaging is based on the property of elements with an odd atomic weight to align the spin

axes of the nuclei along a constant external magnetic field (figure 13.7). A brief electromagnetic pulse can be used to perturb the orientation of the spin axes. When the pulse is turned off, the nuclei return to their original orientation as defined by the external magnetic field. This process is accompanied by release of energy in the form of electromagnetic waves. The frequency of the emitted waves is different for different atoms; another characteristic parameter is the time of relaxation of the nuclei to the original state. These parameters are influenced not only by the type of atom but also by its physicochemical environment. Magnetic resonance imaging is superior to other techniques with respect to its ability to differentiate among tissues, but is also the most expensive.

13.8. NEUROANATOMICAL TRACING

A widely used method of tracing neuronal projections is based on the phenomenon of **fast axonal transport.** Large intracellular particles travel in both directions, from the cell body to the axon terminal (**anterograde** transport) and from the axonal terminals to the cell body (**retrograde transport**). The purpose of fast axonal transport is delivery of substances to the nerve endings and

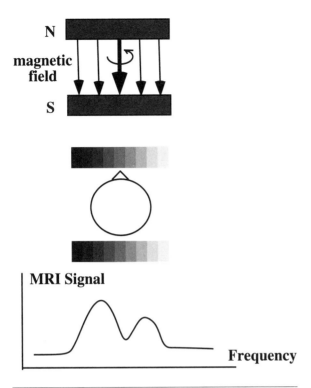

MRI Signal

Frequency

Figure 13.7 Magnetic resonance imaging is based on the ability of elements with an odd atomic weight to align their spins along an external magnetic field. If the field is perturbed, spin alignment is violated. When the perturbation is turned off, the spins return to the previous alignment and emit radio waves in the process. The frequency of the waves and the time it takes the nuclei to come to a lower energy state are specific to the element. Using a magnetic field that changes in space allows one to identify the location of certain elements.

removal of materials from the terminals to the cell body for further removal or reuse. This phenomenon can be used in combination with radiography if a transportable substance is labeled with radioactive amino acids or sugars. Alternatively, specific substances can be employed that are later seen as shades or colors after an appropriate histochemical analysis. One substance frequently used for tracing neuronal projections is horseradish peroxidase, which is transported in the retrograde direction.

13.9. MAJOR BRAIN STRUCTURES

The time has come to move up to the anatomy of the most complex and mysterious part of the central nervous system, the **brain.** I would like to apologize up front for the fact that many brain structures have more than one name, that one and the same structure can be a member of different larger brain compartments, and that there are many systems for identifying structures. It would take tens of pages to present all the nomenclature, and this is not the purpose of the book. There are detailed books on

neuroanatomy where one can find all this information. Here I will use the least confusing (from my very subjective point of view) names for brain structures and not mention all the alternative names.

Both the spinal cord and the brain are protected by bony encasements: the vertebral column protects the spinal cord, and the **cranium** protects the brain. The neural tissue does not come into contact with the surrounding bony structures; it is separated from them by a protective membrane consisting of a number of **meninges** (figure 13.8). The central nervous system is bathed in **cerebrospinal fluid,** which circulates within hollow ventricles of the brain, the **central canal** of the spinal cord, and the **subarachnoid space** that surrounds the whole central nervous system.

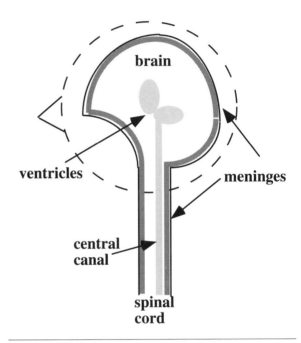

Figure 13.8 The central nervous system consists of the spinal cord and the brain. Both are bathed in the cerebrospinal fluid and are surrounded by meninges.

The central nervous system is characterized by a huge metabolic rate that requires a continuous supply of oxygen and nutrients; the brain receives about 20% of the resting cardiac output even though its weight is only about 2% of the total weight of the body. Consequently the brain is very sensitive to the lack of oxygen and the presence of drugs and toxins. There is a barrier between the cerebrospinal fluid and blood (the **blood-brain barrier**) that plays an important role in maintaining the homeostasis of the central nervous system. This barrier is rather impenetrable to substances soluble in water because of the polar nature of water, but it can be penetrated by lipidsoluble substances. Note that the presence of the bloodbrain barrier has both positive and negative consequences.

The barrier protects the central nervous system from potentially hazardous substances such as toxins. On the other hand, it also prevents water-soluble drugs from crossing the barrier and getting to their target cells.

Problem 13.5

You need a water-soluble substance to reach a group of neural cells. Suggest a method (or methods) of delivering it across the blood-brain barrier.

Let us travel "up" from the spinal cord and make note of anatomical structures within the central nervous system. Most of the illustrations will be schematic. However, first take a look at a general picture showing an MRI image of the main structures of the central nervous system inside the human head (figure 13.9).

At its "upper" (rostral) end, the spinal cord merges with the **medulla,** which is an elongated, bulbous structure about 1 in. long (figure 13.10). Starting from the rostral end of the spinal cord and continuing though the medulla, there is a complex network of neural cells and fibers called the **reticular formation.** Actually, the reticular formation continues rostrally to the medulla and goes into the **midbrain.** Inside the medulla is a space called the **fourth ventricle,** connected at its caudal end to the central canal of the spinal cord and at its rostral end to the **aqueduct.** There are several important nuclei within the medulla. Some transmit information from the periphery to other brain structures (**nucleus gracilis** and **nucleus cuneatus**), while others (**nucleus ambiguus** and

hypoglossal nucleus) are origins of some of the **cranial nerves.** The medulla plays a very important role in the **autonomic function** of the human nervous system, that is, in maintaining an adequate level of functioning of vital internal structures such as the heart, lungs, circulatory system, and digestive system. Most of the autonomic function proceeds without any conscious awareness. The medulla houses three vitally important nuclei: the **cardiac center,** the **vasomotor center,** and the **respiratory center.** It also contains control centers for a number of voluntary and involuntary activities such as sneezing, coughing, vomiting, and swallowing.

The next distinct structure, rostrally to the medulla, is the **pons** (figure 13.11), which looks like a round bulge on the underside portion of the brain. The pons contains more nuclei associated with cranial nerves as well as two centers participating in the control of respiration, the **apneustic** and the **pneumotaxic areas.**

Just behind the medulla and the pons is the second-largest brain structure, the cerebellum (figure 13.12), which deserves a special chapter with respect to its structure, connections, and functions. The cerebellum consists of **two hemispheres** and a central area called the **vermis.** Three pairs of bundles of neural fibers support the cerebellum and provide it with means of communication with the rest of the brain. These bundles are called **peduncles** and are termed **superior, middle,** and **inferior peduncles.** The pons and the cerebellum are sometimes addressed as the **metencephalon.**

Let us return to the main path and continue moving up. At its rostral end, the pons borders the **midbrain** or **mesencephalon.** The mesencephalon (figure 13.13) is a

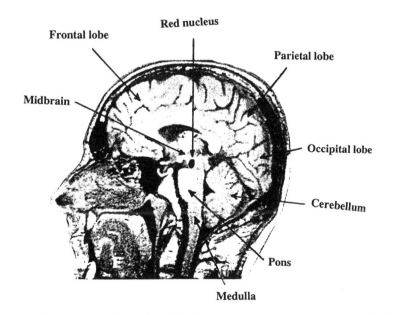

Figure 13.9   Major structures of the rostral part of the central nervous system are shown on this sagittal section of the human head. Adapted, by permission, from A. Gironell, J. Marti-Fabrega, J. Bello, and A. Avila, 1997, "Non-Hodgkin's lymphoma as a new cause of non-thrombotic superior sagittal sinus occlusion," *Journal of Neurology, Neurosurgery, and Psychiatry,* 63: 121. © 1997 BMJ Publishing Group.

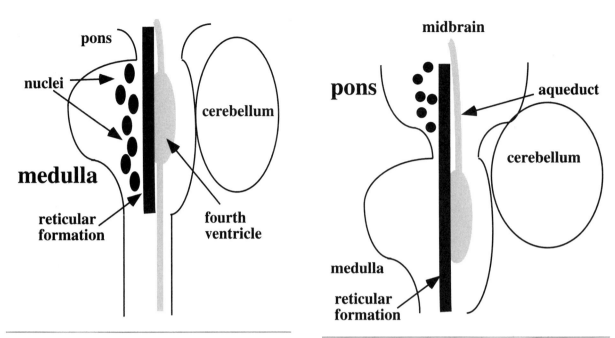

Figure 13.10   At its rostral end, the spinal cord borders the medulla. The medulla contains a number of important nuclei, the caudal portion of the reticular formation, and the fourth ventricle. At its rostral end, the medulla borders the pons.

Figure 13.11   The pons is located between the medulla and the midbrain. It contains white fiber tracts (both ascending and descending) as well as several nuclei including those of cranial nerves V to VIII.

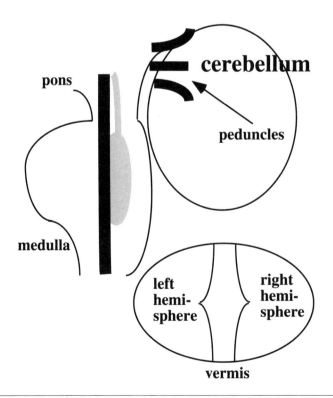

Figure 13.12   The cerebellum lies just behind the medulla and the pons. It consists of two hemispheres and a central area (vermis). The cerebellum is supported by three pairs of peduncles (bundles of neural fibers).

short section of the brainstem that contains several important nuclei as well as the **aqueduct** connecting the third and fourth ventricles. In particular, the midbrain contains the **corpora quadrigemina,** four small hills on the dorsal portion of the midbrain. These hills are also termed **colliculi.** The two upper hills, the **superior colliculi,** play an important role in vision and visual reflexes, while the two lower hills, the **inferior colliculi,** play an important role in the processing of auditory information. The **red nucleus** is located deep within the midbrain and will be interesting to us as a potentially very important structure for the generation of voluntary movements. The **substantia nigra** is located ventrally to the red nucleus and is also very important for motor control. Its possible role will be considered in detail in the chapter on **basal ganglia.** The mesencephalon also contains the **cerebral peduncles,** composed of neural tracts connecting the cerebrum with the rest of the brain.

The next brain structure is the **diencephalon** (figure 13.14), which is almost completely surrounded by the cerebral hemispheres. Inside the diencephalon is a cavity formed by the third ventricle. Four major structures can be found in the diencephalon: the **thalamus, hypothalamus, epithalamus,** and **hypophysis.**

The thalamus occupies about 80% of the total volume of the diencephalon. The thalamus and its nuclei play an important role in **sensory-motor integration,**

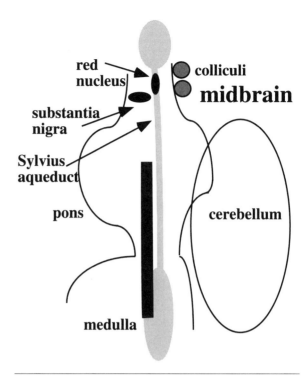

Figure 13.13   The midbrain (mesencephalon) contains four elevations called colliculi: two superior colliculi and two inferior colliculi. It also contains two major nuclei, the red nucleus and substantia nigra, as well as the Sylvius aqueduct.

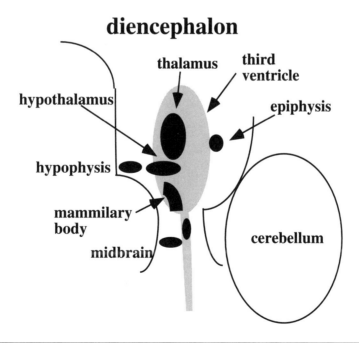

Figure 13.14   The diencephalon is almost completely surrounded by cerebral hemispheres. It contains the thalamus, hypothalamus, hypophysis, and epiphysis (the pineal gland). Inside the diencephalon is the third ventricle.

and their function will be considered in more detail later.

The **hypothalamus** is located below the thalamus and consists of several groups of nuclei. It plays an important role in the autonomic and limbic (emotional) functions of the body. In particular, it participates in control of **cardiovascular function,** regulation of **body temperature,** regulation of **water and electrolyte balance,** control of **gastrointestinal activity,** regulation of **sleep,** regulation of **sexual function,** production of certain **emotional responses** (such as anger, fear, and pleasure), and control of **endocrine function.** So, despite its small size, the hypothalamus may be considered the center of control of autonomic activity.

The hypothalamus is part of the **limbic system,** which is a group of neural fiber tracts and nuclei forming a circle around the brainstem (figure 13.15). The limbic system includes the hypothalamus, the **fornix** (which is a fiber tract), the **hippocampus,** the **amygdaloid nucleus,** and the **cingulate gyrus** of the **cerebral cortex.** This system is involved in emotional reactions such as anger, hunger, and sexual drive. Let us single out the **hippocampus,** whose role is apparently not limited to emotional reactions. According to widespread belief, the hippocampus plays a major role in short-term **memory** and consolidation of information from short-term to long-term memory. The role of the hippocampus in memory-related processes will be further discussed in the chapter on memory.

Two structures of the diencephalon are major endocrine glands that, like other endocrine glands, control certain body functions with the help of chemical substances, that is, **hormones.** The **epithalamus** lies in the dorsal area of the diencephalon and includes the **pineal gland** or **epiphysis.** Somewhat ventrally and rostrally to the mesencephalon lies the **pituitary gland** or **hypophysis,** which is round and has a diameter of about 0.5 in. The endocrine functions will not be discussed in this textbook.

Problem 13.6

You observe a substantial increase in the volume of the third ventricle. What kind of pathological brain changes can you suspect in the patient?

Now we come to the largest part of the brain, the **cerebrum** (figure 13.16), which also has another name, the **telencephalon.** The cerebrum consists of **two hemispheres** that are separated by the **longitudinal fissure** and are connected by a large tract of neural fibers called the **corpus callosum** and by the **anterior commissure.** Each hemisphere contains a **central cavity** formed by lateral ventricles and filled with cerebrospinal fluid. The surface layer of the cerebrum is referred to as **cerebral cortex.** It is a few millimeters deep and consists of gray matter. The cerebral cortex has a characteristic grooved and folded surface. The folds and grooves are called **convolutions;** their elevated parts are called **gyri,** while the depressed parts are called **sulci.** The presence of convolutions greatly increases the area of the cortex. Under the cortex lies the thick white matter of the cerebrum consisting of dendrites, myelinated axons, and neuroglia. The white matter provides much of the connecting network among various areas of the cerebrum.

Each hemisphere is divided by **fissures** into five **lobes.** Four of them, the **frontal, parietal, occipital,** and **tem-**

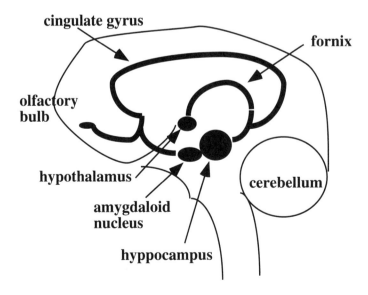

Figure 13.15   The limbic system includes the hypothalamus, the fornix, the hippocampus, the amygdaloid nucleus, and the cingulate gyrus of the cerebral cortex.

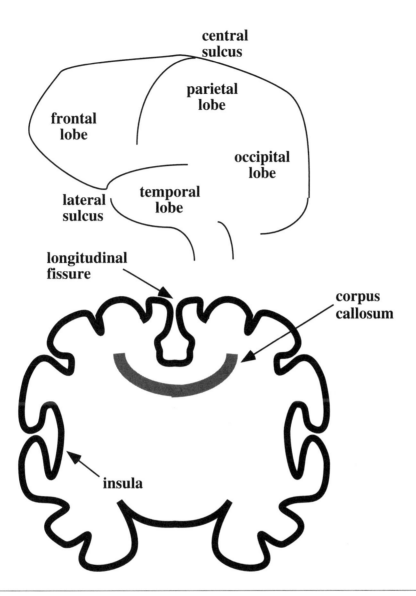

Figure 13.16 The cerebrum consists of two hemispheres connected by the corpus callosum and by the anterior commissure. Each hemisphere is divided by fissures into five lobes: frontal, parietal, occipital, temporal, and insula.

poral lobes, appear on the outer surface of the hemisphere, while the fifth one, called the **insula,** is located deeper in the cerebrum and is covered by portions of the frontal, parietal, and temporal lobes. The frontal lobe forms the anterior portion of each hemisphere and is separated from the parietal lobe by the **Rolando fissure** or **central sulcus.** The parietal lobe is separated from the occipital lobe by the **parieto-occipital fissure.** The temporal lobe lies laterally and somewhat below the frontal and parietal lobes and is separated from them by the **lateral sulcus** or **sylvian fissure.**

The cerebrum has many very important functions, including those related to motor coordination and perception. It certainly deserves a separate chapter.

Within the white matter of the cerebrum lie **basal ganglia** (figure 13.17). Three of the nuclei of the basal ganglia lie deep in the cerebrum, laterally to the thalamus. The phylogenetically oldest nucleus is the **globus pallidus,** which is also called the **paleostriatum.** The globus pallidus consists of two parts, internal (GP_i) and external (GP_e). These parts have different connections with other brain structures. Two nuclei, the **caudate nucleus** and the **putamen,** form the **neostriatum** (or just **striatum**). They are separated from each other by the **internal capsule.** The other two nuclei of the basal ganglia, the **subthalamic nucleus** and the **substantia nigra,** are located in the midbrain. The basal ganglia play a very important role in the generation of voluntary movements. Their dysfunction may lead to various motor disorders including Parkinson's disease and Huntington's chorea. The basal ganglia will be discussed in detail further in this text.

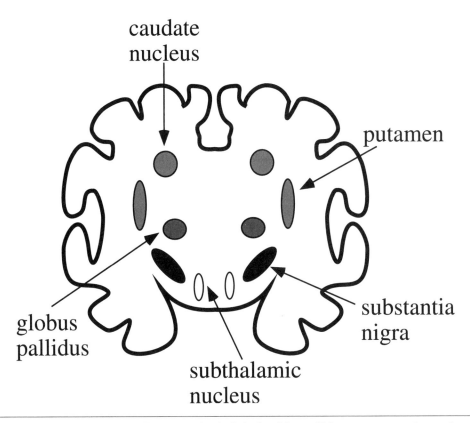

Figure 13.17   Basal ganglia represent pairs of structures that include the globus pallidus, putamen, caudate nucleus, substantia nigra, and subthalamic nucleus.

Chapter 13 in a Nutshell

Methods of brain study provide information about excitatory and inhibitory processes in the brain (single-neuron recording, EEG, and evoked potentials), about the physical properties of brain tissues (x-ray and CT), about anatomical connections among groups of neurons (neuroanatomical tracing), or about the rate of metabolic processes in the brain as reflected by blood flow (MRI and PET). The central nervous system is bathed in cerebrospinal fluid; it consists of the spinal cord, the medulla, and the brain. The brain contains numerous nuclei (groups of neurons) whose function ranges from control of internal body processes, to control of voluntary movements, to control of purely mental processes. The function of most brain structures is poorly understood. Most likely, external functions of the organism emerge as a result of an interaction of many neural structures.

CEREBRAL CORTEX

Key Terms

anatomy of the cortex

hemisphere asymmetry

Brodmann areas

motor and premotor areas

motor body maps

corticospinal tract

neuronal population studies

cortical inputs and outputs

The cerebral cortex (as well as other major brain areas) is an inconceivably complex structure whose function and interaction with other brain areas are likely to be multi-faceted and ambiguous. A wealth of information has been accumulated about the cortex, and this book will only scratch the surface of all this knowledge. Most of the conclusions drawn about the cortex are tentative; thus some statements in this chapter may not be accepted by all the researchers working in this area. It is impossible to do justice to all the work on the cortex in one textbook chapter, so I apologize for not mentioning the names of many colleagues whose studies have significantly influenced the present understanding of this fascinating structure.

14.1. CEREBRAL HEMISPHERES

The cerebral cortex is a part of the brain that is traditionally associated with **"higher nervous activity"** including perceiving and interpreting sensory information, making conscious decisions, and controlling voluntary movements. The formation of such notions as "motor task," "motor goal," "accuracy requirements," "intention," and "will" is also assumed to be based on processes within the cerebral cortex or with an important contribution from it.

Views of the cerebral hemispheres from the side and from above are shown in figure 14.1. These illustrations show the main gyri and sulci that are used as landmarks to define the location of various cortical areas.

The two **hemispheres** of the cerebrum are not identical, and they differ significantly in their functions. In particular, the speech function has been found to be localized in one of the hemispheres that is commonly called **dominant.** The left hemisphere is dominant in about 96% of right-handed persons and in about 70% of left-handed persons. Note that the **cerebrospinal tract** goes on its way from one side of the body to the other, so that the right hemisphere controls movements of the left side of the body. Therefore, in 96% of right-handed persons, movements of the preferred hand are controlled by the dominant hemisphere, while in 70% of left-handed persons, movements of the preferred hand are controlled by the nondominant hemisphere. Most of the studies of hemispheric asymmetry were performed on so-called **split-brain** patients. In some cases of epilepsy, the corpus callosum and anterior commissure are surgically cut so that there is no direct exchange of information between the hemispheres. The behavior of split-brain subjects does not look different from that of healthy people. However, the differences become apparent when sensory information is manipulated in such a way that the hemispheres receive different information. This can be done by placing objects in the left or right visual field, using different auditory stimuli to the left and right ears, and so on. It is commonly stated that the dominant hemisphere takes the responsibility for analytical information processing, particularly that involving symbolic information (such as in mathematics), while the right hemisphere

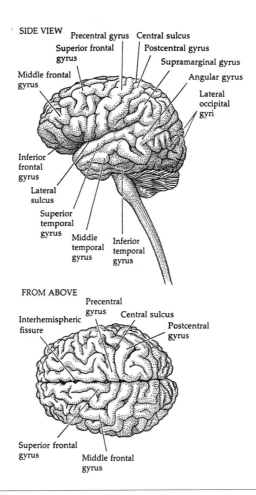

Figure 14.1 Two views of the cerebral cortex show the major sulci and guri.
Reprinted, by permission, from S.W. Kuffler, J.G. Nicholls, and A.R. Martin, 1984, *From neuron to brain,* 2nd ed. (Sunderland, MA: Sinauer Associates, Inc.), 570.

is more emotional and intuitive. This may be true, however, only for split-brain cases, while normally the exchange of information between the hemispheres is such that all functions are based nearly equally on both hemispheres.

Problem 14.1

If you had a choice, would you prefer to be left-handed or right-handed, left-hemisphere dominant or right-hemisphere dominant? Why?

I will be considering similarities across the hemispheres rather than differences, because at our present level of understanding, control of motor function is organized similarly on both sides.

14.2. STRUCTURE OF THE CEREBRAL CORTEX

Cerebral cortex contains two major types of neural cells (figure 14.2). These are **pyramidal** and **stellate** (or gran-

ule) cells. The cortex has a characteristic **layer structure** that can be seen in vertical sections. The uppermost layer is called the **molecular layer.** It is composed mostly of axons and apical dendrites and contains only a few cell bodies. Next is the **external granular layer,** containing a large number of small pyramidal and stellate cells. It is followed by the **external pyramidal layer,** containing mostly pyramidal cells. The next layer, the **internal granular layer,** is composed of stellate and pyramidal cells. The fifth layer, the **ganglionic layer,** contains large pyramidal cells. And the last and sixth layer, the **multiform layer,** consists of various neurons many of whose axons leave the cortex.

The stellate cells play the role of interneurons within the cerebral cortex; that is, their axons do not leave the cortex. The axons of pyramidal cells leave the cortex and form its most conspicuous output. Some of the dendrites of pyramidal cells are oriented toward the surface of the cortex and may reach the molecular level. Other dendrites are oriented horizontally in layers 2, 3, and 4, and may be a few millimeters long.

Input signals (afferents) to cortical neurons come mainly from **thalamic nuclei** and also from other corti-

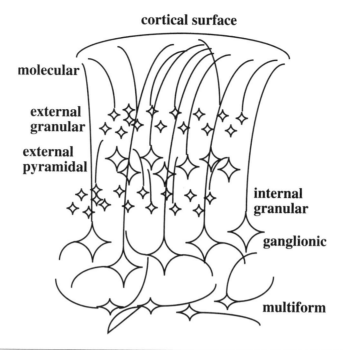

Figure 14.2 Cerebral cortex demonstrates a characteristic multilayer structure seen in a vertical section.

cal neurons. Thalamic nuclei play the role of a relay, transmitting information from peripheral afferents, the cerebellum, and the basal ganglia. Thalamic inputs make synaptic connections mostly in layer 4, which contains many stellate cells with vertically oriented dendrites that make synapses on pyramidal cells. So, output (pyramidal) cells receive sensory information that has been processed in both the thalamus and the cortex. The vertical (column) input-output organization is typical for the cortical structures. It is combined with intercolumn connections with the help of horizontally oriented dendrites.

Frontal cortical areas are particularly involved in processes associated with voluntary movements. It seems most natural to use the classical mapping of the cortex suggested by Brodmann in the beginning of this century (figure 14.3). It is certainly unrealistic to consider all 52 areas suggested by Brodmann, so we will focus on those on the frontal part of the cortex. Brodmann's areas 4 and 6 contain the main motor areas of the frontal cortex. They border area 8, the frontal eye field (on the anterior border), and area 3, the primary sensory cortex (on the posterior border).

14.3. PRIMARY MOTOR AND PREMOTOR AREAS

Area 4 or the precentral cortex is known as the primary motor area. It contains giant output cells (**Betz cells**), particularly in zones with projections to the leg muscles. The axons of these cells run in the corticospinal tract. They actually account for only a fraction of axons in the cerebrospinal tract (about 3%). The famous neurosur-

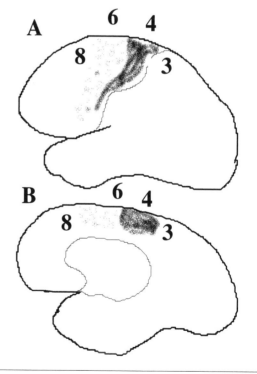

Figure 14.3 Brodmann divided the cerebral cortex into more than 50 areas. Areas 4 and 6 are of particular importance for control of movements. A: Lateral view; B: medial view.

geon Penfield used electrical stimulation of the cortex in patients during brain surgery. He was the first to discover that the primary motor cortex is organized **somatotopically;** that is, it contains a **motor map** of the body. Electrical stimulation of certain areas of the primary motor cortex induces local muscle contractions in certain specific parts of the body. If peripheral body parts are drawn on corresponding cortical areas, it looks as if a distorted human figure were drawn on the surface of the primary motor area, resembling some of the drawings by Pablo Picasso (figure 14.4). Damage of the primary motor area can induce paralysis, complete or partial (paresis), that is frequently associated with the so-called **upper motor neuron syndrome,** including uncontrolled spasms and an increased resting level of muscle contraction **(spasticity).**

Motor effects can also be induced by electrical stimulation of Brodmann's area 6, which lies anterior to area 4. These sections are called the **premotor areas.** The premotor areas contain two major zones termed the **premotor cortex** (on the lateral surface of the hemisphere) and the **supplementary motor area** (on the superior and medial areas of the hemisphere). Stimulation in these areas requires higher magnitudes of current to induce movements. Such stimulation induces more complex movements that frequently involve a number of joints. The supplementary motor area also contains a full map of the body. Damage to the premotor cortex impairs the ability to use external cues (e.g., visual) to control

movements, while damage to the supplementary motor area impairs the ability to construct movements based on internal motor memory. It was also reported to affect the ability of animals to use bimanual coordination to achieve certain motor goals. However, more recent studies by a Swiss scientist, M. Wiesendanger, challenged this conclusion by demonstrating that relative timing of arm movements in bimanual tasks does not suffer in animals with a damaged supplementary motor area.

Problem 14.2

How can you interpret the fact that stimulation of the premotor areas requires higher currents than stimulation of the primary motor cortex in order to induce visible muscle contractions?

14.4. INPUTS TO MOTOR CORTEX

Inputs from the spinal cord, basal ganglia (namely, globus pallidus), and cerebellum project onto the **ventrobasal nuclei** of the thalamus. These in turn make pro-

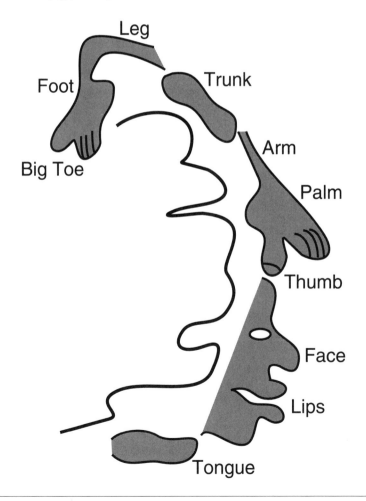

Figure 14.4 A "homunculus" representing the effects of electrical stimulation of the primary motor area.

jections onto the primary motor area, supplementary motor area, and premotor area (figure 14.5). Figure 14.5 oversimplifies the actual picture of thalamocortical projection, which is characterized by considerable overlaps.

Another major source of inputs to motor cortex is other cortical areas. A large proportion of cortico-cortical inputs come from parietal areas (figure 14.5), which receive input signals related to perception of relative position and movement of body segments (**kinesthesia**). Parietal areas also participate in the understanding of speech and in the verbal expression of thoughts and emotions. In particular, primary motor cortex receives inputs from area 2 of the postcentral gyrus and from lateral area 5. Area 5 (and also area 7b) projects to the supplementary motor area. The motor cortex also receives inputs from frontal areas including the cingulate cortex and prefrontal areas. These areas are involved in responses related to emotions, reasoning, planning, memory, and verbal communication. Note that conclusions about the involvement of certain brain areas in specific types of behavior are questionable and are based on circumstantial evidence such as disruption of a function in cases of a localized brain pathology or injury.

Problem 14.3

Suggest an alternative explanation for the finding of an impairment of a function following localized brain damage.

14.5. OUTPUTS OF MOTOR CORTEX

Output projections of motor cortex were extensively studied by two American scientists, Evarts and Asanuma, with the aid of electrical stimulation. In animals, direct stimulation through microelectrodes has been widely employed. In humans, a method of transcranial magnetic stimulation has recently been used that involves placing a wire coil on top of the head. Changing the electrical current in the coil leads to a changing magnetic field that can be relatively accurately focused on various brain structures. The changing magnetic field, in turn, leads to local electrical currents, bringing about activation of brain neurons in the same manner as with direct electrical stimulation. The method of magnetic stimulation is certainly superior to other methods because it is noninvasive and is not accompanied by any painful sensations. However, it cannot assure the precisely localized stimulation that can be achieved with the use of microelectrodes.

The output of the cortical motor areas (figure 14.6) includes projections to basal ganglia, the cerebellum (mediated by pontine nuclei), the red nucleus, the reticular formation, and the spinal cord (the corticospinal tract). The **corticospinal tract** contains about one million axons, approximately half of which come from the primary motor cortex while others originate mostly from the supplementary motor area. There are direct projections of cortical neurons to α-motoneurons (particularly for motoneurons controlling finger movements),

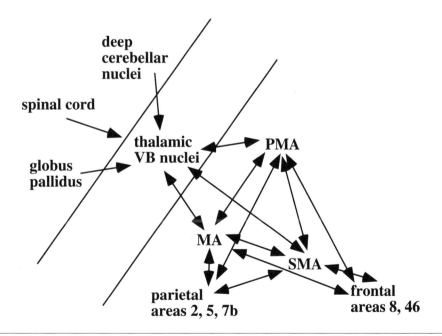

Figure 14.5 Inputs to motor cortex from the spinal cord, basal ganglia, and cerebellum are mediated by ventrobasal nuclei of the thalamus. Major projections from other cortical areas include those from the parietal cortex and certain frontal areas. MA: Primary motor area; SMA: supplementary motor area; PMA: premotor area.

γ-motoneurons, and interneurons. Note that there are two corticospinal tracts, coming from the left and the right hemisphere. Approximately at the level of the medulla, these tracts switch sides (this place is called **decussation**) so that the tract from the right hemisphere travels on the left side of the spinal cord and innervates movements of the left limbs, while the tract from the left hemisphere travels on the right side of the spinal cord and innervates movements of the right limbs.

The axons of pyramidal neurons form a part of the corticospinal tract called the **pyramidal tract.** The activity of pyramidal tract neurons has been examined during relatively simple movements, for example, flexion or extension in a joint, mostly in experiments on monkeys. If a monkey is trained to make a simple movement in response to a sensory stimulus, the first changes in the muscle activity (EMG) occur at a delay (latency) of about 150 ms. Changes in the activity of pyramidal neurons can be seen up to 100 ms prior to the EMG changes. These changes are more tightly coupled with the EMG than with the sensory stimulus, suggesting that they actually induce the movement. The magnitude of changes in the firing rate of pyramidal neurons is more closely related to the magnitude of force produced by the animal than to the position of the joint during the response.

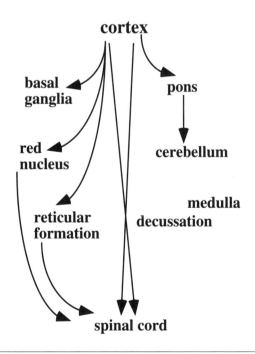

Figure 14.6 Outputs of the motor cortex include projections to basal ganglia, to the cerebellum (via the pons), to the red nucleus, to reticular formation, and to the spinal cord. Corticospinal tracts from the left and right hemispheres change sites at the level of the medulla (decussation).

> ### Problem 14.4
> Does the last finding prove that pyramidal neurons control muscle force? Why?

The behavior of small and large pyramidal cells is somewhat similar to that of small and large α-motoneurons in the spinal cord. Small cells are more likely to maintain a constant firing level when a joint maintains a posture against a constant load. They are also more involved in small movements or small adjustments of muscle force and therefore are likely to be particularly important for precise movements. Large pyramidal cells are recruited during substantial changes in muscle force.

> ### Problem 14.5
> What principle does the behavior of small and large pyramidal cells seem to follow?

More careful, later studies by Humphrey and his colleagues have shown that there are two subpopulations of cortical neurons. One subpopulation shows reciprocal changes in activity during movements in the opposite directions (e.g., flexion and extension). The other subpopulation changes its activity with a change in co-contraction of agonist and antagonist muscles that modifies apparent joint stiffness without causing a major change in the net joint torque and/or joint movement. There is, however, considerable overlap among these groups, just as among virtually all other groups of neurons identified in brain structures. Remember that earlier we considered a hypothesis of movement control that was based on two variables—one related to joint equilibrium position and the other to joint apparent stiffness. The presence of two subpopulations of cortical cells provides indirect support for this view.

14.6. PREPARATION FOR A VOLUNTARY MOVEMENT

Voluntary movements are associated with a certain EEG pattern that can be recorded at different locations on the scalp (figure 14.7). Changes in the resting EEG pattern can be seen as early as 1.5 s prior to the first signs of changes in the background muscle activity. These changes represent a slow shift of the EEG that is called *Bereitschaftpotential* or **readiness potential.** Readiness potential is typically negative, although there are reports of positive readiness potentials in certain special conditions or certain special subject populations. Readiness potential is followed by a relatively small **motor potential.** Note that during unilateral movements, readiness potential is seen over both hemispheres while the motor potential is seen only above the hemisphere contralateral to the movement.

The relatively long duration of the readiness potential looks surprising. Apparently we are able to make a decision to move and to start a movement in a much shorter time than 1.5 s. Actually, the shortest reaction time to a visual or auditory stimulus is just over 100 ms.

Problem 14.6

Suggest an explanation for the difference between the typically short reaction times and rather long readiness potential.

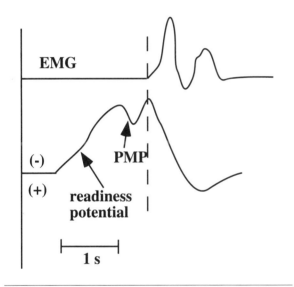

Figure 14.7 A slowly rising negative potential can be seen beginning up to 1.5 s prior to a voluntary movement (negativity in EEG records is typically shown upward). It ends up with a small positive potential (premotor positivity, PMP).

14.7. NEURONAL POPULATION VECTORS

An exciting series of studies was performed recently by A. Georgopoulos and his colleagues in investigations of the behavior of large populations of neurons in the primary motor cortex (and later, in other areas). In these experiments, monkeys were trained to perform hand movements to visual targets that might appear in different parts of the screen; that is, they performed movements in different directions. A large number of neurons were recorded with chronically implanted electrodes. The changes in the firing level of each neuron demonstrated a peak during movements in a certain, preferred direction (figure 14.8). Movements in directions close to the preferred one were accompanied by slightly lower increases in the resting activity. Move-

ment in the opposite direction could lead to a suppression of the resting activity.

Each neuron was associated with a unitary vector in the direction for which it demonstrated the largest increase in its resting activity. Then the animal performed movements in different directions, and all the neurons were recorded for each movement direction. If a neuron demonstrated an action potential in a time interval just prior to the movement, its unitary vector was drawn. If the neuron demonstrated two or three action potentials, two or three vectors were summed up, and so forth. Then all the vectors were summed up across all the neurons. The results of this procedure are shown in figure 14.9. Note that the **population vector** points in a direction that is very close to the direction of the movement. A change in movement direction in response to a change in the position of the visual stimulus is accompanied by a rotation of the population vector from the first to the second target. It looks like magic!

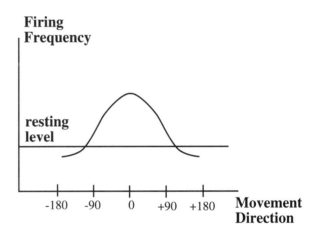

Figure 14.8 A cortical neuron demonstrates a cosine-like dependence of its firing frequency on the direction of voluntary movement. For this particular neuron, the preferred direction is 0°.

Actually, the procedure itself is largely responsible for the result, which can be obtained for any array of units (neurons or non-neurons) that possess two features, that is, (1) if their activity is related to movement direction by a cosine function and (2) if they cover the whole range of movement directions. In particular, if we record EMGs of all the limb muscles during the same task, the results will be very similar. The same thing may happen if we record and process in a similar fashion the activity of muscle spindle endings or Golgi tendon organs.

Problem 14.7

Why? Can you prove it?

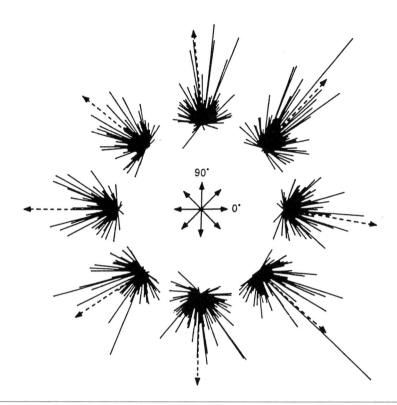

Figure 14.9 For each movement direction, activity vectors for all the neurons were summed up. The resulting vector points in the direction of the movement.

Reprinted, by permission, from A.P. Georgopoulos, R. Caminiti, J.F. Kalaska, J.T. Massey, 1982, "Spatial coding of movement direction by motor cortical populations," *Journal of Neuroscience*, 2: 1527-1537.

These results, by themselves, do not prove that the population of neurons in the cortex controls movement direction. This is an example of a very important distinction between correlation and causation.

Later this same experiment was performed with the modification that the monkeys were required to move not in the direction of the target but in another direction shifted by a constant angle value from the target. This procedure apparently requires a mental calculation (or a **mental rotation**) in order to produce movement in the required direction. In this task, the monkeys demonstrated a considerably larger delay between the stimulus and the initiation of a response; apparently this was related to the task complexity. Recording the activity of a population of cortical neurons revealed that the population vector rotated from the direction of the stimulus to the movement direction during the prolonged preparatory period. These very elegant experiments strongly suggest that cortical neurons participate in processes encoding direction of voluntary movement.

Chapter 14 in a Nutshell

The cerebral cortex consists of two hemispheres connected by the corpus callosum and anterior commissure. The two hemispheres are different in their apparent functions; the hemisphere that controls speech is called dominant. The cerebral cortex is commonly associated with such functions as perceiving and interpreting sensory information, making conscious decisions, and controlling voluntary movements. The cortex has a characteristic layer structure; it is divided into areas associated with certain functions. The principle of somatotopy can be seen in a number of cortical areas, both motor and sensory. Electrical stimulation of the motor area induces movements in muscles of the body at a short latency and low strength of stimulation. The premotor cortex and supplementary motor area also play an important role in the generation of movements. These areas receive main inputs from thalamic nuclei and also from other cortical areas. The corticospinal tract contains fast-conducting axons some of which terminate directly on spinal motoneurons while others terminate on spinal interneurons. Groups of cortical neurons can demonstrate firing patterns related to the direction of an intended voluntary movement. Disorders of the motor cortex can lead to spasticity and paralysis.

CHAPTER 15

THE CEREBELLUM

Key Terms

anatomy of the cerebellum

neuronal structure of the cerebellum

cerebellar nuclei

Purkinje cells

cerebellar inputs and outputs

cerebellar disorders

The **cerebellum** contains more neurons than the rest of the brain. It is also probably the favorite structure for different kinds of modeling because of its unusually regular cellular structure, which looks as if it had been wired purposefully by a Superior Designer. However, the present knowledge about the role of the cerebellum in various functions of the body is meager and fragmented. There have been quite a few theories about the role of the cerebellum in voluntary movements. It has been assumed to be a timing device assuring correct order and timing of activation of individual muscles, or a learning device participating in acquisition and memorization of new motor skills, or a coordination device putting together components of a complex multi-joint or multi-limb movement, or a comparator comparing the errors emerging during a movement with a "motor plan," or all these devices taken together. However, most of these theories are reformulations of experimental findings based on observations of movement impairments in patients with cerebellar disorders or in animals with an experimental "switching off" of a portion of the cerebellum.

Problem 15.1

Why can you not conclude that an area of the brain controls a certain function if the function is disrupted when the brain area is removed or turned off?

Let us consider, step by step, the anatomy and physiology of the cerebellum, keeping in mind the aforementioned hypotheses on its function.

15.1. ANATOMY OF THE CEREBELLUM

The cerebellum consists of a gray outer mantle (the **cerebellar cortex**), internal white matter, and three pairs of nuclei. The human cerebellum has **two hemispheres** and a midline ridge that is called the **vermis** (figure 15.1). Three pairs of nuclei are located symmetrically to the midline. These are the **fastigial,** the **interposed** (consisting of the **globose** and **emboliform** nuclei), and the **dentate** nuclei. Three pairs of large fiber tracts, called cerebellar **peduncles** (inferior, middle, and superior peduncle on each side), contain input and output fibers connecting the cerebellum with the brainstem. The cerebellum receives many more input fibers (afferents) than it has output fibers (efferents); the ratio is about 40:1.

Two deep **transverse fissures** divide the cerebellum into three **lobes** (figure 15.2). The primary fissure on the upper surface divides the cerebellum into **anterior** and **posterior** lobes, while the posterolateral fissure on the underside of the cerebellum separates the posterior lobe from the **flocculonodular** lobe. Smaller fissures subdivide the lobes into lobules, so that a sagittal section of

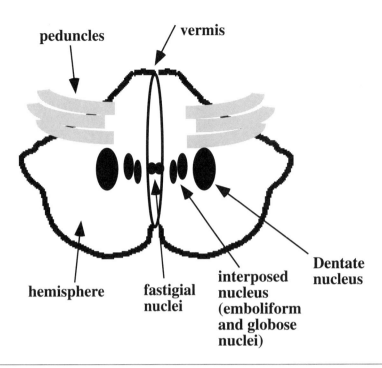

Figure 15.1   The cerebellum consists of two hemispheres and a medial area called the vermis. The cerebellum is connected to other neural structures by three pairs of peduncles. The figure shows a dorsal view of the cerebellum so that the peduncles and cerebellar nuclei are obscured (shown by black areas).

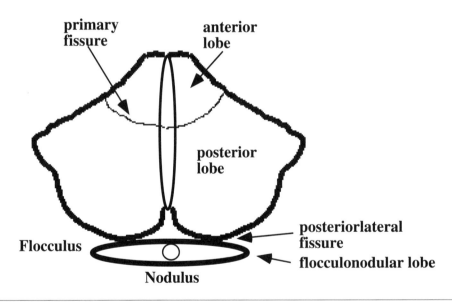

Figure 15.2   The cerebellum is divided into three lobes: the anterior lobe, the posterior lobe, and the flocculonodular lobe.

the cerebellum looks like a tree with branches on the white matter stem.

The **cerebellar cortex** is a relatively simple-looking structure consisting of three layers and five types of neurons (figure 15.3). From the surface down, there are the **molecular layer,** the **Purkinje cell layer,** and the **granular layer.** The outermost molecular layer is mostly composed of the axons of **granule cells** called **parallel fibers.** This layer also contains **basket cells** and **stellate**

cells that function as interneurons within the cerebellum. They receive inputs from parallel fibers and inhibit **Purkinje cells.** The intermediate, Purkinje cell layer contains the largest neurons in the brain, called Purkinje cells. These cells are inhibitory (their mediator is GABA) and are the only output elements of the cerebellum. The dendrites of the Purkinje cells are oriented outward, toward the molecular layer, forming large dendritic trees oriented in one plane perpendicular to the long axis of the folium.

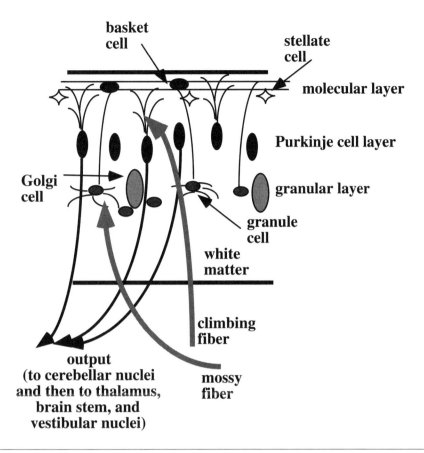

Figure 15.3 Cerebellar cortex consists of three layers and five types of neurons. Inputs to the cerebellum are carried by mossy fibers (from inferior olives) and climbing fibers (from pontine nuclei, vestibular system, and the spinal cord). The only output system of the cerebellum is the axons of Purkinje cells.

The Purkinje cells send their axons downward, through the white matter, to cerebellar or vestibular nuclei. The innermost, granular layer contains mostly densely packed small, granule cells and a few larger, **Golgi cells** at its outer border. The Golgi cells receive inputs from parallel fibers and inhibit granule cells.

Figure 15.3 is very schematic and does not do justice to the beauty of the cerebellar neurons. Figure 15.4 shows more realistic pictures of individual cerebellar cells. Note, in particular, the amazing dendritic tree of the typical Purkinje cell.

The granular layer contains structures called **glomeruli** (figure 15.5), where cells from the granular layer make synaptic contacts with the bulbous expansions of afferent, mossy fibers. A single glomerulus consists of an incoming mossy fiber, clusters of small dendrites (called rosettes) from a few dozen granule cells, and the axons of Golgi cells. A single mossy fiber may innervate many glomeruli.

15.2. CEREBELLAR INPUTS

Two excitatory afferent systems act as inputs to the cerebellum. These are **mossy fibers** and **climbing fibers**

(figure 15.6). The mossy fibers originate from a variety of brainstem nuclei and from neurons in the spinal cord whose axons form the **spinocerebellar tract.** The spinocerebellar tract conveys somatosensory information. Its projections are organized somatotopically; that is, they may be represented as another distorted human figure drawn on the cerebellar surface (this time it looks more like the creation of a primitivist artist). Actually, there are two somatotopical maps of the entire body in two areas of the spinocerebellum, one in the anterior lobe and the other in the posterior lobe (figure 15.7). Note the opposite orientation of the projections in figure 15.7. This figure is again an oversimplification; actual somatotopic maps can be quite fragmented.

Mossy fibers make excitatory synapses on the granule cells. The axons of the granule cells ascend into the molecular layer, where each axon splits into two and joins the system of parallel fibers. Each granule cell receives inputs from many mossy fibers (this is an example of **convergence** of neural information), while each mossy fiber innervates a few hundred granule cells (this is an example of **divergence**). Each Purkinje cell receives inputs from numerous parallel fibers (up to 200,000).

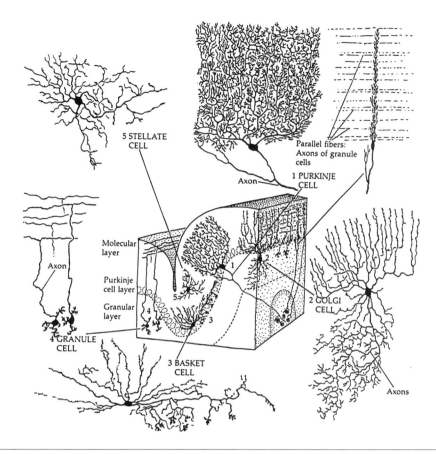

Figure 15.4   A more realistic drawing of individual cerebellar neurons.

Reprinted, by permission, from S.W. Kuffler, J.G. Nicholls, and A.R. Martin, 1984, *From neuron to brain,* 2nd ed. (Sunderland, MA: Sinauer Associates, Inc.), 11.

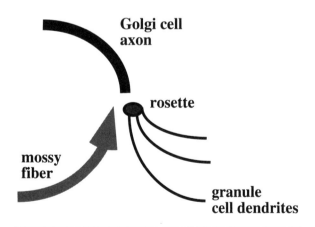

Figure 15.5   A single glomerulus consists of an incoming mossy fiber, clusters of small dendrites (called rosettes) from a few dozen granule cells, and the axons of the Golgi cells.

The climbing fibers originate in the medulla, in the **inferior olivary nucleus.** Their axons enter the cerebellar cortex and wrap around the soma and proximal portions of the dendrites of Purkinje cells. Their synapses are excitatory and very strong. Each Purkinje cell receives synaptic inputs from only one climbing fiber, which forms more than a hundred synapses on the soma and the dendrites of the Purkinje cell it innervates. One climbing fiber may innervate a few Purkinje cells. A single action potential in a climbing fiber always induces a complex action potential in the Purkinje cells it innervates; that is, its action is obligatory.

Problem 15.2

Can you present another example of obligatory action of a presynaptic neural fiber?

15.3. CEREBELLAR OUTPUTS

Purkinje cells provide the only output of the cerebellum. In response to a single excitatory input, a Purkinje cell may produce either a single action potential (a simple spike) or a sequence of events consisting of a large action potential followed by a few smaller action potentials (figure 15.8) (a complex spike). Complex spikes are commonly induced by excitatory inputs from the climbing fibers, while simple spikes may be induced by spa-

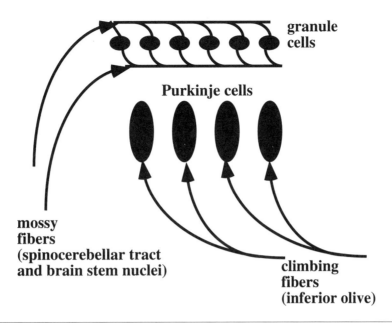

Figure 15.6 Excitatory inputs to the cerebellum are provided by mossy fibers and climbing fibers. Mossy fibers originate from the spinocerebellar tract and from brain stem nuclei; they excite granule cells. Climbing fibers originate from the medulla (inferior olive); they make synapses on Purkinje cells.

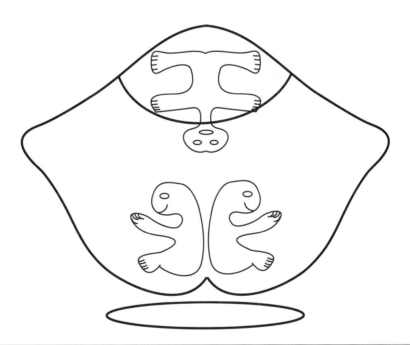

Figure 15.7 Somatotopical projections on the cerebellar surface (another homunculus!).

tial and temporal summation of the postsynaptic potentials generated by inputs from the mossy fibers.

Problem 15.3

Is the existence of simple and complex spikes a violation of the all-or-none principle? How can this be?

Purkinje cells are characterized by a very high frequency of discharge (up to 80 Hz), even when the animal is at rest. Thus, the cerebellum always provides a tonic inhibitory input to other structures. During active movements, Purkinje cells may demonstrate discharge at a rate of a few hundred hertz, while their strongest inputs (the climbing fibers) are firing at frequencies under 1 Hz.

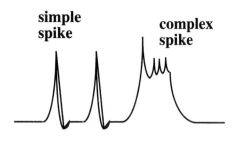

Figure 15.8   In response to a single excitatory stimulus, a Purkinje cell may generate either a single action potential (a simple spike; in response to a mossy fiber input) or a larger action potential followed by a few smaller ones (a complex spike; in response to a signal from climbing fibers).

The activity of Purkinje cells is modulated by three types of inhibitory interneurons: the stellate, the basket, and the Golgi cells. The stellate cells make inhibitory synapses within the molecular layer, on the dendrites of nearby Purkinje cells. The basket cell axons run perpendicular to the parallel fibers, and make inhibitory contacts on the bodies and proximal dendrites of relatively distant Purkinje cells. As a result, if a beam of parallel fibers is activated, it activates a group of Purkinje cells and a group of basket cells. The basket cells inhibit the activity of Purkinje cells just outside the beam of the parallel fibers, thus sharpening the difference between the levels of activity of the Purkinje cells (figure 15.9).

The Golgi cells are excited by the parallel fibers and make inhibitory connections with the dendrites of granular cells, within the glomeruli, decreasing their response to an excitatory input from the mossy fibers.

Problem 15.4

Can you interpret the function of the stellate, basket, and Golgi cells in terms of negative or positive feedback?

The axons of the Purkinje cells make inhibitory synapses on neurons within the **cerebellar** and **vestibular nuclei.** The output fibers of these nuclei transmit signals from the cerebellum to other structures within the brain and the spinal cord.

All three pairs of cerebellar nuclei make projections to the thalamus and, from there, to the cerebral cortex. They also make connections in various midbrain and brainstem nuclei, as well as in the spinal cord. Most of the cerebellar output is provided by the **interpositus** and **dentate nuclei.** Their axons run in one tract that crosses the midline at the level of the midbrain and divides into an ascending and a descending branch. The descending axons innervate the reticular formation in the pons and the medulla, while the ascending axons innervate the red nucleus as well as a ventrolateral part of the thalamus

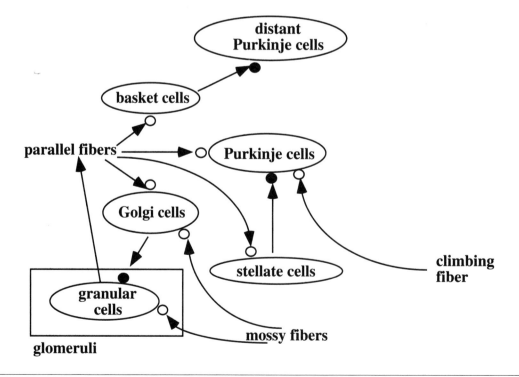

Figure 15.9   Stellate cells make inhibitory synapses on the dendrites of Purkinje cells. Parallel fibers activate Purkinje, basket, stellate, and Golgi cells. Basket cells inhibit relatively distant Purkinje cells. Golgi cells inhibit granular cells, decreasing their response to mossy fibers.

that receives inputs virtually only from the cerebellar nuclei. This area is sometimes called the "cerebellar thalamus." It mediates cerebellar projections to the cerebral cortex. Most of the cerebellar projections are in areas 4 and 6 of the cerebral cortex, that is, in the areas related to control of voluntary movements. A portion of the red nucleus neurons make projections to the inferior olive, which makes projections to the cerebellum (the climbing fibers). So a complete loop is formed: olives—cerebellum—cerebellar nuclei—red nucleus—olives—cerebellum. . . .

Problem 15.5

Can you infer from what you know whether the olives—cerebellum—cerebellar nuclei—red nucleus—olives loop is positive feedback or negative feedback?

15.4. RELATION OF CEREBELLAR ACTIVITY TO VOLUNTARY MOVEMENT

Cerebellar neurons do not make direct connections with spinal neurons; thus, their activity is less likely to be related to certain specific patterns of muscle activity. Experiments on monkeys have demonstrated a considerable scatter in the timing of changes in the background activity of neurons in the cerebellar nuclei with respect to movement initiation. During single-joint (wrist) movements, on average, neurons of the dentate nuclei change their activity simultaneously with motor cortex cells, prior to changes in the activity of the interpositus or the fastigial nuclei. However, during whole-arm reaches, changes in the background activity are seen in the fastigial neurons. Tentative conclusions from these observations are that firing of the dentate neurons is related to the initiation of a voluntary movement whereas interpositus neurons fire mostly with respect to the actual movement course, while fastigial activity may be related to the presence or absence of a postural component within a motor task. Other observations supporting these conclusions involve (a) the relation of interpositus neuron activity to EMG timing during locomotion in cats and (b) the responsiveness of dentate neuron activity to perturbations that lead to arrest and resumption of locomotion. Furthermore, cooling the dentate nuclei (which leads to a reversible switching off) brings about an increase in the reaction-time delay (a movement in response to a visual stimulus) accompanied by an increase in the delay of motor cortical neuron firing.

A number of researchers have tried to investigate the relation between the discharge rate of cerebellar neurons and movement parameters such as muscle force, joint velocity, movement amplitude, movement direction, and so on. These studies provided unclear and sometimes controversial data. In several studies, interpositus neurons demonstrated a relation to muscle force or EMG but not to movement velocity or direction, while dentate neurons did not demonstrate a correlation with any of the movement parameters mentioned. Other studies have shown that Purkinje cells in monkeys are activated in a reciprocal fashion during flexion or extension forces but that their activity is suppressed when both flexors and extensors are activated simultaneously. A tentative conclusion from this series is that Purkinje cell activity is related to suppression of the activity of antagonist muscles.

15.5. NEURONAL POPULATION VECTORS

The method of Georgopoulos for studying the behavior of populations of neurons in the motor cortex was applied to cerebellar neurons as well. Remember that the method is based on finding a "preferred direction" for each neuron (a direction of movement corresponding to its highest discharge frequency) and calculating a sum of the vectors for all the neurons active during the initiation of a movement in a certain direction. As already mentioned, single cerebellar neurons do not show a clear correlation between their discharge rate and movement direction. However, application of the method to a large population of neurons has shown a good correspondence between the population vector and movement direction (figure 15.10). This figure looks much more noisy and "hairy" than similar figures for motor cortical neurons, but the sum of all the vectors points more or less in the direction of the movement. This result was obtained for populations of Purkinje cells, dentate neurons, and interpositus neurons. Taking into account our previous discussion of the advantages and limitations of this method, we may conclude that these results prove only that cerebellar neuron activity has a weak relation to movement direction while other factors (not controlled in the experiments) are probably more important.

15.6. THE EFFECTS OF CEREBELLAR LESIONS

Cerebellar lesions produce rather different effects in different animals. In cats and dogs, such lesions are reported to produce an increase in muscle tone (whatever this is!). The increased tone is particularly strong in limb and neck extensor muscles, leading to a typical picture of **extensor rigidity.** These effects may be seen after

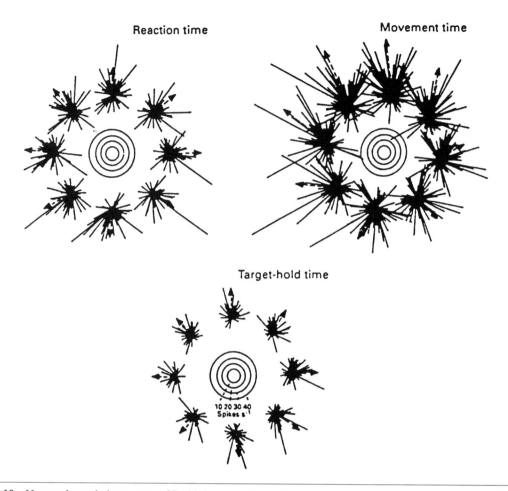

Figure 15.10   Neuronal population vectors of Purkinje cells, interpositus, and dentate nuclei point close to the direction of the movement, although with a larger scatter than population vectors of cerebral cortical neurons.

Reprinted, by permission, from P.A. Fortier, J.F. Kalaska, and A.M. Smith, 1990, "Cerebellar neuronal activity related to whole-arm reaching movements in the monkey," *Journal of Neurophysiology,* 62: 198-211.

ablation of only the anterior cerebellar lobes. The rigidity is not decreased by cutting the dorsal roots, which means that it does not depend on stretch reflexes (or any other reflexes from proprioceptors). Thus, it is assumed to be primarily attributable to an increase in the excitability of α-motoneurons and is termed **alpha rigidity.** The mechanism of extensor rigidity is assumed to be based on an increase in the activity of the vestibulospinal tract that originates in **Deiters' nucleus** (a vestibular nucleus), which normally receives inhibitory inputs from the anterior cerebellar lobes. Cerebellar lesions in these animals also have effects on the activity of the fusimotor system; these effects are inhibitory and lead to a depression of the stretch reflexes. The effects of cerebellar lesions are followed by the relatively quick recovery of a normal extensor tone and stretch sensitivity, which takes a few days.

In primates, there is a smaller cerebellar input to Deiters' nucleus. Possibly this is the reason for the lack of direct effects of cerebellar lesions on the excitability of α-motoneurons. So most of the effects of cerebellar

lesions on movements are assumed to be mediated by an action on the fusimotor system. Such lesions lead to a depression of muscle tone **(hypotonia)** that recovers very slowly or may not recover at all. There are also deficits in the rate and force of voluntary muscle contractions as well as a low-frequency tremor that is sometimes termed **cerebellar tremor** (about 3-5 Hz). The deficits are particularly pronounced during movements that involve a postural component. One tentative (and rather nonspecific) conclusion from these observations is that the cerebellum is responsible for providing balance between activation of the α- and the γ-motoneuronal systems.

In animal experiments, reversible local cooling is frequently used to study the effects of local lesions on movements. Local cooling of the dentate and interpositus nuclei in monkeys leads to motor deficits resembling those seen in patients with cerebellar disorders. During single-joint movements, typical changes include

1. an increase in reaction time;

2. an increase in movement distance (target overshoot, **hypermetria**) accompanied by a prolonged agonist EMG burst and a delayed antagonist EMG burst;

3. an interruption of the rhythm of an oscillatory movement due to an increase in time spent at the turning points;

4. segmentation of slow movements, which become jerky and demonstrate a 3-5 Hz tremor;

5. perturbation-induced alternating EMG patterns in the flexor-extensor muscles leading to joint oscillation (figure 15.11); and

6. during the tracking of a visual target, a jerkiness of movement and an apparent loss of the ability to use velocity-related information.

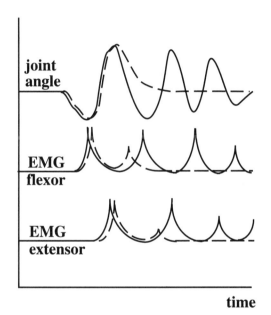

Figure 15.11 After a cerebellar lesion, a perturbation of a joint may lead to an alternating EMG pattern in the joint flexors and extensors, and a joint oscillation. Dashed lines: before the lesion; solid lines: after the lesion.

Note, however, that all the deficits mentioned are relatively mild and typically allow the animal to accomplish the task, albeit in a clumsy manner.

The deficits become much more pronounced when multi-joint movements are performed. Cooling the fastigial nuclei brings about the inability to sit, stand, or walk, leading to frequent falls. Cooling the interpositus nuclei leads to a severe 3-5 Hz tremor, particularly pronounced during targeted movements (**action tremor**). Cooling the dentate nuclei leads to a major overshooting of targets and loss of the ability to use the precision grip for food retrieval.

So one may conclude that the cerebellum may be much more involved in coordination of many muscles than in control of simple, single-joint systems.

In humans, cerebellar disorders are accompanied by ataxia of voluntary movements, that is, a decomposition of movement into a number of jerky segments. This is typically accompanied by prolonged reaction time and the other symptoms described for monkeys in experiments with local cooling. A number of terms are used for description of motor abnormalities in cerebellar disorders:

1. **Kinetic tremor** represents oscillations seen during voluntary movement.

2. **Intentional tremor** represents large oscillations seen when the arm approaches a target.

3. **Postural tremor** is seen when a limb maintains a constant position.

4. **Dysmetria** refers to the inability to achieve a required final position; it may include overshoots (hypermetria) and undershoots (hypometria).

5. **Dysdiadochokinesia** is an inability to perform movements at a certain constant rhythm.

6. **Hypotonia** is a decrease in resistance to passive joint motion.

Problem 15.6

Can you suggest a definition for hypotonia at the level of mechanisms?

---

7. **Asynergia** is an impairment in interjoint coordination. This may include disorders of gait and stance (particularly when the medial zone of the cerebellum is damaged).

Cerebellar disorders are also seen at the level of facial muscles, leading to slurring of speech and nystagmus (repetitive jumps of the eyes).

The tendon tap leads, in cerebellar patients, to a pendular reflex, that is, to slowly decaying oscillations in the joint following a single tap. Tonic vibration reflex is suppressed.

Problem 15.7

Suggest an explanation for the suppressed tonic vibration reflex in cerebellar disorders.

Patients with cerebellar disorders show **impaired learning** of some motor tasks. Similar impairment can be seen in monkeys in experiments with cooling of cerebellar structures. More specifically, when a healthy human or an animal wears prisms that distort visual perception, the vestibulo-ocular reflex (which maintains the axis of the eyeball in a constant position during head movements) adapts quickly. This adaptation is absent in cases of cerebellar disorders.

There is a never ending debate about whether the cerebellum is the site of **learning.** The regular and relatively simple cellular structure of the cerebellum is very attractive for modelers. Many of these models are built on an assumption that learning is based on changing synaptic weights (efficacy of individual synapses). This assumption is far from obvious and actually is likely to be wrong!

Some of these models are based on a principle similar to the **holographic principle** in physics. That is, if two signals coming from different sources to one synapse coincide in time, the synapse "remembers" the event and changes its state permanently. For example, climbing fibers can modify the effectiveness of the synapses that parallel fibers make on Purkinje cells (figure 15.12).

Problem 15.8

Can you give a reason why basing memory on synaptic weight is unrealistic?

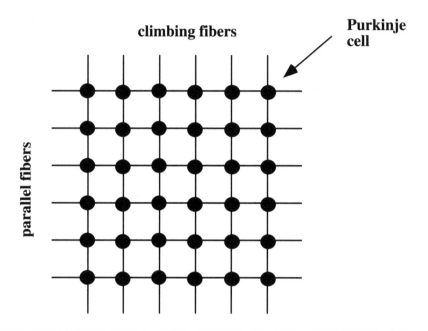

Figure 15.12   If an action potential in a climbing fiber and another action potential in a parallel fiber arrive simultaneously to a Purkinje cell, the cell may "remember" this event with the help of a chemical mechanism changing the synaptic efficacy or with the help of a postsynaptic mechanism.

Chapter 15 in a Nutshell

The cerebellum contains more neurons than the rest of the brain. It has a unique regular cellular structure. The human cerebellum has two hemispheres and a vermis. Three pairs of cerebellar nuclei are located symmetrically to the midline: the fastigial, the interposed, and the dentate nuclei. Three pairs of large fiber tracts, called cerebellar peduncles, contain input and output fibers connecting the cerebellum with the brainstem. Inputs into the cerebellum come through mossy and climbing fibers from a number of brain nuclei and from the spinal cord; the inputs represent a mixture of ascending and descending signals. Cerebellar output is always inhibitory; it is generated by Purkinje cells that project on vestibular and cerebellar nuclei. Lesions of the cerebellum lead to gross motor disorders that can include rigidity, tremor, hypotonia, dysmetria, and asynergia. Motor learning is particularly affected in cases of cerebellar lesions. The cerebellum has been implicated in such diverse functions as memory and coordination of multi-joint and multi-limb movements.

CHAPTER 16

THE BASAL GANGLIA

Key Terms

anatomy of the basal
    ganglia

inputs and outputs

direct and indirect loops

basal ganglia in control of
    movements

dysfunctions of the basal
    ganglia

Parkinson's disease

Huntington's chorea

The basal ganglia consist of five large subcortical nuclei that do not receive direct inputs from, and do not send direct outputs to, the spinal cord. The importance of the basal ganglia for control of voluntary movements had been assumed mostly on the basis of clinical observations. Basal ganglia disorders may bring about quite different clinical pictures ranging from excessive involuntary movements to movement poverty and slowness, although without paralysis. Because of these clinical observations, in the past it was supposed that the basal ganglia were major components of the so-called **extrapyramidal system,** which was thought to participate in control of movements in parallel to and largely independently of the **pyramidal** (corticospinal) system. This classification is not satisfactory, however, because the pyramidal and extrapyramidal systems are not independent; rather they cooperate in movement control. Furthermore, other brain structures, such as the thalamus and red nucleus, also participate in control of movement, and their lesions induce motor disorders. The function of the basal ganglia is not limited to controlling movements; these structures have a role in cognitive and emotional functions. So I will consider the basal ganglia as a part of a complex system that is important for a number of functions served by the brain.

16.1. ANATOMY OF THE BASAL GANGLIA

Three of the nuclei of the basal ganglia lie deep in the cerebrum, laterally to the thalamus (figure 16.1). The phylogenetically oldest nucleus is the **globus pallidus,** which is also called the **paleostriatum.** The globus pallidus consists of two parts, internal (GP_i) and external (GP_e). These parts have different connections with other brain structures. Two nuclei, the **caudate nucleus** and the **putamen,** form the **neostriatum** (or simply **striatum**). They are separated from each other by the **internal capsule.** The other two nuclei of the basal ganglia, the **subthalamic nucleus** and the **substantia nigra,** are located in the midbrain. The substantia nigra is the largest nucleus of the human midbrain. It is divided anatomically into two parts; its dorsal region is called **pars compacta,** and its ventral region is called **pars reticulata.** The pars reticulata and GP_i are the major output structures of the basal ganglia.

The striatum is organized into modules called **striosomes** and **matrix** (these appear to be analogous to the column organization of cortical neurons). Striosomes are islands of relatively densely packed cells that are parts of a larger, less densely packed compartment called the matrix.

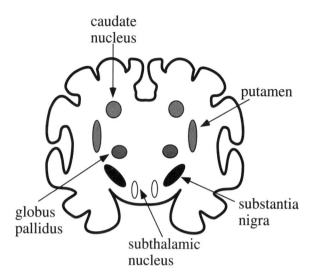

Figure 16.1 The basal ganglia consist of five paired structures that include globus pallidus, putamen, caudate nucleus, subthalamic nucleus, and substantia nigra.

16.2. INPUTS AND OUTPUTS OF THE BASAL GANGLIA

The basal ganglia receive their major input from areas of the cerebral cortex (figure 16.2). Inputs from different cortical areas are kept quite separate while they flow through the loops involving the basal ganglia (this is sometimes called the **topographic principle**). For example, within the motor circuit, inputs from the arm, face, and leg areas are kept separate throughout the basal ganglia. Most of the output of the basal ganglia returns back to the cortex through the thalamus (figure 16.3).

Cortical neurons make projections on the striatal neurons; these projections are **glutamatergic.** Striatal neurons, in turn, project onto both segments of the globus pallidus and onto the pars reticulata of the substantia nigra, using **GABA** as the mediator. Projections to the internal pallidum and to the substantia nigra form the so-called **direct pathway** through the basal ganglia. Neurons in these structures make projections directly onto the ventrolateral thalamus and from there back to the cortex. Striatal projections to the external pallidum form the **indirect pathway** (figure 16.4). There are very few projections from the external pallidum to the thalamus. Most of the external pallidum output is directed toward the subthalamic nucleus, which then projects to the pallidum and to the substantia nigra (using glutamate as the mediator), which in turn project via the thalamus to the cortex. So the indirect pathway goes through the subthalamic nucleus, which is bypassed by the direct pathway.

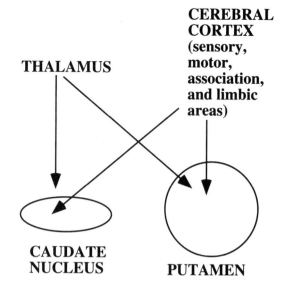

Figure 16.2 The caudate nucleus and putamen (structures of the striatum) are sites of almost all afferent inputs to the basal ganglia. Much of the input comes from different areas of the cerebral cortex; other input comes from nuclei of the thalamus.

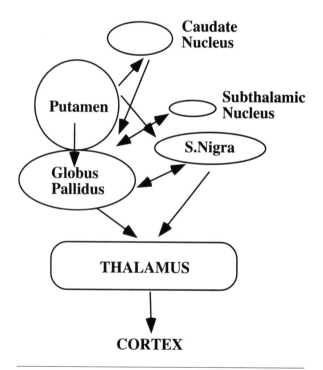

Figure 16.3 All the nuclei of the basal ganglia are interconnected. The major output (efferent) pathway originates from the globus pallidus (internal segment) and the substantia nigra (pars reticulata). These nuclei project on thalamic nuclei, and then back to cortex.

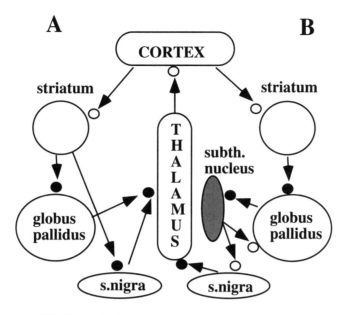

Figure 16.4 The direct (A) and indirect (B) loops involving the basal ganglia. The direct pathway goes from cortical neurons to the striatum, then to both segments of the globus pallidus and to the pars reticulata (substantia nigra), then to the thalamus, and back to the cortex. The indirect pathway goes from the cortex to the striatum, then to the external pallidum, then to the subthalamic nucleus (which then projects to the pallidum and to the substantia nigra), and then, through the thalamus, back to the cortex. Inhibitory connections are shown by filled circles; excitatory connections are shown by open circles.

There is also a smaller projection of the external pallidum and the substantia nigra to the midbrain. In particular, projections to the superior colliculi play an important role in oculomotor control.

Note that GABA-ergic projections are inhibitory while glutamatergic projections are excitatory. Thus, the direct pathway involves two excitatory and two inhibitory connections (figure 16.4), resulting in an excitation of cortical neurons (positive feedback). The indirect pathway involves three excitatory and three inhibitory projections with a net inhibitory effect on cortical neurons (negative feedback). It is not clear, however, whether the same cortical cells are targets of both the direct and the indirect loops.

Problem 16.1

Imagine that the indirect loop targets cortical cells laterally to those targeted by the direct loop. Suggest a functional importance of such an organization.

The reader should pay particular attention to the role of another mediator, **dopamine,** in the basal ganglia, since Parkinson's disease is associated with a dysfunction of dopaminergic loops. Within the basal ganglia, the caudate nucleus and the putamen receive dopaminergic inputs,

mostly from the pars compacta of the substantia nigra. The location of the dopaminergic synapses on the target neurons makes them probable candidates as regulators of the effectiveness of cortical inputs to the same cells. It is actually not clear whether the dopaminergic synapses are excitatory or inhibitory; there is a possibility that they may be excitatory for the cells of the direct pathway and inhibitory for the cells of the indirect pathway.

Problem 16.2

How can one and the same mediator be excitatory for some neurons and inhibitory for others?

16.3. MOTOR CIRCUITS INVOLVING THE BASAL GANGLIA

Figure 16.5 illustrates major paths originating from different areas in the cortex, passing through the basal ganglia and the thalamus and terminating back in the cortex. Inputs to the basal ganglia may originate in different cortical areas such as the motor cortex, the premotor area, the supplementary motor area, the somatosensory cortex, and the superior parietal cortex (which lies dorsally to the somatosensory areas). The projections from the

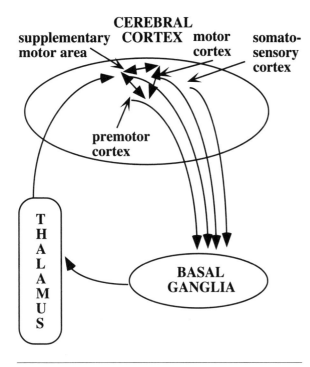

Figure 16.5 Major pathways originating from different cortical areas and involving the basal ganglia. Both direct and indirect loops contribute to the motor circuit of the basal ganglia. Most of the thalamic projections to the cortex are directed to the premotor cortex and supplementary motor area. These areas have connections with each other (mostly inhibitory) and with the motor cortex, and all of them project directly to brainstem motor centers and to the spinal cord.

somatosensory cortical areas to the putamen are organized somatotopically; that is, one more primitive drawing of a human figure may be found on the surface of the putamen. This somatotopy is preserved in the projections from the putamen to both internal and external segments of the globus pallidus. Both direct and indirect loops participate in the motor circuit of the basal ganglia; they are both mediated by thalamic neurons. Most of the thalamic projections to the cortex are directed at the premotor cortex and supplementary motor area. These areas have connections with each other (mostly inhibitory) and with the motor cortex, and all of them project directly to brainstem motor centers and to the spinal cord.

Most somatosensory and motor areas of the cortex project exclusively to the matrix, while many striosomes receive inputs from **limbic structures.** Remember that limbic structures include the hypothalamus, the fornix, the hippocampus, the amygdaloid nucleus, and the cingulate gyrus of the cerebral cortex and are believed to be involved in such elements of behavior as attention and emotion (chapter 13). Striosomes that receive projections from limbic structures, in turn, project on dopaminergic cells in the midbrain. Midbrain neurons project back upon the matrix and striosomes. The latter projections may

modulate the effectiveness of cortical inputs to the same neurons. Thus, this circle provides means for the brain to change the effectiveness of transmission in the basal ganglia motor loop on the basis of attentional and emotional factors.

16.4. ACTIVITY OF THE BASAL GANGLIA DURING MOVEMENTS

Animal studies have shown that, at rest, there is substantial activity of neurons in the globus pallidus and in the pars reticulata of the substantia nigra (at frequencies of about 50-100 Hz), while neurons in other structures of the basal ganglia are rather quiet. Neurons in GP_i fire at a relatively constant high rate, while neurons in GP_e demonstrate high-frequency, burstlike activity.

Problem 16.3

Suggest a functional reason for the neurons in the globus pallidus to have a high rate of activity at rest.

Many neurons in the basal ganglia show phasic modulation of their firing frequency during voluntary movements of the contralateral side of the body. Some of these neurons show a correlation of their firing frequency with such movement parameters as velocity, force, and amplitude. Discharge patterns of other neurons, however, are both movement and context dependent.

An important feature of changes in the firing patterns of cells in the basal ganglia is that they occur rather late. Thus, in reaction-time tasks, the majority of the cells show changes in their firing after the movement initiation. Note that many neurons of the motor cortex change their firing prior to movement initiation. So it is possible to conclude that neurons of the basal ganglia do not initiate movements under these experimental conditions and are related more to control of movements that are already under way.

Another important characteristic of the basal ganglia neurons is that their firing correlates more closely with movement direction than with forces that are necessary to perform a movement.

Problem 16.4

What result would you expect to get if you performed a study of the neuronal population vectors within the basal ganglia that was similar to the studies in cortical and cerebellar neuronal populations?

There are several hypotheses about the function of basal ganglia in motor control:

1. The basal ganglia disinhibit areas of the motor system (for example, cortical motor areas) and thus *allow movement to occur.*
2. The basal ganglia turn off the ever present postural activity, thus allowing a voluntary movement to occur.
3. The basal ganglia are involved in *sequencing movement fragments* or various movements.
4. The basal ganglia *do a number of things* in parallel that are related to movement.

Problem 16.5

Which of these hypotheses seem more (or less) likely than the others? Why?

16.5. EFFECTS OF LESIONS OF THE BASAL GANGLIA

Animal Studies. Since the basal ganglia are located deep in the brain tissue, it is very hard to produce lesions in them without affecting the surrounding structures and/or neural pathways. So many of the observations in animals should be taken with a grain of salt. Local lesions of the globus pallidus (commonly performed with a **local cooling** technique or with neurotoxic agents) lead to movement disorders rather similar to those observed in patients with **Parkinson's disease.** In particular, the animals become slow in reaction time and especially movement time, the amplitude of movements decreases, the movement trajectories become more variable, and a co-contraction of antagonist muscles is typically seen during attempts at simple movements. Stimulation of the globus pallidus during the course of a movement (i.e., when its neurons normally change their firing) leads to changes in movement duration and in the accompanying EMG patterns. This implies, in particular, that even delayed firing of neurons of the basal ganglia is able to produce changes in a movement that is already under way.

Relatively recently, a neurotoxic drug has been discovered that brings about symptoms very similar to those of Parkinson's disease in humans. This drug (MPTP) has allowed researchers to induce experimental "Parkinson's disease" in monkeys and study the effects of various experimental therapies. In particular, MPTP leads to an increase in the resting firing level of neurons in the internal globus pallidus and a decrease in the resting firing rate of neurons in the external globus pallidus. Moreover, neurons of the globus pallidus increase their response to peripheral inputs while losing their selectivity to different inputs.

Basal Ganglia Diseases in Humans. The best-known consequence of basal ganglia dysfunctions is Parkinson's disease, which will be discussed in detail later. I will now mention only the four basic symptoms of Parkinson's disease, which resemble the effects of lesions of the basal ganglia and particularly the effects of MPTP in animals. The four basic symptoms are

1. **bradykinesia** (slowness of movements including prolonged reaction time),
2. **tremor** (involuntary, oscillatory movements at a frequency of about 4-6 Hz),
3. **rigidity** (an increased resistance to external joint movement), and
4. **postural deficits.**

In combination, these symptoms contribute to the overall pattern of movements of patients with Parkinson's disease, which includes a shuffling gait, stooped posture, trembling of the hands, and slow and frequently ineffective voluntary movements.

The basal ganglia contain about 80% of total dopamine in the brain, while their weight is only about 0.5% of the total weight of the brain. So the basal ganglia are the site of the most vigorous dopaminergic activity. Parkinson's disease is associated with a dramatic reduction in the dopaminergic activity and is commonly treated with a drug (**L-dopa**) that is an immediate precursor of dopamine and can cross the blood-brain barrier.

Problem 16.6

What can you tell about L-dopa based on the fact that it can easily cross the blood-brain barrier?

Let us speculate about what consequences one can expect from a deficit of dopamine given what we know about the connections within the basal ganglia and between the basal ganglia and other brain structures. The pars compacta of the substantia nigra has a dopaminergic innervation of the striatum (figure 16.6). Therefore a deficit in dopamine can lead to a decrease in dopaminergic excitation of the internal pallidum (smaller activity in the direct pathway) and an increase in inhibition of the external pallidum. Via the indirect pathway, the decrease in the activity of the external pallidum leads to a disinhibition (an increased activity) in the subthalamic nucleus and consequently to an additional excitation of the internal pallidum. As a result, the ultimate thalamic output to the cortex is reduced. This may account for the slowness and poverty of movements in Parkinson's disease.

Chorea and Ballism. Chorea and ballism are examples of the **hyperkinesias,** that is, disorders characterized by excessive movements. Chorea is a major symptom of **Huntington's disease;** it involves involuntary, irregular, and purposeless movements. Such movements are

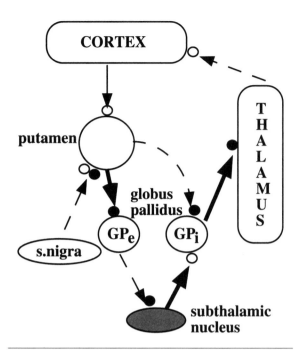

Figure 16.6 The lack of dopamine can lead to a decrease in the input from the thalamus to the cortex due to changes in the action of both direct and indirect pathways. Broken lines show weaker connections; bold lines show strengthened connections.

relatively slow and relatively small in amplitude as compared to those of ballism. Other symptoms of this disease involve slurred speech, which slowly becomes incomprehensible and eventually stops altogether, and distorted facial expressions. Cognitive function and the ability to reason deteriorate as well. Pathological analysis at early stages of Huntington's disease shows a se-

lective loss of GABA/enkephalin projections from the striatum to the external pallidum. This may be expected to lead to a disinhibition of the external pallidum and an increased inhibition of the subthalamic nucleus (the indirect pathway). A smaller output of the subthalamic nucleus leads to a smaller inhibitory output of the internal pallidum, leading to a disinhibition of the thalamic output to the cortical cells. This may be a reason for chorea.

Ballism (hemiballism, if the disorder is limited to one side of the body) is a consequence of a lesion of the subthalamic nucleus and is characterized by uncontrollable, rapid movements of the contralateral limbs (most commonly, the contralateral arm). Movements in cases of ballism and chorea may look rather similar.

Problem 16.7

How can you explain ballism assuming that it is produced by a dysfunction of the subthalamic nucleus?

Torsion Dystonia. Torsion dystonia is a pathological state characterized by twisted, sustained postures of the neck, trunk, or limbs. Most frequently it affects the neck and is called torticollis. Other frequent cases of torsion dystonia involve the so-called writer's cramp (or musician's cramp, or typist's cramp), in which the symptoms are limited to one limb and particularly affect precision movements. In most cases of torsion dystonia, no brain abnormalities can be found. However, in some cases these symptoms have been related to lesions of the basal ganglia.

Chapter 16 in a Nutshell

The basal ganglia consist of five pairs of subcortical nuclei that include the globus pallidus, the caudate nucleus, the putamen, the subthalamic nucleus, and the substantia nigra. Two feedback loops, direct and indirect, connecting the motor cortex with the thalamus, pass through the basal ganglia. The role of the basal ganglia in voluntary movements is unclear. They may be involved in the processes of movement initiation and sequencing of movement fragments. Dysfunction of the basal ganglia can lead to major motor disorders including hypokinesias and hyperkinesias. Parkinson's disease has been associated with a decrease in dopamine production by the substantia nigra. Huntington's chorea and ballism have been associated with selective loss of GABA/enkephalin projections from the striatum to the external pallidum. Basal ganglia have also been implicated in cases of dystonia.

CHAPTER 17

ASCENDING AND DESCENDING PATHWAYS

Key terms

basic properties of neural pathways

topographic organization

sensory pathways

inputs into the spinal cord

dorsal column pathway

spinothalamic tract

spinocerebellar tracts

spinoreticular tract

motor pathways

pyramidal tract

rubrospinal tract

vestibulospinal tracts

reticulospinal tract

propriospinal tracts

17.1. BASIC PROPERTIES OF NEURAL PATHWAYS

In this chapter we will consider how sensory information is transmitted from its peripheral sources to the spinal cord and brain structures, as well as how command signals get back to the periphery, to muscles, for example. Typical speed of information transmission within the central nervous system is of the order of a few tens of meters per second, which means that transmission delays are not negligible and may create a bottleneck for some types of behavior, particularly those involving very fast movements. This speed, however, is much higher in mammals with their myelinated nerves than in reptiles, for example. So one of the greatest scientists of our century, Nicholai Bernstein, suggested, as a joke, that the dinosaurs disappeared because they were eaten alive by the early mammals that were fast enough to bite a chunk of meat and run away during the time it took the unfortunate dinosaur to feel the bite and react to it.

Problem 17.1

How long will it take for a dinosaur whose body (from the foot of a hindlimb to the brain) is 20 m long to react to a bite if the speed of action potential conduction is 5 m/s?

It is important to remember that individual pathways do not correspond to individual functions (figure 17.1). Each functional system, sensory or motor, uses information carried by a number of anatomically distinct pathways whose contribution can vary depending on the type of activity in which the system is involved. This feature of functional systems is closely related to the fact that each system contains synaptic relays that do not simply transmit incoming information, but also process it. Relay nuclei may receive several inputs, so that information coming along individual pathways is processed and integrated. The best-known relay is the thalamus, which receives both sensory and motor information, processes it, and sends it to the brain cortex.

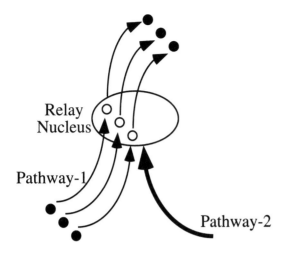

Figure 17.1 Typical features of pathways within the central nervous system involve the presence of synaptic relays, integration of information from different pathways, and topographic organization.

Sensory pathways display a feature called topographic organization that is preserved throughout the central nervous system. This feature means that neighboring receptor cells project to neighboring cells in relay nuclei, which in turn project to neighboring cells in other nuclei, ending up by projecting to neighboring cells in the corresponding sensory area of the cortex (figure 17.1). Similarly, descending (motor) pathways that originate from neighboring cells of a motor cortical area (or another brain structure) project onto motoneurons that induce contractions of muscles controlling movements of neighboring body segments. As a result, there are many **motor maps** and **sensory maps** within the central nervous system. Violations of topographic organization can be seen in central connections among brain structures.

17.2. AFFERENT INPUT TO THE SPINAL CORD

Let us start from the peripheral side. Sensory (afferent) fibers enter the spinal cord through the dorsal roots (figure 17.2). Some of them branch at the entrance into an ascending and a descending branch that make synapses in nearby segments of the spinal cord. Thick fibers typically make synapses deeper in the gray matter. For example, primary muscle afferents may terminate anywhere starting from Rexed's lamina V to lamina IX. The smallest unmyelinated fibers, including those involved in nociception (type C), terminate in the superficial Rexed's laminae I and II. Other fibers terminate in intermediate layers as shown in figure 17.2.

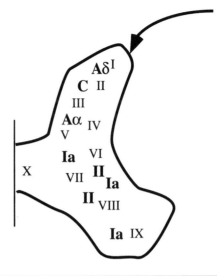

Figure 17.2 Afferent fibers enter the spinal cord through the dorsal columns. Small, unmyelinated fibers (Aδ, C) typically terminate in Rexed laminae I and II. Larger sensory fibers terminate in laminae III-IV, while muscle afferents (Ia, II) terminate anywhere from lamina V to lamina IX.

Problem 17.2

On the basis of figure 17.2, suggest which fibers can make monosynaptic connections on α-motoneurons.

17.3. DORSAL COLUMN PATHWAY

The dorsal columns of the spinal cord carry information from sensory neurons in the spinal ganglia to the brain (figure 17.3). These neurons have a T-shaped axon whose central branch joins the **dorsal column pathway.** In particular, the dorsal column pathway contains the axons of the primary muscle afferents. Note that these fibers originate from the original sensory cell and are therefore called **first-order afferent fibers.**

The dorsal column pathway also contains the axons of **second-order sensory neurons,** that is, neurons of the spinal cord that receive sensory information, process it, and deliver already processed information to the brain. Another group of neurons, whose axons travel in the dorsal column pathway, are those that transmit information between segments of the spinal cord. They are called **propriospinal** neurons. Some of these neurons are actually first-order sensory cells whose axons branch and send one of the branches to other spinal segments.

The ascending fibers of the dorsal column pathway terminate in the **cuneate** and **gracilis** nuclei in the medulla. Afferents from the legs travel in the gracile fasciculus and terminate in the gracilis nucleus, while afferents from the arms travel in the cuneate fasciculus and

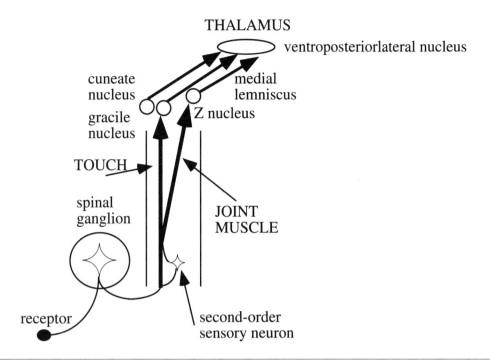

Figure 17.3 The dorsal columns of the spinal cord carry information from sensory neurons in the spinal ganglia to the brain. The ascending fibers of the dorsal column pathway terminate in the cuneate and gracile nuclei in the medulla (sense of touch). From the medulla, these signals travel to the ventroposterior-lateral nucleus of the thalamus via the medial lemniscus. On its way, the medial lemniscus crosses the midline of the body. Articular and group I muscle receptors travel in the dorsolateral funiculus and make a relay in nucleus Z before joining the medial lemniscus.

terminate in the cuneate nucleus. From the medulla, these signals travel to the **ventroposterior-lateral nucleus** of the thalamus via the **medial lemniscus.** On its way, the medial lemniscus crosses the midline of the body, so that signals from the left part of the body are received by the right ventroposterior-lateral nucleus.

Problem 17.3

What kind of sensory deficit can be expected from a combined trauma of the right gracilis nucleus and right ventroposterior-lateral nucleus?

17.4. SPINOCERVICAL PATHWAY

The spinocervical tract carries the axons of second-order sensory neurons that convey nociceptive information as well as information related to touch. This tract terminates in the cervical nucleus, which consists of columns of neurons in the first and second cervical segments. The axons of these neurons form the cervicothalamic tract, which also ascends to the ventroposterior-lateral nucleus via the medial lemniscus. The spinocervical tract is prominent in cats but is rather small in monkeys and humans. However, the next tract to be consid-

ered is very prominent in humans and is much smaller in cats.

17.5. SPINOTHALAMIC TRACT

The spinothalamic tract consists of the axons of neurons whose bodies lie in the dorsal and intermediate parts of the gray matter. The axons cross the midline at the segmental level and travel along the contralateral side of the spinal cord in the ventrolateral funiculus (figure 17.4). This tract conveys the sensations of touch, pressure, temperature, and pain. Its axons go through the medulla and the pons directly to the ventroposterior-lateral nucleus of the thalamus. Its fibers send branches to the reticular formation on their way.

The three tracts mentioned convey sensory information to the thalamus, which is the sensory center of the brain. There the information is additionally processed and sent to the brain cortex.

17.6. SPINOCEREBELLAR TRACTS

The cerebellum receives information from peripheral sensory receptors by means of several tracts. These include the dorsal, ventral, and rostral spinocerebellar tracts,

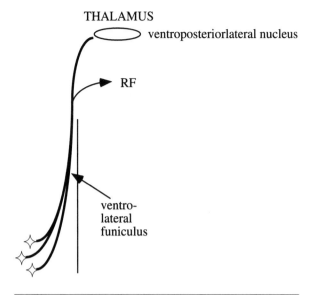

Figure 17.4 The spinothalamic tract consists of the axons of neurons whose bodies lie in the dorsal and intermediate parts of the gray matter. The axons cross the midline and travel along the contralateral side of the spinal cord in the ventrolateral funiculus. This tract conveys the sensations of touch, pressure, temperature, and pain. Its axons go directly to the ventroposterior-lateral nucleus of the thalamus sending branches to the reticular formation (RF).

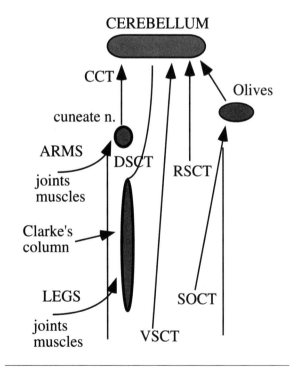

Figure 17.5 The cerebellum receives information from peripheral sensory receptors by means of the dorsal (DSCT), ventral (VSCT), and rostral (RSCT) spinocerebellar tracts, the cuneocerebellar tract (CCT), and the spino-olivary-cerebellar tract (SOCT).

the cuneocerebellar tract, and the spino-olivary-cerebellar tract (figure 17.5).

Fast-conducting afferents from muscle and joint receptors (groups Ia and Ib) make monosynaptic connections on spinal neurons within the nucleus dorsalis or Clarke's column. This column, in humans, lies on the dorsal surface of the spinal cord and extends from the T1 to L2 spinal segments. The fast-conducting, myelinated axons of the neurons of Clarke's column form a major portion of the dorsal spinocerebellar tract. This tract also receives contributions from cutaneous touch and pressure receptors and from the secondary muscle spindle afferents. However, there is virtually no convergence of information from muscle receptors and cutaneous receptors. The neurons within Clarke's column have rather small receptive fields; in other words, they convey information that is location specific (and may be modality specific as well). Note that Clarke's column starts only at the T1 level, which means that the dorsal spinocerebellar tract conveys information only from the hindlimbs, not from the forelimbs. The axons of neurons in Clarke's column travel in the ipsilateral lateral column of the spinal cord. The analogue of the dorsal spinocerebellar tract, with basically the same properties but from the forelimb, is known as the cuneocerebellar tract. Peripheral afferent fibers project on the cuneate nucleus, whose neurons send their axons to the cerebellum.

The ventral and rostral spinocerebellar tracts contain smaller axons of spinal neurons that mostly receive afferent input from the flexor reflex afferents and a small contribution from the primary muscle afferents. The information is much more mixed in these tracts as a result of a widespread convergence. The ventral tract conveys information from the hindlimbs (legs), while the rostral tract conveys information from the forelimbs (arms). Note that the axons of the ventral spinocerebellar tract cross the midline and ascend in the contralateral lateral fasciculus, while the axons of the rostral tract do not cross the midline.

Inferior olives receive information from spinal afferents either directly (via the spino-olivary tract) or indirectly (using a relay in the dorsal column nuclei). The axons of the neurons of inferior olives project on the contralateral cerebellar nuclei and also enter the cerebellar cortex, as climbing fibers.

17.7. SPINORETICULAR TRACT

The spinoreticular tract runs parallel to the spinothalamic tract up until the brainstem, where the axons of the spinoreticular tract make synapses on the dendrites of neurons of the reticular formation, particularly in the medulla and in the pons. The lateral reticular nucleus receives a somatotopically organized projection, mostly from the flexor reflex afferents, and sends its axons to the cerebellar nuclei and the cerebellar cortex (as mossy fibers).

The spinovestibular and spinotectal projections are believed to be relatively small, and their function is not well understood.

Thus, most ascending pathways to the brain structures end up in the thalamus or the cerebellum, which then distribute peripheral information, already in a processed form, to other brain structures. Eventually a decision is made to generate a command to the periphery on the basis of sensory information and of internal brain processes that are sometimes loosely described as "will" or "intention." Now we will turn to pathways that deliver commands to the executive organs, that is, to muscles.

17.8. PYRAMIDAL TRACT

The **pyramidal tract** is probably the neurophysiologists' favorite descending tract; it has received much more attention than all the other descending tracts taken together. Its name originates from the **medullary pyramids** in which the fibers of this tract run. The human pyramidal tract consists of about one million fibers. Most of them are myelinated (more than 90%) and conduct at different velocities. Only about 2% of these fibers conduct at velocities over 50 m/s.

Problem 17.4

What is the range of diameters of the 2% of fibers in the pyramidal tract that are the fastest conducting?

The pyramidal tract (figure 17.6) consists of two major groups of axons. The first group includes the axons of cortical neurons that go down to the spinal cord. These axons are known as the **corticospinal tract.** Some fibers leave the pyramidal tract while it is passing the pyramids, or even somewhat earlier, and innervate the motor nuclei of the cranial nerves. These fibers are called the **corticobulbar tract.**

In monkeys, about 60% of the pyramidal tract fibers come from frontal motor areas of the cortex while the other 40% originate from the primary somatosensory areas and parietal cortex. The bodies of the neurons whose axons run in the pyramidal tract are mostly located in cortical layer 5. These include, in particular, the giant, pyramidal-shaped Betz cells.

Most of the fibers of the pyramidal tract cross the midline of the body at the brainstem level (**decussation of pyramids**) and travel in the contralateral dorsolateral column of the spinal cord to all the spinal levels. A smaller number of fibers do not cross the midline and descend

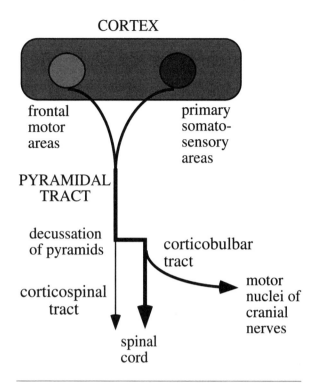

Figure 17.6 The pyramidal tract consists of two major groups of axons. Axons of the first group go down to the spinal cord (corticospinal tract). Some fibers leave the pyramidal tract and innervate the motor nuclei of the cranial nerves (corticobulbar tract).

within the ventromedial part of the spinal cord. The uncrossed fibers innervate mostly axial muscles, that is, those involved in rotation of the trunk. These two parts of the pyramidal tract are known as the **lateral corticospinal tract** and the **ventral corticospinal tract.**

Corticospinal neurons project to many different neurons in the spinal cord including α- and γ-motoneurons, Renshaw cells, Ia-interneurons, and other interneurons. In cats, there are very few monosynaptic connections of pyramidal tract axons with α-motoneurons. The number of such connections is much larger in primates, particularly for motoneuron pools controlling the muscles of the forearm and the hand. In humans, the method of transcranial stimulation was used to study the projections of the corticospinal tract to many muscles throughout the body. The findings have suggested that there are likely to be monosynaptic connections of this tract with α-motoneurons of virtually all the muscles.

Problem 17.5

How can you decide whether or not a projection of one cell to another is monosynaptic if you study corticospinal projections in humans?

17.9. RUBROSPINAL TRACT

The axons of neurons in the red nucleus that descend to the spinal cord form the **rubrospinal tract** (figure 17.7). This tract has been well studied in cats, but not in humans. It consists of axons of different diameters corresponding to a wide range of conduction velocities up to 120 m/s (higher than in the pyramidal tract). The tract crosses the midline (decussates) close to its origin and descends through the contralateral brainstem, giving branches to other brain structures including the interpositus nucleus of the cerebellum, the olives, and the vestibular nuclei. In the spinal cord, the rubrospinal tract lies somewhat lateral and ventral to the lateral corticospinal tract. Some spinal interneurons actually receive inputs from both tracts.

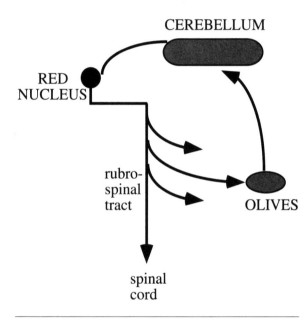

Figure 17.7   The rubrospinal tract crosses the midline (decussates) close to its origin and gives branches to brain structures including the interpositus nucleus of the cerebellum, the olives, and the vestibular nuclei. It is part of the cerebellum—red nucleus—olive—cerebellum loop.

Electrical stimulation of the red nucleus in cats induces a di- or tri-synaptic excitation of contralateral flexor motoneurons and an inhibition of extensor motoneurons. There are no monosynaptic connections to α-motoneurons in cats, but such connections are present in monkeys and probably also in humans.

The red nucleus is suspected of playing a very important role in control of voluntary movements; an American neurophysiologist, Jim Houk, suggested a hypothesis of motor control that considers the red nucleus a vital contributor to the process of formulating motor commands in terms "understandable" to the spinal cord struc-

tures. The major input to the red nucleus comes from the ipsilateral dentate nucleus, while its output goes through the olives to the cerebellar cortex. So the red nucleus is part of the loop consisting of cerebellum—red nucleus—olive—cerebellum.

17.10. VESTIBULOSPINAL TRACTS

Almost all the information about the vestibulospinal tracts also comes from cat experiments. Neurons in Deiters' nucleus (which is also called the lateral vestibular nucleus) give rise to the **lateral vestibulospinal tract** (figure 17.8). There axons run ipsilaterally in the ventrolateral columns of the spinal cord and terminate mainly in laminae VII and VIII of the spinal cord. Another, smaller tract, the **medial vestibulospinal tract,** consists of the axons of neurons mainly in the medial vestibular nucleus. Vestibular nuclei receive their major inputs from the labyrinth and the cerebellum. Vestibulospinal projections are assumed to play an important role in control of neck muscles, and monosynaptic projections have been found from the vestibular nuclei to the motoneurons controlling neck muscles.

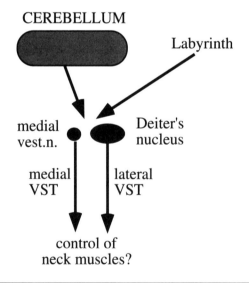

Figure 17.8   Vestibular nuclei receive main inputs from the cerebellum and labyrinth. Deiters' nucleus gives rise to the lateral vestibulospinal tract, while the medial vestibular nucleus is the origin of the medial vestibulospinal tract.

17.11. RETICULOSPINAL TRACT AND OTHER DESCENDING TRACTS

The reticulospinal tract originates from the **medium tegmental field** (an area in the bulbar reticular formation).

This area includes several nuclei such as the **giganto-cellular nucleus,** the **paragigantocellular nucleus,** and the **pontine reticular nucleus.** The major part of this tract goes down the **ipsilateral ventral funiculus** of the spinal cord. Unlike other descending tracts, this one does not have a somatotopic organization. It makes connections in laminae VII and VIII of the spinal cord. There is also a crossed reticulospinal tract that travels in the dorsolateral funiculus together with the corticospinal and rubrospinal tracts. The reticulospinal tract is suspected of bringing about the startle reaction. This reaction is observed in response to an unexpected loud auditory stimulus and consists of a short-lasting contraction of many muscles of the face, trunk, and limbs at a variable latency of the order of 150 ms.

Let me mention two other descending tracts. The **tectospinal tract** comes from neurons in the superior colliculus. It decussates in the midbrain and terminates mostly at the level of cervical segments, probably contributing to the control of neck muscles. The superior colliculus receives a major input from the cortical visual areas, so this tract may play a role in head orientation with respect to visual stimuli.

The **interstitiospinal tract** comes from neurons in the interstitial nucleus in the rostral part of the midbrain. It terminates in approximately the same areas of the spinal cord as the vestibulospinal tract.

17.12. PROPRIOSPINAL TRACTS

By definition, **propriospinal neurons** are those that have a soma in one spinal segment and an axon terminating in another spinal segment. Some of these neurons have relatively short axons and provide connections over neighboring segments, for example within the cervical and the lumbar enlargements. Other neurons have long axons that travel to remote spinal segments.

Most propriospinal neurons receive a strong peripheral input and a relatively weak supraspinal input. The most extensively studied exception is the C3/C4 propriospinal system, which consists of neurons whose body is located at the C3/C4 spinal level and whose axons travel down the spinal cord. Most of the axons make projections in the C6-T1 levels; a minority travel down to the lumbar region, where they may participate in coordinating the activity of the forelimb and hindlimb muscles. This system receives strong, monosynaptic corticospinal projections and weaker excitatory projections from other descending tracts. The neurons of the system project to motoneurons controlling different muscles of a forelimb (arm) and thus may be involved in the organization of synergies, that is, coordinated contractions of many muscles. The C3/C4 propriospinal neurons also receive local projections from inhibitory interneurons, which in turn receive inputs from both peripheral afferents and supraspinal systems.

Chapter 17 in a Nutshell

Neural pathways provide means for information exchange and integration among nuclei within the central nervous system. Neural pathways display a topographic organization that is preserved through the relay nuclei leading to many motor maps and sensory maps. Afferent (sensory) information enters the spinal cord through the dorsal roots and is delivered to brain structures via the dorsal column pathway, spinothalamic tract, spinocerebellar tract, and spinoreticular tract. The thalamus sends sensory information to other brain structures including the brain cortex. Descending pathways carry motor signals through the pyramidal and extrapyramidal systems. The pyramidal tract contains corticospinal and corticobulbar fibers. Most of its fibers cross the midline at the brainstem level. The uncrossed fibers innervate mostly muscles involved in rotation of the trunk. Other important descending tracts include the rubrospinal, the vestibulospinal, and the reticulospinal tracts. The rubrospinal tract is viewed as an important part of the system for control of voluntary movements. Vestibulospinal projections are assumed to play an important role in the control of neck muscles. Propriospinal tracts participate in information exchange among spinal segments.

CHAPTER 18

MEMORY

Key Terms

types of memory

habituation of reflexes

learning

conditioned reflexes

Pavlov's theory

neuronal/synaptic
hypothesis of memory

memory retrieval

plasticity

hippocampus

Korsakoff's syndrome

spinal memory

Mechanisms of memory are rarely in the center of attention of researchers studying voluntary movements. This is surprising, because most motor control theories have an implicit or even explicit memory component. When a person performs a reaching movement to a target without looking at the target, he or she certainly relies on memory (and current kinesthetic information) to generate appropriate commands to effectors and to correct these commands if the movement happens to be inaccurate. The important role of memory is obvious for any skilled movement and for the process of motor learning. However, in most motor control hypotheses, memory is considered an external component that comes from obscure "higher centers," is very reliable, and is absolutely beyond our present comprehension. Unfortunately, this pessimistic view is not very far from the truth. However, in this chapter we will consider a few aspects of memory as a transition from the structure-based World III to the behavior-based World IV.

Two groups of phenomena can be termed **memory.** The first (memory-1) is very broad and includes storage of a trace of an event for some time after the event has ended. According to this definition, when a person picks up a rock from the ground, an indentation in the ground represents a memory-1 of the rock. Apparently, many of the phenomena of everyday life satisfy this criterion, including those relating to both animate and inanimate objects. The second group of phenomena (memory-2)

implies the possibility of an active process of memory retrieval; that is, a trace of a past event is there, but it is not obvious and requires effort or a specific stimulus to be brought to the surface. According to this definition, a scar on a soldier's face is not by itself a memory-2 (it is a memory-1), but his recollections of the event that gave him the scar are. When researchers speak about human memory, they commonly imply this second group of phenomena associated with information selection, storage, and retrieval.

The difference between the two groups is not that sharp; in particular, it is probably not easy to separate them by the animate-versus-inanimate characteristic. For example, muscle reaction to a central command signal may depend on the history of its previous contractions, that is, on past events. Is this memory-1 or memory-2? On the other hand, what kind of memory resides in the hard drive of a personal computer? And what about the RAM?

18.1. DESCARTES' DUALISM AND CELLULAR MECHANISMS OF MEMORY

There are two extremes in dealing with the phenomena of learning and memory. The first is represented by **Descartes' dualism.** Rene Descartes considered mind

152

(and all the attributes of mind such as the ability to learn and memorize, as in memory-2) to be a uniquely human feature rather independent of the body, including all its material components. The second view is **reductionism,** which considers all the features of human behavior to be unambiguously reflected in measurable physical properties of neurons and their connections (synapses). Within the reductionist approach, learning and memory reside in changes in the biochemistry and/or morphology of synapses between neurons. This approach looks much more "scientific" in that it assumes a possibility of localizing and measuring these changes and thus pinning memory down to a substrate. In general, experimental science hates to deal with something that cannot be precisely measured. However, not everything in nature happens according to the desires of experimentalists. For example, the Heisenberg principle of indeterminicity states that it is impossible to measure precisely both the location and impulse of a particle, the errors becoming particularly prominent when one deals with small particles such as neutrinos or photons, for example. Researchers working in experimental physics have eventually accepted this fact, albeit not without quite a few years of reluctance. Now, the physicists are not driven into depression by the fact that they are unable to define the position of an electron with infinite precision. They are rather happy to have a whole new area of study that requires new, specific methods of analysis and promises new insights into the physical foundations of our world. So, if a theoretical view does not allow us to pin down a phenomenon to a substrate, this by itself does not mean that the view is wrong.

The complex system approach to human studies suggests that, until proven otherwise, a function of a complex system is an emergent property of all the elements of the system and cannot be assigned to certain changes in individual neurons and synapses. This view differs from the pure dualism of Descartes by making "mind" an emergent property of the "body" rather than an absolutely independent entity. For example, the temperature of a bowl of water is defined by the average energy of the molecules within the bowl; that is, it is their emergent property. On the other hand, it can be considered an independent, "external factor" that affects individual molecules.

Problem 18.1

When you look at a great painting, you feel emotions reflecting the ideas of the artist who died a long time ago. What happens in your brain according to the dualist, reductionist, and complex system views?

Problem 18.2

A great Canadian neurosurgeon and scientist, Wilder Penfield, stimulated areas of the brain in his patients during surgery, and the patients reported bright recollections of events from their lives. What can you conclude about the role of these areas in memory storage and retrieval?

18.2. HABITUATION OF REFLEXES

At the beginning of this century it was known that repetitive activation of simple spinal reflexes causes them to become smaller or to require larger stimuli. This effect has been termed **habituation.** Habituation may last considerable amounts of time; thus it represents storage of information within the central nervous system (CNS) and may be considered an example of memory-1. Habituation can be seen in human experiments such as those with the startle reaction (a phasic motor reaction to an unexpected loud auditory stimulus), which decreases in magnitude when the stimulus is applied again and again.

18.3. LEARNING AND MEMORY

There is a distinction between **learning** and **memory.** Learning is an ability to change with experience, while memory is an ability to maintain this change over time.

In physics, the term **hysteresis** means that a physical system can display different behaviors depending on its immediate history. There are effects of hysteresis in elements of the human motor system, in particular in muscles. For example, imagine that an isolated muscle is being stimulated at a constant rate by an external stimulator (figure 18.1). Muscle length is being changed very slowly (so that we can ignore the dependence of muscle force on velocity), and muscle force is measured. If the muscle is stretched, its force will change along curve-1, while if the muscle passes through the same values of length while being shortened, its force changes along curve-2. This means that muscle force depends not only on its length but also on its history.

Problem 18.3

Give a couple of examples of hysteresis from everyday life.

18.4. TYPES OF LEARNING

Commonly, learning phenomena are classified into associative and nonassociative.

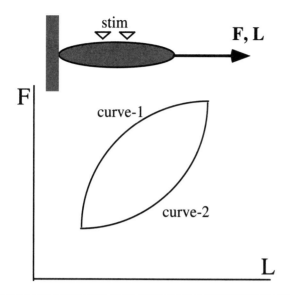

Figure 18.1 An isolated muscle is being stimulated at a constant rate and strength. Muscle force will depend on muscle length. During slow stretching and slow shortening, the muscle will display different dependences F(L). This behavior is called hysteresis.

Associative learning involves creating a relation between two stimuli. Typical examples include **classical conditioning** and **operant conditioning.** In operant conditioning, a relation between an action by the animal and an external stimulus (commonly, a food reward) is being learned; that is, the role of one of the stimuli is played by the animal's own behavior. Classical conditioning involves a special group of phenomena termed **conditioned reflexes.** These will be considered in more detail later.

Nonassociative learning occurs when the CNS learns certain properties of a stimulus, that is, adjusts its response when the properties of the stimulus are repeated. For example, habituation of reflexes is seen when parameters of the stimulus are kept constant during successive applications of the stimulus. On the other hand, if a novel stimulus occurs, it may increase the response to a continuously repeated stimulus. This phenomenon is called **sensitization.**

18.5. CONDITIONED REFLEXES

It is known that having food in one's mouth leads to salivation, which is particularly strong if the food is dry. Food stimulates the mucous membrane of the mouth; this stimulation is transferred by sensory nerves to the salivatory brain center, which reacts to the stimulation with a command to the salivary grands. This phenomenon occurs even in the smallest cubs. Such inborn mechanisms are termed **unconditioned** or **inborn re-**

flexes. A famous Russian physiologist, Ivan Pavlov, discovered that if a hungry dog each day hears a bell or a whistle, or sees a light bulb of a certain color turning on, or experiences some other such event half a minute prior to feeding, after many days of repetition of this pattern the animal gradually starts to salivate, not when it gets the food, and not even when it sees the food—but when the additional signal is turned on. It is clear that in such a case the experimenter witnesses the birth of a new version of the salivation reflex elaborated with artificial means. This is not an inborn, general reflex, as the inborn salivation reflex is, but a reflex reflecting an enrichment of the personal experience of the dog. These reflexes are termed **conditioned** in contrast to the inborn, unconditioned reflexes.

Pavlov suggested a theory of brain functioning based on an interaction among unconditioned and conditioned reflexes. This theory considered the brain as a purely reactive organ whose behavior is defined by environmental stimuli, while human (or animal) behavior was seen as the process of "equilibrating" the body with the environment. Unfortunately for this theory, and fortunately for human beings (as well as many other animals), higher animals are not purely reactive systems but instead are actively exploring the environment, formulating their needs, and trying to satisfy these needs rather than waiting for appropriate stimuli for conditioned reflexes from the environment. Activity is the driving force of the functioning of the human brain.

This was understood only in the 1960s by the great Russian scientist, Nicholai Bernstein, who formulated the goals of behavior as overcoming the environment rather than equilibrating the body with it. Bernstein created the **physiology of initiative** (which has been inaccurately referred to in Western publications as **physiology of activity**), a whole new field of study that tries to explain behavior based on the internal needs and goals of an animal (or a human), which are commonly in conflict with stimuli from the environment.

Bernstein created the physiology of initiative largely based on his earlier studies of the process of automation of labor and athletic movements. He found out that in the process of movement automation, the variability of movement trajectories and other characteristics was not eliminated. Movements did not become identical or machinelike, although the ultimate motor outcome became highly reproducible. For example, during such movements as shaving with a sharp razor blade or shooting at a target, success of the ultimate precise outcome depends on fractions of millimeters or angular seconds. Only the high variability of the behavior of individual elements of automated movements allows people to reach such high accuracy during repetitions in conditions of ever present unexpected forces. Therefore, memory traces of such movements cannot represent "movement formulas" such as combinations of patterns of muscle forces, muscle activation levels, or joint trajectories. As will be discussed in chapter 21, researchers in the area of motor control have not been able to agree on the physical or physiological nature of control variables used by the CNS during natural voluntary movements. However, it is safe to say that skill formation is an active process of the CNS, a process whose implications for the neurophysiology of memory have not been adequately explored.

Problem 18.4

Pavlov built "towers of silence" in which his dogs were deprived of any stimuli except those used for conditioned reflexes. Predict the behavior of the dogs on the basis of the theory of conditioned reflexes and the physiology of initiative.

Another typical procedure used for studies of memory in animals is **operant conditioning.** It includes rewarding an animal (with a small portion of a favorite food) for correct behavioral responses. The response may be under apparent control by the animal, for example in choosing the correct turn while running in a maze, or it may not, for example during spinal reflex responses. However, even the simplest, monosynaptic spinal reflexes can "learn" and store memory traces in operant conditioning experiments, as was shown in ingenious studies by J. Wolpaw and his group. Thousands of repetitions may be required, but the animal's CNS eventually learns to "control" an apparently uncontrollable event such as the amplitude of a monosynaptic response.

18.6. SHORT-TERM AND LONG-TERM MEMORIES

Two overlapping categories of memory have been identified in humans. The first is termed **short-term memory.** Its effectiveness usually lasts a few minutes or hours. Special memory **consolidation** processes are invoked to explain the process of conversion of short-term memories into **long-term memories,** which can last years, up to a lifetime (figure 18.2). There are many clinical cases, mainly different types of brain trauma, that lead to a memory loss or deficiency. In particular, some patients lack the ability to consolidate short-term memory. They demonstrate normal ability to maintain short-term memories but lose them when their attention is distracted. There are also cases in which a trauma leads to loss of memories related to events that happened for some time period prior to the trauma (**retrograde amnesia**) or for some time period immediately following the trauma (**anterograde amnesia**).

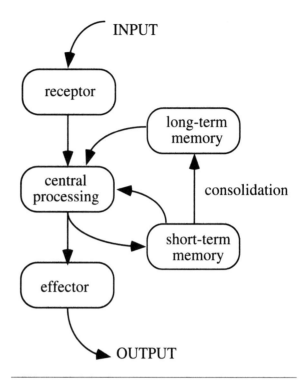

Figure 18.2   Processing of a sensory stimulus may lead to creation of a short-term memory trace in parallel with production of an effector (motor) output. Short-term memory can be consolidated into a long-term memory. Both short-term and long-term memories can participate in processing future incoming sensory stimuli and forming an effector response.

The process of consolidation depends on the context in which a memorized event occurs, as well as on the number of repetitions of presentation of the event. For example, highly emotional events have a higher chance of being consolidated into long-term memory, sometimes even after a singular presentation. More boring things, like the contents of the present book, require repetition and effort to be remembered.

18.7. NEURONAL/SYNAPTIC MECHANISMS OF MEMORY?

If one considers memory as an emergent property of many neurons pertaining to many neuronal structures, it is obvious that searching for a neuronal or synaptic location for a certain memory is doomed to failure. In particular, in classical experiments by Karl Lashley, a learned motor task in rats was preserved even after surgical removal of up to 98% of the cortical areas related to the task. Moreover, it did not matter which 2% of the areas were spared by the surgical procedure. These observations suggested that memory was a distributed phenomenon.

There was a theory, advanced in the 1930s by a great neuroscientist, Lorente de No, that short-term memory was based on so-called **reverberating circuits,** that is, chains of neurons that give rise to a certain pattern of activity sustained in time and space (figure 18.3). This theory was not confirmed, however, in experiments that failed to find repeated bursts of activity in anatomically identified closed loops.

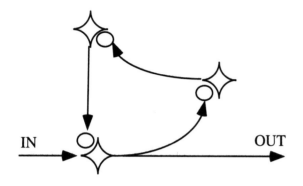

Figure 18.3 An example of a simple reverberating circuit. Note that the activity in the circuit will persist until some crucial substances are depleted. Open circles show excitatory synapses.

An alternative theory suggests that short-term memory results from modifications of neuronal ion channels and mediator receptors leading to a change in presynaptic mediator-release mechanisms and/or in postsynaptic sensitivity to the mediator. It is based on numerous observations of synaptic changes that may last a relatively short time (under 1 s). These changes may be responsible for such short-lasting events as visual afterimage, which can be perceived after a brief presentation of a bright object. Longer-lasting synaptic changes have also been described, including **long-term potentiation, long-term depression, and activity-dependent presynaptic facilitation.** These changes may be relevant to information storage over time; however, their relation to human memory is rather speculative.

Other theories of short-term memory are based on assumptions of the creation of new neuronal pathways or the synthesis of new proteins. Their experimental support, however, is meager. Protein synthesis has also been implicated in the process of consolidation of short-term memories into long-term memories.

Similar problems emerge with phenomena of motor memory. This is so, in particular, because the researchers do not know how hypothetical control variables are represented and stored in the CNS. It is commonly and rather arbitrarily assumed that motor memory resides in synapses. These assumptions have been typically based on experiments that compared certain neurophysiological changes to behavior. However, behavioral patterns may reflect many factors that are not directly related to

memory, such as the level of attention, the state of the effectors, and others.

The use of synapses for storing long-term memory looks very uneconomical. Using a synapse in remembering an event renders that synapse occupied and useless for future memories. As a result, numerous "disposable synapses" are required to memorize a single event. The amount of memory of an adult suggests that even the astronomical number of synapses within the CNS might be insufficient if such a crude and straightforward mechanism were used. Apparently, memorizing an event requires *a pattern of activity in complex neuronal formations whose organization and neuronal composition may vary.*

One of the most ubiquitous features of human voluntary movements is their **variability.** Even the most skilled movements demonstrate different kinematic profiles, different muscle force patterns, and different muscle activation patterns in successive trials. The variability of patterns of skilled movements suggests that there is a comparable variability in the afferent signals from proprioceptive receptors. Hence, one is safe in assuming that virtually all the neurons in the body will demonstrate somewhat different patterns of activity during repetitions of even the simplest motor task. This is the strongest argument that a control pattern for a skilled movement cannot be represented as a combination of activity of a number of individual neurons induced by stable changes in individual synapses.

18.8. RETRIEVAL OF MEMORY

To store a memory is not enough; one needs to have means to retrieve it. Some of the features of memory retrieval in humans make human memory quite unlike computer memory. In computers, memory is organized in a sequential fashion; that is, memories are stored under specific addresses, and one needs to know the exact address in order to access a memory. In animals, even a small amount of information, sometimes distorted, is enough to retrieve a correct memory (remember the experiments by Lashley). This happens because memory in animals is distributed and its retrieval is content based.

One example of distributed memory from inanimate nature is presented by holography (figure 18.4). Holography is a physical method of storing three-dimensional images of objects on a photographic plate. It uses an interaction of two light beams to store the information; one of the beams plays the role of a "key," and the information (the other beam) can be restored only with the aid of the key beam. An interesting feature of holography is that it allows storage of many images on one plate as long as they were recorded using different key beams. Another feature making holography similar to human memory is

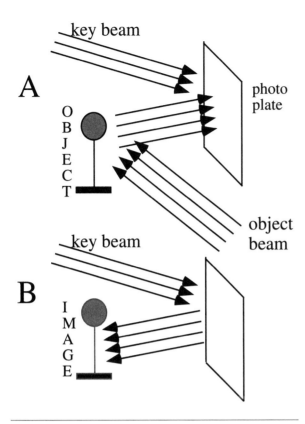

Figure 18.4 Holography creates an image (a memory) of an object on a photographic plate with the help of two light beams, the object beam and the key beam (A). One plate can store a number of images using different key beams. If the plate is illumined by a key beam, an image of the corresponding object will emerge (B).

that a small piece of the plate is enough to restore the whole picture, although the quality of the restored image will certainly suffer. A number of models of memory have been based on the holographic principle and the anatomy of certain brain structures, such as the cerebellum.

18.9. GENETIC CODE AS AN EXAMPLE OF MEMORY

There is an everlasting **nature-versus-nurture** debate on how much of human abilities and destiny are preprogrammed genetically and how much can be changed by experience. Genetic code is a way in which information is transferred over generations, and it may certainly be considered an example of a very long-term memory. Part of the genetic code carries information that is common among all human beings. Not only the number of legs, arms, eyes, and noses, but also the prewiring of the structures within the CNS have not changed much during thousands of years of human civilization. Another aspect of the code, however, makes all persons different in both appearance (height, color of hair, etc.) and abilities. The

last statement may sound politically incorrect. However, it is well known that some people are talented in music while others have problems whistling a simple tune even after extended practice; the same is true for such diverse activities as playing chess, studying mathematics, writing poetry, playing basketball, and so on. Furthermore, observations in twins suggest that even if they are separated at birth, they are likely to have very similar mental abilities. There are human subpopulations with a higher percentage of slow muscle fibers who may be expected to be very good, for example, at long-distance running, while there are other subpopulations with a higher percentage of fast fibers who are likely to be much better at a 100 m dash or at jumping. These "predictions" are certainly probabilistic; that is, they show a shift of a nearly normal distribution of a certain feature within a subpopulation, while individuals within each subpopulation may display quite diverse abilities.

18.10. PLASTICITY IN THE BRAIN

The flexibility (plasticity) of the projections within the CNS represents one of its most remarkable features and is likely to contribute to the processes of motor learning and adaptation to trauma. Since the classical works of Lashley in the 1930s, it has been proposed that brain injury may lead to a dramatic topographic reorganization in adjacent areas that may, in particular, significantly contribute to recovery after stroke. Changes in peripheral afferent inflow have been shown to induce changes in the receptor field sizes and locations in brain cortex of the cat. Somatosensory cortical representations in monkeys have been shown to change after specific training of one hand and after digit amputation or fusion. Central nervous system plasticity is not limited to grossly changed pathological states or to supraspinal structures, as demonstrated by the previously mentioned experiments showing changes in monosynaptic reflexes after prolonged operant conditioning.

Neurological reorganization of descending control signals after a below-knee amputation in humans was demonstrated with transcranial magnetic stimulation. In this study, stimuli at optimal positions of the coil over the scalp recruited a larger percentage of α-motoneurons controlling the muscles in the residual leg. These muscles could also be activated from larger areas of the scalp than could the muscles on the intact side. Similar results, also in human subjects, have been reported after an upper limb amputation.

18.11. KORSAKOFF'S SYNDROME

Chronic alcoholism and associated changes in metabolism lead in some patients to a complex of symptoms called **Korsakoff's syndrome** or psychosis. These patients demonstrate severe memory deficits. Studies of memory deficits in such patients have revealed that the deficit is due, at least partly, to defective encoding at the time of learning rather than to defective retrieval mechanisms. These patients do much better if they are provided with prompts or partial cues. Memories that can be retrieved with the help of such prompts are termed priming, and they are commonly intact even in patients with severe memory losses. Patients with Korsakoff's syndrome exhibit pathological changes in the mammillary bodies of the hypothalamus and in the medial dorsal nucleus of the thalamus, suggesting that these structures are also involved in the mechanism of memory.

18.12. POSSIBLE ROLE OF HIPPOCAMPUS IN MEMORY

Patients with a hippocampal lesion may learn to solve a complex mechanical puzzle as quickly and successfully as unimpaired persons. However, later they do not remember solving the puzzle or working with it. So there are two types of memory involved in this procedure, one of which is apparently unimpaired in these patients while the other one is impaired. The first type of memory is called **reflexive.** It accumulates slowly through repetitions of many trials and does not depend crucially on such cognitive processes as comparison and evaluation. Many perceptual and motor skills are examples of reflexive memory. The second type of memory is called **declarative.** It depends on cognitive processes such as evaluation, comparison, and inference and can be established after a single event. In particular, it involves restoring a whole event based on small bits and pieces, such as restoring a celebration that occurred a month ago upon seeing a bunch of balloons.

As demonstrated by the example just mentioned, the hippocampus is important for storage of declarative memory. There is evidence that hippocampal neurons show a plasticity that may form the basis for associative learning. Figure 18.5 illustrates, in a very schematic way, how major excitatory pathways into the hippocampus interact. These include the **perforant fiber pathway,** which runs from the **subiculum** to the granule cells in the hilus of the **dentate gyrus; the mossy fiber pathway,** which runs from the granule cells to the pyramidal cells in the CA3 area; and the **Schaeffer collateral,** which runs from the CA3 area to the pyramidal cells in the CA1 area. It was shown that a brief high-frequency train of electrical stimuli applied to one of the three major excitatory pathways may produce a stable excitatory postsynaptic potential in the hippocampal neurons that could last for hours, even days and weeks. This phenomenon was termed **long-term potentiation** (LTP). It immediately became the leading candidate for memory substrate.

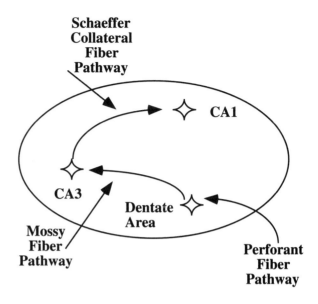

Figure 18.5   The hippocampus is a leading candidate for storage of declarative memory. The hypothetical memory mechanism is based on the phenomenon of long-term potentiation (LTP). LTP requires simultaneous activity in several excitatory fibers. It is associative in the area CA1 but not in CA3.

Long-term potentiation has a few interesting features: (1) more than one input fiber needs to be active to bring about LTP—that is, cooperativity is required; (2) input fibers and the postsynaptic neuron need to be active together to lead to LTP—that is, it is associative; and (3) LTP is specific to the pathway that induced it. The molecular mechanisms underlying LTP have been extensively studied recently, leading to a suggestion that there may be a molecular grammar for learning and memory.

There are problems, however, with the hypothesis that LTP in the hippocampus or other mechanisms involving stable changes in synapses are a memory substrate. Some of these issues were discussed in an earlier section.

18.13. SPINAL MEMORY

A study of spinal memory in rats was performed by Lev Latash, who used as a model the phenomenon of stable asymmetry of monosynaptic reflexes (see chapter 8) induced by destruction of one cerebellar hemisphere. After this surgical procedure, the asymmetry of the descending signals induced an asymmetry of the H-reflexes seen in the left and right hindlimb. Within this study, a second surgery was performed, somewhat later, involving a total transection of the spinal cord at an upper thoracic level. This second surgery apparently eliminated the asymmetry of the descending signals that had been the original cause of the H-reflex asymmetry. However, the asymmetry of reflexes continued to persist after the total spinal transection if the time interval between the two surgeries was sufficiently long.

Let us consider hypothetical sources of the reflex asymmetry after the second surgery. These could theoretically involve traces of the first surgery (memory) stored either in **motoneurons,** or in **presynaptic afferent terminals,** or in **interneurons** controlling the monosynaptic reflex arc. Experiments with warming up after deep local cooling demonstrated an initial restoration of reflexes without asymmetry followed by restoration of the asymmetry. These observations, together with experiments using pharmacological agents, pointed at interneurons as the site of long-term changes underlying the asymmetry (probably inhibition of inhibitory interneurons). Note that after the spinal transection, presynaptic influences to interneurons were removed; therefore the site of memory traces must be **postsynaptic,** probably using macromolecules within the cell bodies.

There may be major differences between the phenomena of memory in the spinal cord and that in the brain; however, these observations show that memory can be based on mechanisms that do not involve stable changes in synapses.

Chapter 18 in a Nutshell

The effects of memory can be seen at various levels, from hysteresis in muscle behavior, to habituation of reflexes, to classical or operant conditioning, to skill acquisition. Pavlov's theory considers animal behavior as a combination of inborn and conditioned reflexes. It views motor skill acquisition as a process of "beating a trail." Bernstein's physiology of initiative emphasizes the principle of activity and views motor skill acquisition as an active search process. Short-term memory lasts up to a few hours; its contents can be moved to long-term memory as a result of a consolidation process. Reflexive memory accumulates slowly through repetitions of many trials and does not depend crucially on cognitive processes. Declarative memory depends on cognitive processes such as evaluation, comparison, and inference and can be established after a single event. Memories are distributed over a substrate; their retrieval displays features resembling those of holographic pictures. Neuronal mechanisms of memory are unknown. Long-term potentiation in the hippocampus is frequently viewed as the neuronal mechanism of memory, implying synapses as the storage site. This view is rather controversial. Memory can be seen at the spinal level, where its site is likely to be postsynaptic.

Self-Test Problems

1. What kind of motor problems can you expect to see in a person in whom the left Deiters' nucleus was completely destroyed?

2. A person has a tumor in the second ventricle. What kind of pathological sensory-motor effects can be expected?

3. The output of the cerebellum is suddenly increased 10-fold. What kind of motor effects can you expect?

4. A subject is asked to imagine performance of a motor task, for example, a fast arm movement. No actual movement or change in the muscle activation levels occurs. In which structures of the central nervous system would you expect to see changes in the background activity of the neurons? In which structures would you expect to see no changes in the neuronal activity?

5. When you listen to music, unexpected bright memories can occur. Take a philosophical position (reductionist, or dualist, or complex systems) and suggest a neurophysiological mechanism for this effect.

6. After a spinal cord injury at a midthoracic level, a person can send voluntary commands to leg muscles but does not have sensation in the legs. Which sections of the spinal cord are likely to have been damaged and which ones are likely to have been spared by the trauma?

Recommended Additional Readings

Bloedel JR (1992). Functional heterogeneity with structural homogeneity: How does the cerebellum operate? *Behavioral and Brain Sciences* 15: 666-678.

Georgopoulos AP (1986). On reaching. *Annual Reviews in Neuroscience* 9: 147-170.

MacKay DM (1966). Cerebral organization and the conscious control of action. In: Eccles JC (Ed.), *Brain and Conscious Experience,* pp. 422-445. New York: Springer-Verlag.

Kutas M, Donchin E (1980). Preparation to respond as manifested by movement-related brain potentials. *Brain Research* 202: 95-115.

Partridge LD, Partridge LD (1993). *The Nervous System: Its Function and Its Interaction with the World.* Cambridge, MA: MIT Press. Chapter 9.

Rothwell JR (1994). *Control of Human Voluntary Movement.* 2nd ed. London: Chapman & Hall. Chapters 7, 9, 10, 11.

WORLD IV

BEHAVIORS

CHAPTER 19

POSTURAL CONTROL

Key Terms

vertical posture

vestibular system

role of vision

preprogrammed reactions

anticipatory postural
    control

synergy

effects of vibration on
    posture

19.1. VERTICAL POSTURE

The fact that human beings are able to maintain **vertical posture** is in itself a miracle. One would have hard time imagining a mechanical system that is less stable in the field of gravity. Sometimes during analysis of control of the vertical posture, the human body is modeled as an **inverted pendulum** (figure 19.1), which is not easy to equilibrate, especially in the presence of external perturbations and changes in its orientation with respect to the field of gravity. However, the problem is much more complicated because of the presence of a

number of joints along the axis of the pendulum. In physics, stability of a mechanical system in the field of gravity requires that the projection of its center of mass fall within the area of support (figure 19.2). The area of support for a human being is relatively small (of the order of 1 ft²), requiring fine-tuning of interaction between movements in different joints along the body in order to maintain the equilibrium.

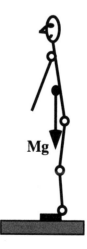

Figure 19.2 The human body has a number of joints along its vertical axis. Maintaining equilibrium in the field of gravity requires the projection of the center of mass to fall within the area of support.

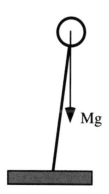

Figure 19.1 The human body in the field of gravity can be modeled as an inverted pendulum, which is inherently very unstable.

Problem 19.1

Can one maintain postural equilibrium if the projection of the center of mass is beyond the limits of the area of support?

Another miraculous phenomenon is that we can perform limb movements without falling down. Assessments of the dynamic forces during natural limb movements suggest that they are more than sufficient to destroy the fragile postural equilibrium. And, finally, there are no words adequate to express the profound awe experienced by motor control physiologists when they see a walking person. A multi-link inverted pendulum can walk and run and even maintain vertical posture during stumbling!

These fantastic features of the hypothetical system controlling vertical posture did not escape attention of Bernstein, who formulated a number of problems and approaches that remain in the center of contemporary research. Bernstein suggested that programming of a voluntary movement must include two distinct components—the first related to the movement itself and the second related to maintenance of the vertical posture. Bernstein also considered maintenance of the vertical posture as an illustration of his concept of **synergies,** that is, built-in coordinated combinations of motor commands to a number of joints leading to a desired common goal (e.g., not falling down). Synergies were viewed by Bernstein as building blocks for movements that could be scaled and combined according to a particular motor task. The presence of synergies is assumed to simplify the control of vertical posture solving, at least partially, the problem of mechanical redundancy, which will be addressed in chapter 21.

Several aspects of postural stability need to be discussed. Proper balance requires integration of information from various sources, including **vestibular system** information, visual information, and proprioceptive information. I will start with the role of the vestibular and ocular systems in postural control and then discuss the contribution of signals originating from proprioceptors in urgent corrections of posture.

19.2. VESTIBULAR SYSTEM

The sense of balance is one of the least prominent in our consciousness. Humans become aware of it only in extreme situations when balance is seriously endangered. The vestibular system of the brain and inner ear provides signals related to the relative orientation of the head with respect to the direction of the field of gravity. Its peripheral organs are found in the vestibule of the inner ear; their most important structures are the semicircular canals and the labyrinth.

The bony **labyrinth** consists of several cavities in the temporal bone; within these cavities is the membranous labyrinth, which is filled with **endolymph,** an unusual extracellular fluid whose ion composition resembles that of intracellular fluid. The membranous labyrinth is surrounded by the **perilymph,** whose ion composition is close to that of the cerebrospinal fluid. Ion pumps provide the unusual ion composition of the endolymph so that its potential is +80 mV with respect to the surrounding endolymph. Hair cells within the inner ear have an intracellular potential of –60 mV, which adds up to 140 mV of electrical driving potential.

The construction of the inner ear is quite intricate (figure 19.3). Both ends of each of the **semicircular ducts** are in the **utricle;** one end, which dilates before joining the utricle, is called the **ampulla.** An area with thickened epithelium within the ampulla is called the **ampullary crest.** In this region, specialized receptor cells, the **vestibular hair cells,** are located. They are innervated by peripheral ends of bipolar sensory neurons in the **ampullary nerve.** The ampullary crest is covered by a gelatinous, diaphragm-like mass called the **cupula.** When the head is rotated, the force is created by the inertia of the fluid in the semicircular ducts. This force acts on the cupula, producing a displacement of the hair cells of the ampullary crest that eventually leads to a change in the level of activity in nerve fibers innervating these receptors.

Problem 19.2

Why do we need three semicircular ducts? Could we possibly do with one or two? What about four?

This receptor apparatus is very sensitive and can detect acceleration as small as $0.1°/s^2$. Note that physical displacements of the cupula are less than 10 nm, in other words, comparable to those produced by low-amplitude sound in the auditory system.

A portion of the floor in the utricle is also thickened and contains hair receptors. This zone is called the **macula.** The macula is covered with a gelatinous substance containing crystals of calcium carbonate called **otoliths.** The macula is nearly horizontal when the head is held vertically. If the head is tilted or accelerated in a certain direction (linear acceleration), the otoliths deform the gelatinous substance, which in turn bends the hair cells, generating action potentials.

So, hair cells in the semicircular ducts respond to angular acceleration in specific directions, while hair cells in the utricle respond to linear acceleration in all direction.

One can separate the **dynamic** and the **static function** of the vestibular system. The dynamic function is principally mediated by the receptors in the semicircular ducts; it allows us to track head rotations in space and plays an important role in the reflex control of eye movement. The static function is mediated mostly by the hair

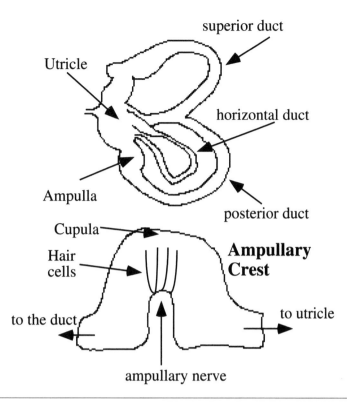

Figure 19.3 Both ends of each of the semicircular ducts end in the utricle. One end dilates before joining the utricle; this area is called the ampulla. An area with thickened epithelium within the ampulla is called the ampullary crest. In this region, specialized receptor cells, the vestibular hair cells, are located. They are innervated by peripheral ends of bipolar sensory neurons in the ampullary nerve. The ampullary crest is covered by a gelatinous, diaphragm-like mass called the cupula.

cells in the utricle and the saccule (another saclike structure of the inner ear). It enables humans to monitor the absolute head position in space and plays a very important part in postural control. The cell bodies of neurons innervating vestibular receptors are located in the **vestibular ganglion** (also called **Scarpa's ganglion**). These neurons are bipolar. One branch of each axon goes to the peripheral receptors (hair cells), while the other branch travels in the eighth cranial nerve and terminates in the brainstem.

The **vestibular nuclei** occupy a substantial part of the medulla. This complex includes four nuclei (figure 19.4): the **lateral vestibular nucleus** (also known as **Deiters' nucleus**), the **medial vestibular nucleus,** the **superior vestibular nucleus,** and the **inferior vestibular nucleus.** In addition to signals from vestibular receptors, Deiters' nucleus receives inputs from the cerebellum and the spinal cord.

Problem 19.3

Which cerebellar cells project onto Deiters' nucleus? Can these projections be excitatory or inhibitory?

Neurons of the dorsal portion of this nucleus send their axons into the **lateral vestibulospinal tract,** which terminates ipsilaterally in the central horns and has a profound facilitatory effect on both α- and γ-motoneurons innervating limb muscles. This tonic input is likely to play a major role in producing the background activity of the anti-gravity muscles.

The medial and superior vestibular nuclei play an important role in oculomotor control mediating **vestibulo-ocular reflexes.** (Note that voluntary control of eye movements is independent of the vestibular system.) Their input originates mostly from receptors within the semicircular ducts and is mostly dynamic. Both nuclei send the axons of their neurons into the **medial longitudinal fasciculus,** a tract running to the rostral parts of the brainstem. The inferior vestibular nucleus receives information from both vestibular receptor cells and the vermis of the cerebellum. Its efferent fibers contribute to the **medial vestibulospinal tract,** which terminates bilaterally in the cervical spinal cord and participates in reflex control of neck muscles, and to the vestibuloreticular pathways.

19.3. THE ROLE OF VISION IN POSTURAL CONTROL

Vision provides one of the most reliable sources of information for the human brain. When visual information

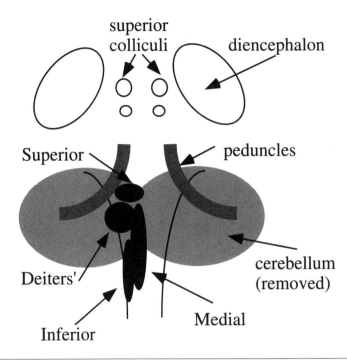

Figure 19.4 Vestibular nuclei include the lateral vestibular nucleus (also known as Deiters' nucleus), the medial vestibular nucleus, the superior vestibular nucleus, and the inferior vestibular nucleus.

comes into conflict with information of another modality, people tend to "believe" their eyes, not the other source of information. This happens, for example, when a person looks at his/her limb during high-frequency, low-amplitude vibration of a muscle within the limb. Without visual information, the vibration frequently leads to strong illusions of limb motion, sometimes bringing about sensations of anatomically impossible joint positions. If one looks at the limb, however, the illusions become much less pronounced and commonly disappear.

The system for postural control is also strongly dependent upon visual information. For example, all possible indexes of postural stability become worse if the subject is standing with eyes closed. In particular, there will be an increase in body sway during quiet standing, larger deviations of the **center of mass** in response to postural perturbations, and larger postural deviations induced by vibration of postural muscles (which we will consider later).

Movement of the visual background is well known to produce **illusions** of movement of the observer. For example, if a person is sitting in a train that has stopped at a station, and the train on the next track starts to move slowly, the person has the feeling that the stopped train is moving in the opposite direction. If a person stands and looks at a screen that is displaying a certain pattern, an accelerated movement of the pattern toward the subject induces a sensation of moving forward and a corresponding sway of the body backward (figure 19.5). Similarly, a movement of the pattern away from the subject induces body sway forward.

Usually there are limits to the extent to which the human brain "believes" any one of the sources of information used for postural control. Thus, an illusion created by a flow of information along one of the channels is kept down or may even be eliminated by information coming from other sources. In order to create a really strong illusion, one needs to manipulate synchronously all three major sources of information related to body position and orientation—vestibular, visual, and proprioceptive. Disney World uses such methods in simulation rides during which the viewers are seated in comfortable chairs that can be tilted synchronously with changes of an image projected on the large screen. I strongly recommend that all readers take one of these rides!

19.4. THE ROLE OF PROPRIOCEPTION IN POSTURAL CONTROL

One of the major sources of information about the role of signals from proprioceptors in postural control is observations of postural disturbances when proprioceptive signals are distorted. Some of the effects of high-frequency, low-amplitude muscle vibration were discussed earlier, including the tonic vibration reflex and changes in other reflex responses. These effects may also be observed at the level of postural control. They are related to

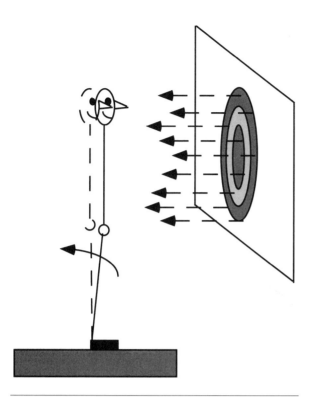

Figure 19.5 If a standing subject looks at a screen that displays a certain pattern, an accelerated movement of the pattern toward the subject induces a sway of the body backward.

the unusually high level of activity of muscle spindles induced by the vibration. Let me note again that muscle vibration applied to a muscle tendon can "drive" virtually all the spindles of the muscle. The central nervous system is confused by this proprioceptive information and may interpret it as signaling an increase in muscle length.

If the vibration is applied to a postural muscle, an illusory increase in its length is further interpreted as a change in body orientation. This illusory body sway is compensated for by an actual change in body position. For example, vibration of the Achilles tendon leads to central overestimation of the length of the triceps muscles (an illusory body sway forward) that is "corrected" by an actually observed body sway backward. These effects are termed **vibration-induced fallings** (VIFs). They are very strong if the subject is standing with eyes closed. Vibration of the Achilles tendon may even lead to actual falling backward, so this experiment requires that an experimenter stand behind the subject to prevent injury. If the subject opens his/her eyes, the effects of vibration are attenuated and may even disappear.

Similar effects on body posture can be observed during vibration of other postural muscles, as well as of muscles whose contribution to postural control may not be so obvious. For example, vibration of neck muscles induces similar illusions with respect to the position of the head.

Illusory deviations of the head may further lead to vestibular illusions, and ultimately, to postural adjustments similar to VIFs observed during vibration of leg muscles.

19.5. ANTICIPATORY AND CORRECTIVE POSTURAL ADJUSTMENTS

We have already noted that voluntary arm movements performed by a standing person are sources of **postural perturbations** (figure 19.6). Two major sources of postural perturbations are associated with fast voluntary movements. First, a change in the body geometry leads to a change in the projection of the center of mass, which may move outside the area of support and thus needs to be corrected. Second, during arm movements, inertial forces and mechanical joint coupling create torque changes in numerous joints of the body, including those involved in postural control.

Therefore, voluntary movements, particularly fast ones, are virtually always associated with changes in the activity of postural muscles. Some of these changes occur prior to the movement itself and can be addressed as **anticipatory postural adjustments.** Their assumed role is to minimize perturbations of the vertical posture that would otherwise be induced by the movement. Accordingly, one may expect anticipatory postural adjustments to initiate an acceleration of the body that would oppose the expected perturbation due to an intended limb

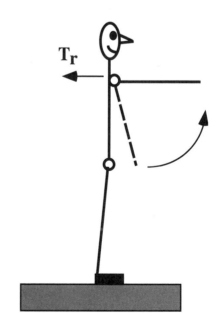

Figure 19.6 A fast arm movement by a standing person is a source of strong postural perturbation because of the joint coupling. A fast shoulder flexion creates reactive torques (Tr) that try to push the body backward.

movement. Mechanical consequences of anticipatory postural adjustments can actually be observed as displacements of the center of pressure of the body on the support surface. These adjustments are apparently prepared by the central nervous system before the actual perturbation occurs (i.e., in a feedforward manner) and therefore are frequently suboptimal. Another group of reactions in postural muscles occur later, in response to signals from proprioceptors about an actual perturbation. This group can be considered **compensatory reactions** to balance perturbations induced by the intended movement (or by other factors; e.g., in laboratories, unexpected platform rotations or translations are commonly used as sources of controlled postural perturbations). Their latency is rather small, of the order of 60-80 ms; so they can be considered an example of preprogrammed reactions, which we discussed in chapter 12.

Figure 19.7 shows a typical pattern of postural adjustments associated with a fast bilateral shoulder flexion (arm movement forward). Note that changes in the background activity of postural muscles occur prior to a visible increase in the activity of the "prime mover," that is, a muscle that is assumed to initiate the required arm movement (deltoid muscle, in our case; this point is marked with dashed lines). These changes lead to a displacement of the center of pressure. One can also see later corrective reactions in the activity of postural muscles that occur about 100 ms after the surge in the deltoid EMG.

There are clear differences in the mode of control and function between these two groups of associated changes in the activity of postural muscles. Anticipatory reactions are initiated by the subject; the later, compensatory reactions are initiated by sensory feedback triggering signals. Anticipatory reactions try to predict postural perturbations associated with a planned movement and to minimize them, while compensatory reactions deal with actual perturbations of balance that occur due to suboptimal efficacy of the anticipatory components. So, both anticipatory and compensatory reactions are assumed to be preprogrammed, and they differ in their relative timing with respect to the limb movement and method of triggering, feedforward or feedback.

Problem 19.4

What changes in anticipatory and corrective postural reactions do you expect to observe if one and the same perturbation is applied many times?

It seems that predictability of an upcoming perturbation is insufficient by itself to bring about anticipatory postural adjustments. In particular, if a perturbation is delivered by an experimenter according to a precisely predictable pattern, for example, is timed synchronously with a metronome, the subject is still unable to generate anticipatory postural adjustments. Recent studies have demonstrated that an action by a standing person, even a minimal action triggering a postural perturbation, is necessary and sufficient for bringing about these adjustments. However, if an unusually minor action triggers a large perturbation, the amplitude of the adjustment is frequently scaled with respect to the magnitude of the action rather than with respect to the magnitude of the perturbation, even if the perturbation is fully predictable. For example, if a person shoots a rifle, the rebound commonly leads to a strong postural perturbation. One needs to be an experienced marksman to be able to generate anticipatory postural adjustments that would compensate for this predictable and relatively standard perturbation. These observations are rather counterintuitive and suggest that the human brain may be not as smart as people used to think.

Problem 19.5

Suggest an example from everyday life in which postural adjustments are scaled with respect to an action rather than with respect to an expected perturbation.

There are several lines of defense against unexpected or uncompensated postural perturbations. The first is **peripheral elasticity** of muscles, tendons, and other tissues. Any displacement of a joint creates elastic forces resisting the displacement. The second line of defense is the **stretch reflex** with its phasic and tonic components. It also demonstrates elastic properties and contributes to the damping of external perturbations, although at a certain reflex delay. However, these two mechanisms are not enough to provide equilibrium of the body in the field of gravity. The next defensive mechanism has a longer delay and belongs to the group of **preprogrammed reactions.** It is more powerful and more flexible that the first two mechanisms. Specifically, in certain situations the nervous system may "wish" to increase the level of activity of a muscle that is shortened by an external perturbation. This can be done with the help of the mechanism of preprogramming.

Preprogrammed corrective reactions are frequently described as combinations of muscle activation patterns (EMGs) specific for a given perturbation (cf. chapter 12). The earliest of these reactions appear at a latency of less than 100 ms, suggesting their preprogrammed rather than voluntary nature. They are thought to be triggered by multimodal sensory inputs with an important contribution from proprioceptive, visual, and vestibular receptors. Some of these reactions seem to be rather general, for example, coactivation of the an agonist-antagonist muscle pair stabilizing the joint irrespective of the direc-

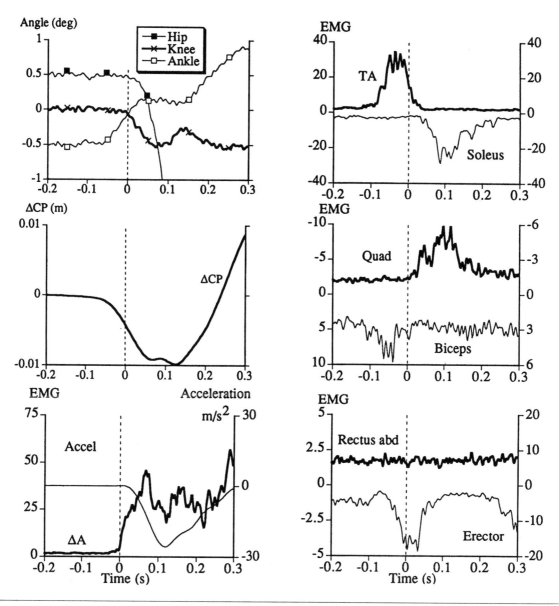

Figure 19.7 A typical pattern of postural adjustments associated with a fast bilateral shoulder flexion. Changes in the background activity of postural muscles (e.g., tibialis anterior [TA], biceps femoris, and erector spinae) occur prior to a visible increase in the activity of the "prime mover" (anterior deltoid, ΔA in the left lower panel). These changes lead to a displacement of the center of pressure (ΔCP, left middle panel) and movements of major leg joints (left upper panel). Later, corrective reactions in the activity of postural muscles occur.

Reprinted, by permission, from M.L. Latash, A.S. Aruin, I. Neyman, and J.J. Nicholas, 1995, "Anticipatory postural adjustments during self inflicted and predictable perturbations in Parkinson's disease," *Journal of Neurology, Neurosurgery, and Psychiatry*, 58: 326-334. © 1995 BMJ Publishing Group.

tion of a perturbation. Other reactions are specific to the type and direction of a perturbation.

There are certain preferred patterns of corrective postural reactions. In particular, an external perturbation of balance in a standing young subject, induced by an unexpected quick rotation or translation of the platform on which the subject stands, typically induces the most prominent changes in the level of activation of ankle flexors and/or extensors, leading to a visible displacement in the ankle joint—the **ankle strategy** (these experiments

were originally performed by Lewis Nashner and his group). A similar perturbation in an elderly subject frequently induces most prominent changes in the activity of hip flexors and/or extensors, the **hip strategy.** Apparently, an ankle movement leads to larger horizontal displacements of the center of gravity as compared to a hip movement of the same amplitude. On the other hand, if an error occurs and a larger or smaller joint rotation is generated, the ankle strategy is likely to lead to a bigger error in the displacement of the center of gravity and consequently to a possibility of falling down. Thus, the ankle strategy seems to be more effective and more challenging, while the hip strategy trades efficacy for safety. There are intermediate patterns of corrective postural adjustments that may also involve the knee joint.

Problem 19.6

Can one see anticipatory and corrective postural adjustments in arm muscles? Give examples.

19.6. THE NOTION OF POSTURAL SYNERGY

Nicholai Bernstein, whose name we have already encountered, introduced the notion of **postural synergy** as a combination of control signals to a number of muscles whose purpose is to assure stability of a limb or of the whole body in anticipation of a predictable postural perturbation or in response to an actual perturbation. Postural synergies may be considered as bricks used by the central nervous system to construct meaningful control

signals to numerous joints and muscles. Later, the notion of synergies was expanded to include **movement synergies,** that is, combinations of control signals whose purpose is to assure a certain movement of a body segment. It has been supposed that the existence of synergies takes part of the computational load off the shoulders of the central nervous system.

A traditional view has been that postural synergies form a separate group of motor programs that can be mixed and matched with the "focal" motor programs. In other words, people are assumed to have two pockets in the brain: one pocket contains programs for a planned voluntary movement (movement synergies), and the other contains sets of appropriate anticipatory and/or corrective reactions (postural synergies) (figure 19.8). An alternative view is that there is only one pocket and that separation of peripheral motor patterns into "focal" and "postural" is done by researchers but not by the brain (figure 19.9). According to the latter view, any movement, even the most local one, involves many more joints than those apparently used to produce the movement. Thus, changes in the activity of postural muscles become not an addition to a motor program but an inherent part of it.

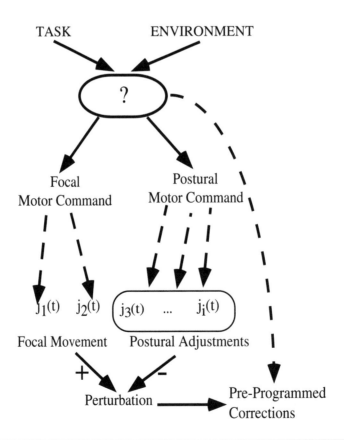

Figure 19.8   According to the traditional view, two motor commands are generated by the central nervous system based on the task and external force field. One is related to the "focal" movement, while the other provides postural stability.

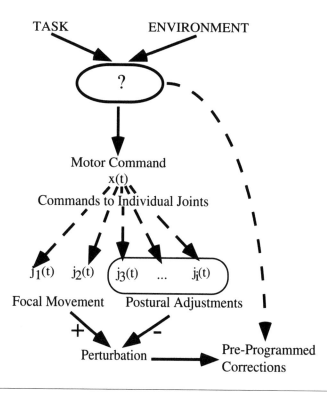

Figure 19.9   A motor command is generated by the central nervous system based on the task and external force field. It is later transformed to commands to individual joints. Some of them may have an apparently postural function while others may be apparently "focal." This classification, however, is made by the researchers, not by the brain.

Chapter 19 in a Nutshell

Human vertical posture is inherently unstable. Voluntary limb movements generate postural perturbations because of joint coupling and changes in body geometry. Postural stabilization is assured through a number of mechanisms including anticipatory postural adjustments, peripheral elasticity of muscles and tendons, muscle reflexes, preprogrammed postural corrections, and voluntary corrections. Postural synergy is a scalable pattern of control signals to a number of muscles whose purpose is to preserve equilibrium. The vestibular apparatus plays a major role in postural equilibrium; it consists of peripheral receptors sensitive to acceleration and vestibular nuclei. Other sensory systems, such as vision and proprioception, also contribute to postural control. Changes in visual or proprioceptive information can lead to postural disturbances.

CHAPTER 20

LOCOMOTION

Key Terms

motor programming
approach to locomotion

central pattern generator

spinal locomotion

gaits

corrective stumbling
reaction

dynamical systems
approach

20.1. TWO APPROACHES TO LOCOMOTION

Locomotion is probably the most common everyday activity of higher animals, including humans. It is defined as a motor action during which the location of the whole body in the environment changes. Lower animals do not locomote, and as a result their activity is limited to a small area in close proximity to the body. Locomotion is a great invention of evolution/creation that expanded the horizons of remote relatives (ancestors) of human beings, allowing them to use qualitatively new strategies of searching for food or escaping potential dangers. One may say that the "invention" of locomotion led to the emergence of a whole new class of motor problems for animals to confront in everyday life, bringing about the emergence/development of new systems of neural control encompassing virtually the entire central nervous system of contemporary higher animals. If it were not for locomotion, humans would probably have continued waiting for a piece of food to emerge by pure chance close enough to their tentacles to be captured and placed into the mouth, or trembled with fear in witnessing a larger tentacle slowly approaching their helpless body.

There are many types of locomotion such as crawling, flying, swimming, hopping, walking, and running. In this book I consider mostly walking and running as the two most common modes of locomotion used by humans. Analysis of work on the possible organization of the central neural structures controlling locomotion clearly reveals two highly influential competing philosophical approaches to the control of voluntary movements. The first may be called **motor programming** and is based, in the case of locomotion, on the notion of a **central pattern generator** (CPG). A hypothetical neural structure, the CPG explicitly generates a rhythmic neural activity that is later transformed into a rhythmic muscle activity leading to a rhythmic behavior, such as locomotion. Note that **rhythmicity** is probably one of the most common and basic features of locomotor behaviors.

Problem 20.1

Some animals can participate in various kinds of locomotion, such as swimming, walking, hopping, crawling, flying, etc. How many CPGs do these creatures have?

The competing approach considers rhythmicity as an emergent feature of a possibly nonrhythmic neural activity and an interaction of the peripheral apparatus (including its connections with the central nervous system) with the environment. This approach has been called the **dynamic systems approach,** or **dynamic pattern generation.** I am going to argue that both approaches

172

have elements of truth but not the whole truth, so that they are not really in competition but can be naturally reconciled.

20.2. CENTRAL PATTERN GENERATOR

The notion of the CPG emerged at the time of active developments in the field of cybernetics and originally represented rather simplified schemes consisting of feedforward and feedback loops that could, by themselves, generate rhythmic activity (a very simple example is presented in figure 20.1). Simply speaking, it is supposed that a CPG involves three types of cells. Cells of two types act at each other, suppressing the activity of the cells of the other type, and also provide output for the executive apparatus (for example, motoneurons of muscles involved in locomotion). It is supposed that these cells fatigue quickly or that they turn off after a brief period of high activity for other reasons. Imagine that one group of cells becomes very active. They will inhibit the other group. After a period of time, cells of the first group will fatigue and turn off, and the other group of cells will be released from the inhibition and become active. This cycle will continue until an external influence turns both cell groups off. It is supposed that neurons of a third type provide input that can suppress or excite cells of the first two groups and also modify relations among them, thus controlling parameters of the behavior produced by the whole system.

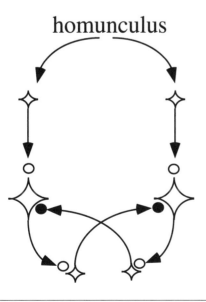

homunculus

Figure 20.1 A simple scheme illustrating the idea of a central pattern generator driven by a "higher center" (a homunculus).

Problem 20.2

How can the system shown in figure 20.1 generate oscillatory output signals? Which parameters of this system are important for the generation of rhythmic behavior?

The position of a CPG within the whole movement-producing system is illustrated in figure 20.2. It is supposed that the CPG is under the control of a smart "higher center" that "knows" where to locomote, when, and how. The CPG also receives inputs from peripheral sensors (in particular, visual receptors, vestibular receptors, and proprioceptors) and possibly other structures within the central nervous system. In particular, afferent inputs into a CPG may bring about changes in the pattern of its activity, leading, for example, to changes in gait (from walking to trotting to galloping). Such changes can also be induced voluntarily, that is, by changing the input from the "higher center" shown in figure 20.2.

This description of a CPG leaves one with a feeling of dissatisfaction because of the loosely defined notion of the "higher center" and the lack of definitions of important variables. This feeling of dissatisfaction was probably one of the major driving forces leading to the development of the alternative approach, dynamic pattern generation, which considers the whole system for movement production, including external forces, as a CPG. We will consider this approach in a later section of this chapter.

Note that the notion of CPG may be applicable not only to locomotion but also to other types of rhythmic activity, such as breathing. Experimental support for the idea of the CPG came from studies of locomotor-like rhythms (and rhythms resembling other activities) generated by the central nervous system of animals whose movements were suppressed by agents such as kurare (a poison suppressing neuromuscular transmission that was originally used by hunters in Central and South America), as well as studies of rhythms generated by isolated preparations. In these investigations, parts of the central nervous system were proven to be able to generate rhythmic changes in the neural activity. The question of the relation of these rhythms to actual locomotor activity remained open for some time, until the end of the 1960s.

20.3. LOCOMOTOR CENTERS

A groundbreaking series of experiments was performed in the late 1960s by a group consisting of Mark Shik, Grigory Orlovsky, and Fyodor Severin in Moscow. These researchers stimulated the **reticular formation** of the midbrain (mesencephalon) of decerebrate cats with an electrical stimulation of a constant

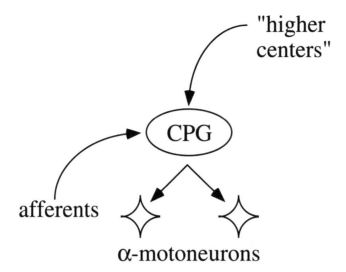

Figure 20.2 A central pattern generator (CPG) can be driven both by descending signals from the "higher centers" and by afferent information. Ultimately, the CPG leads to changes in the patterns of activation of α-motoneuronal pools.

frequency and amplitude. Within the reticular formation they found certain areas whose stimulation led to the emergence of rhythmic locomotor-like movements of the cat's limbs. The frequency of the locomotion was not explicitly related to the frequency of the stimulation, which was about 30 Hz; so a CPG was assumed to be activated by the descending signals generated by the stimulation. An increase in the amplitude of the stimulation could lead to a speeding up of the locomotion and, at a certain level, to a change in the gait (e.g., from walking to trotting). Changing the location of the stimulating electrode allowed these researchers to define an area whose stimulation could induce locomotion (the **mesencephalic locomotor region**).

Later, similar studies involving the stimulation of structures within the upper segments of the spinal cord allowed the researchers to trace the locomotor area to cervical spinal segments revealing the so-called **locomotor strip** (figure 20.3). That the induced locomotor pattern was not associated with an activity in feedback loops from the peripheral proprioceptors was proven in experiments in which similar locomotor-like patterns were recorded in muscle nerves (in the ventral roots of the spinal cord at an appropriate level) in the absence of peripheral muscular activity, which had been blocked by kurare. Let me note that much earlier, a great British physiologist, Graham Brown, had proven that locomotion was possible after deafferentation of a limb, that is, in the absence of reflexes or other feedback effects originating from the limb's proprioceptors.

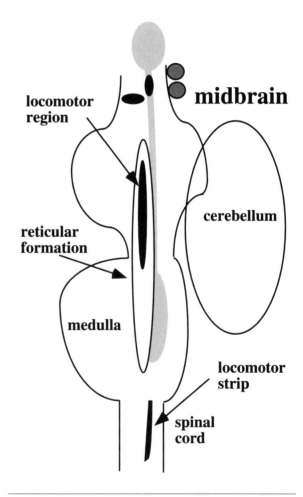

Figure 20.3 An illustration of the mesencephalic locomotor area and the locomotor strip.

20.4. SPINAL LOCOMOTION

Locomotion in **spinal preparations,** that is, in animals whose spinal cord does not receive any signals from the more rostral structures of the central nervous system, has been recognized since the classical studies by Brown and Sherrington at the beginning of this century. If the spinal cord of an animal is cut acutely, a locomotor pattern is typically observed for a few seconds; for example, a chicken whose head has just been cut off runs and even tries to fly. These observations are commonly explained as a "release" of the activity of a spinal CPG from the tonic descending inhibitory influence.

A chronic spinal animal does not display locomotion in the absence of external stimuli or special influences. However, if the limbs of a spinal cat are placed on a treadmill, movement of the treadmill at a constant speed can induce locomotor-like stepping of the limbs. Changing the speed leads to associated changes in the stepping frequency and to shifts in gait from walking to trotting to galloping. Stepping cycles can also be observed in response to certain drugs, for example DOPA, which is better known as a drug often used in therapy of Parkinson's disease (see chapter 26). On the other hand, spinal locomotion can also be observed in an animal in which all the dorsal roots of the spinal cord have been cut, that is, without any afferent inflow. These observations prove that the spinal cord is capable of producing locomotor-like activity even without any sensory feedback. Further experiments, especially those by a Swedish scientist, Stan Grillner, have demonstrated that individual CPGs exist for each limb. During normal locomotion, all the individual limb CPGs are coordinated so as to produce a coherent interlimb pattern.

Recently the existence of a spinal locomotor generator at a lower thoracic-upper lumbar level in humans has been suggested based on observations in patients with a spinal cord injury. In certain conditions, these patients can demonstrate involuntary stepping movements of the legs whereas they are unable to produce such movements voluntarily. In another series of observations, stepping movements were induced in persons with spinal cord injury by an electrical stimulation applied to the spinal cord at the lower thoracic-upper lumbar level.

It can be concluded from the described data that a CPG for locomotion exists in the spinal cord of mammals and is able to produce a coordinated locomotor-like activity in response to both descending stimulation and peripheral input. This activity is insufficient by itself to assure meaningful locomotion, for a number of reasons. First, the animal needs to know where to locomote; that is, it needs signals from visual (or other) receptors carrying **information about the environment,** attractive or dangerous objects, and the like. Second, locomotion is always intimately tied to **control of posture** in the field of gravity. In all the experiments with spinal locomotion, the animals were suspended with a system of belts so that they did not need to support their own weight or worry about losing their balance. Third, normal locomotion is always associated with **perturbations** (e.g., stepping on an uneven area of a surface) that may require urgent corrections.

20.5. GAIT PATTERNS

If a spinal cat is placed on a moving treadmill, its hindlimbs will demonstrate a stable phase relation during induced locomotion. At low speeds of the treadmill, the hindlimbs will be out of phase with each other. As the speed increases, the hindlimbs will preserve the phase relation up to a certain speed, and then the relations among individual limb kinematics will change abruptly as the animal switches from walking to trotting and from trotting to galloping (figure 20.4).

Problem 20.3

What are, from your point of view, the most important limiting factors for the maximal speed of locomotion?

These and some other observations suggested application of ideas from the area of dynamic systems to processes controlling locomotion. According to this approach, oscillatory behaviors can demonstrate changes in the stability properties of their kinematics and phase transitions in response to changes in one or more input variables. In particular, a change in the descending signals (as in experiments by Shik and his colleagues) and in the peripheral information may lead to the emergence of a new stable solution for the system, leading to a new gait pattern.

20.6. CORRECTIVE STUMBLING REACTION

A particular pattern of automatic, reflex-like responses has been observed during cat locomotion associated with overcoming an unexpected obstacle, the **corrective stumbling reaction** (see chapter 12). This pattern could be observed during a weak mechanical stimulation of skin areas of the paw or of the leg (even with an air puff) or

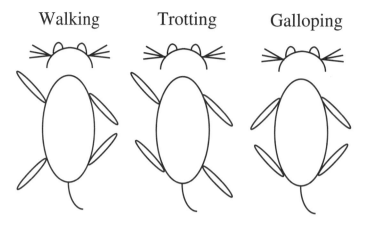

Figure 20.4   An illustration of three major gaits in a quadrupedal animal.

during short episodes of electrical stimulation of skin nerves or dermatomes. Similar patterns have also been seen in humans.

The application of any of these stimuli during the swing phase gave rise to a flexor reaction with hindlimb transfer over a hypothetical obstacle (figure 20.5). The same stimulation applied during the stance phase could give rise to an extensor reaction. The latency of these reactions was higher than the latency of monosynaptic reflexes and lower than the voluntary reaction time. The functional appropriateness of these reactions and their relative independence of the stimulus suggest that they are in fact preprogrammed responses of a mechanism responsible in everyday life for the compensatory reactions during actual stumbling (see chapter 12).

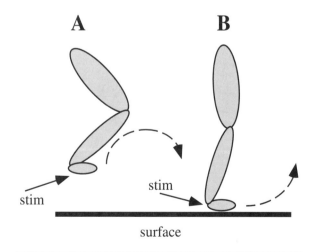

Figure 20.5   The corrective stumbling reaction involves a coordinated adjustment of the walking pattern in response to an external stimulus (mechanical or electrical). It involves different changes in the muscle activation patterns depending on the phase of the step cycle when the stimulus is delivered.

Problem 20.4

When you suddenly step on a nail during walking, preprogrammed reactions are generated (e.g., jumping and cursing). What kind of reaction would you expect to see in a person stepping on a nail while crossing an abyss via a narrow plank?

One can hypothesize that the execution of any functionally important motor task is associated with preprogramming of certain motor patterns, depending on the task and on possible perturbations that can occur during the task execution (see chapter 12). These preprogrammed patterns provide for the very quick initiation of compensatory responses to the perturbation. Because these motor reactions are prepared by the central nervous system prior to an actual perturbation, they always lead to rather crude approximate corrections that can be further corrected with a voluntary action. Locomotion is one of the most commonly used movements in everyday animal and human activity. As such, the mechanism of locomotor movements is well protected with a set of preprogrammed corrections that can be triggered by appropriate proprioceptive stimuli.

Problem 20.5

Give examples of other tasks that are associated with a system of preprogrammed corrections.

20.7. DYNAMIC PATTERN GENERATION

The alternative approach to locomotion (as well as to the generation of other movements) has been pioneered by Scott Kelso and Gregor Schöner and termed the **dynamic**

systems approach or **dynamic pattern generation.**
According to this approach, the system for movement
production—including the central neural structures, the
effectors and their connections with the central structures,
and environmental forces—can be modeled with a nonlinear differential equation. The term **nonlinear** means
that the response of a system, as described by these equations, to an input signal may change disproportionally to
changes in the input signal. Such equations cannot typically be solved analytically. When applied to motor problems, they can describe rather complex behaviors including, in particular, oscillations and changes in relative
coordination. Note that oscillations are typical features
of locomotor movements, while changes in relative limb
coordination describe changes in gaits.

The dynamic systems approach has shown impressive success in its description of certain features of motor coordination, including interlimb and interjoint coordination. There are two major views on the approach.
Some accept it as the only correct approach to voluntary
movement production in humans—the one that ties together events of the inanimate world and biological phenomena. Others see it another example of mathematical
modeling, that is, an example of efforts to address biological problems with tools that have been developed for
other areas of science. It is no surprise that a complex
equation can model complex behavior better than a simple
equation. A major question is whether the equation has
biological relevance—whether its parameters can be assigned physiological meaning. To date, parameters of
equations used within the dynamic systems approach
have not been assigned a measurable physical or physiological meaning; that is, their values are selected rather
arbitrarily in order to make sure that the model produces
desired coordination patterns.

Let us use figure 20.6, which is analogous to a figure
originally published by champions of the dynamic systems approach, Claudia Carello and Michael Turvey, to
illustrate the major difference between the motor programming (or CPG) approach and the dynamic systems
approach. The upper drawing (A) illustrates control of
locomotor of an owl from the motor programming (or
CPG) view. The "owl homunculus" controls all the details of owl movement patterns, as with a marionette.
The middle drawing (B) illustrates the same owl without
any supreme homunculus but with numerous links connecting its elements (connections with external variables
are also implied; note the open eyes of the owl!), in line
with the dynamic systems view. It is supposed that these
links give rise to the equations mentioned, potentially
leading to complex behavioral patterns.

Note that the upper drawing lacks the element of coordination or, more precisely, that all the details of coordination are delegated to the ultimate controller; in other
words, they are assumed to be preplanned by the supreme

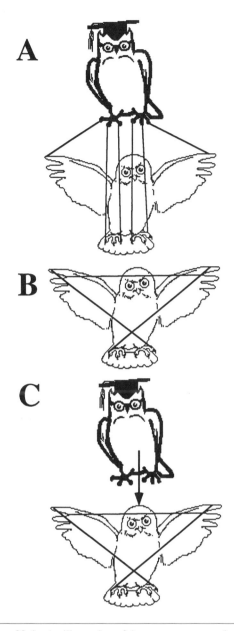

Figure 20.6   An illustration of the motor programming
approach (upper drawing, A), the dynamic pattern generation
approach (middle drawing, B), and a combination of the two
(bottom drawing, C). Note that the upper drawing does not
involve coordination and the middle drawing lacks control.

omnipotent homunculus. This is not very attractive for a
number of reasons, particularly because, as we know,
similar coordination patterns can be observed in spinal
animals that apparently lack any homunculus. Moreover,
assigning all the details of coordination to a smart "black
box" does not solve the problem but rather emphasizes
our inability to deal with it.

The middle drawing illustrates a much more appeal-
ing approach to coordination, which can emerge without any supreme problem solver; but it lacks the element of control. This owl will never be able to change

its behavior based on its own will, only in response to signals from the environment. Remember that earlier (in chapter 18) we discussed the differences between the physiology of initiative and the physiology of reflex-type movements and came to the conclusion that behavior cannot be based exclusively on reactions to external stimuli. Thus, this drawing is also unsatisfactory.

The bottom drawing (C) shows a "hybrid owl" that retains all the coordinative links among its elements but also has an independent descending signal, generated by its upper neural structures, that can be used for movement initiation or modification even if the environment does not dictate it. This descending signal represents one of the important parameters in the equations that describe the coordination. Bernstein's **principle of initiative** states that this input cannot be reduced to reactions to external stimuli. In this respect, its nature remains mysterious.

This may not sound very "scientific," but unfortunately, I am unaware of viable alternatives to the scheme shown in figure 20.6C. Coordination and control can and must coexist in order to allow both active central generation of meaningful movements and adjustment of coordination to control and environmental demands.

Problem 20.6

In classical experiments by Kelso, when the subjects tapped a rhythm with two index fingers, an increase in tapping frequency could lead to an automatic switch from an out-of-phase regime into an in-phase regime. Try to interpret these observations based on the three approaches illustrated by the three parts of figure 20.6.

Chapter 20 in a Nutshell

Locomotion is an activity during which the location of the whole body of the animal in the environment changes. Electrical stimulation of an area in the reticular formation of the midbrain and also of areas in the cervical spinal cord can induce locomotion and lead to changes in gait. Peripheral stimulation of the legs, as well as certain drugs, can lead to gait initiation and changes in a spinal animal preparation. Reflex responses of limb muscles to mechanical stimulation of a paw, or to an electrical stimulation of an afferent nerve in a limb, depend on the phase of locomotion. This pattern is termed a corrective stumbling reaction. Locomotion can be viewed as a result of the activity of a CPG that is under the control of a superior executive structure and can change its activity in response to changes in peripheral information. Alternatively, locomotion can be viewed as an emerging pattern within a complex system that involves central neural structures, peripheral organs, and interaction with the environment.

CHAPTER 21

MULTI-JOINT MOVEMENT

Key Terms

reaching movement	redundancy	control variables
working point	Bernstein problem	supraspinal mechanisms

21.1. GENERAL FEATURES OF TARGETED MOVEMENTS

We will now consider how a unidirectional movement of a limb from a certain initial to a certain final position is controlled. Such movements may be considered basic components of virtually the entire human everyday motor repertoire. Pointing at an object, picking up a cup of coffee, hitting a nail with a hammer—all involve components that may be considered single, unidirectional reaching movements.

First, it is necessary to introduce the notion of the **working point,** that is, a point whose trajectory is most directly related to successful execution of a motor task. During pointing at objects or picking up or manipulating objects, this point may be located on the fingertip(s) or somewhere on the palm. During kicking a football, the working point is somewhere on the tip of the shoe. This point does not even need to be in permanent direct contact with the body. When Michael Jordan of the Chicago Bulls throws a basketball, the task is to get the working point (the basketball) into the basket. In this example, the working point is in direct contact with the player's hand only during the initial segment of its trajectory. In most computer games, the working point is an image of a fighter plane or a superman on the screen, and the player controls it by moving the joystick, without any direct mechanical contact with the working point.

If one asks a naive person to make a movement with the dominant hand from a comfortable position in the work space to another comfortable position, this movement will demonstrate certain features:

1. The trajectory of the endpoint will be nearly straight.
2. The velocity profile of the endpoint will be nearly symmetrical (bell shaped).
3. The acceleration of the endpoint will demonstrate two peaks.
4. Trajectories, velocities, and accelerations of individual joints may demonstrate different properties including reversals in the direction of motion.

If the subject is asked to repeat the same movement several times, there will be relatively high variability of the individual joint trajectories and a lower variability of the endpoint trajectory. These observations date back to the classical studies of blacksmiths by Bernstein in the 1920s. Bernstein's subjects were asked to hit the chisel with the hammer (figure 21.1). They demonstrated highly reproducible trajectories of the tip of the hammer (the working point, which was, by the way, located outside the body!) and much less reproducible trajectories of all the limb joints.

Thus the main conclusion is that the most reproducible feature of the trajectories of multi-joint reaching movements is the lack of reproducibility, which is addressed as **variability.** Variability is a curse of motor control studies that do not investigate it explicitly. Reducing variability is frequently the goal of training

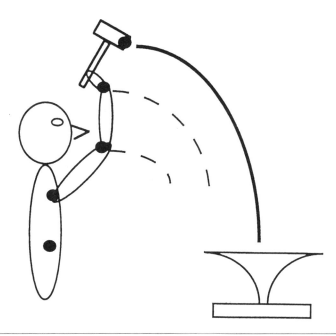

Figure 21.1 When a blacksmith hits the chisel with the hammer, the trajectory of the tip of the hammer is more reproducible than any joint trajectory.
Reprinted, by permission, from M.L. Latash, 1996, How does our brain make its choices? In *Dexterity and its development,* edited by M.L. Latash and M.T. Turvey (Mahwah, NJ: Lawrence Erlbaum Associates, Inc.), 287.

procedures in both "real life" (including the training of athletes or rehabilitation of patients with motor disorders) and the laboratory environment. On the other hand, variability by itself is a fascinating phenomenon that obeys its own laws and demonstrates consistent relations among task and performance parameters. Any theory that aspires to explain how multi-joint movements are controlled needs to have an explanation for the phenomena of variability and flexibility of natural human movements.

Problem 21.1

What can you conclude from the higher variability of individual joints in comparison to the variability of the tip of a tool?

21.2. MAJOR PROBLEMS OF CONTROLLING NATURAL REACHING MOVEMENTS

During reaching movements, the working point is typically located on the hand, and controlling its trajectory in a **body-centered reference frame** means controlling a multi-link chain connecting the hand to the body. If the body moves, and you would like to control a trajectory of the working point in the external, **Cartesian space,** the situation becomes even more complicated. Two ma-

jor sources of complexity emerge when a researcher makes the step from controlling a single joint to controlling a more realistic multi-joint limb. The first source of complexity is related to the more complex biomechanics of the controlled peripheral system. It is due, in particular, to the important roles of new forces, for example, **Coriolis and centrifugal forces,** that are generally ignored during single-joint movement analysis. **Biarticular** muscles provide links between adjacent joints, thus introducing one more important factor into joint interactions. There are also new neurophysiological factors that play roles during multi-joint movements, such as **interjoint** and **interlimb reflexes.**

Problem 21.2

Can you give examples of purely single-joint movements from everyday life? From laboratory experiments?

The second source of complexity is the famous **Bernstein problem** of overcoming excessive **degrees of freedom.** During virtually all voluntary movements, the number of kinematic degrees of freedom (n) for the limb, which can be associated with the number of independent axes of joint rotation summed over all the joints of the limb, is higher than the number of variables (n_0) necessary to execute a motor task or to describe its execution. The latter number is frequently 3, corresponding to the three-dimensional space where we happen to live. Figure 21.2 illustrates Bernstein's problem for a three-joint limb performing a planar movement from an initial to a final position. Note that an infinite number of limb configurations may correspond to the final position of the endpoint.

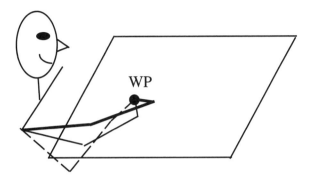

Figure 21.2 There are an infinite number of limb configurations (combinations of joint angles) corresponding to a fixed position of the tip (working point, WP) of a three-joint limb on a plane.

Bernstein's problem is a problem of choice: How does the central nervous system choose which joints to move and over what amplitude in order to occupy a predefined final hand position? This formulation, by the way, implies the nontrivial assumption that the central nervous system plans multi-joint movements in the space of joint angles. Let us keep in mind, however, that the language of motor control is different from the language of individual joint rotations. Thus, the number of control variables manipulated by the central nervous system may be higher or lower than n.

For example, imagine that a person controls the movement of a dot along a straight line with two knobs so that dot position P equals the sum of signals from the knobs:

$$P = x + y$$

where x and y are signals from the knobs (figure 21.3). This is a typical case of redundancy introduced at the level of control (two variables are manipulated to produce a single outcome). On the other hand, imagine that the same two knobs control movements in three joints of the limb shown in figure 21.2:

$$J_1 = x + y$$
$$J_2 = x - y$$
$$J_3 = 3x - 2y$$

where J_{1-3} are displacements of the joints and x and y are signals from the knobs. In this example, the design of the controls eliminates the apparent peripheral redun-

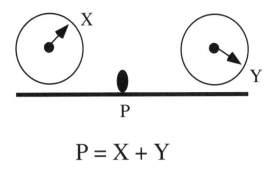

$$P = X + Y$$

Figure 21.3 Controlling the position of a dot on a line with two knobs leads to a problem of redundancy (one equation with two unknowns) at the control level.

dancy of the system: there are exactly two control variables to control a two-dimensional movement of the working point.

There is at least one strong reason to believe that the number of control variables is higher than n_0, so that Bernstein's problem typically does not disappear. The reason is the natural **variability** of movements that has already been mentioned. For example, if an experimenter asks a subject to pick up a matchbox from a table several times (figure 21.4), the trajectories of all the joints and of the working point (the hand) will be different in different attempts. This means that the task does not unambiguously specify a unique solution and that the central nervous system has a choice. So, an adequate formulation of Bernstein's problem would be: How does the central nervous system choose patterns of control variables to match a motor task?

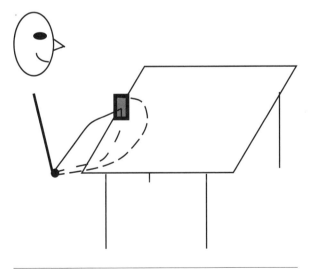

Figure 21.4 Natural motor variability is the strongest reason to believe that the problem of choice is virtually always present for natural movements. Here, different attempts at picking up the matchbox will generate different trajectories of the working point.

Actually, it is possible that the central nervous system does not care about particular combinations of control variables and joint rotations as long as the task is successfully accomplished. Imagine that a person in a grocery store is picking apples from a large bin containing hundreds of pieces of fruit. How does the person's brain choose which fruits to select? The answer probably is that it does not. It allows uncontrolled factors ("noise") to lead to a selection as long as the overall number of apples is correct and no obviously bad fruits are selected. Consider another example in which the conductor of an orchestra of 100 drummers needs to produce a noise level of 100 dB. One solution is to tell each drummer what force to use based on certain criteria, in other words, to eliminate the redundant degrees of freedom explicitly. An alternative solution is to tell each drummer, "Listen to the level of noise. If it is above 100 dB, beat lighter; if it is below 100 dB, beat harder." The second solution does not eliminate the "redundant" degrees of freedom; it uses them. Note that in the second case, the solution will produce a correct outcome even if one of the drummers falls ill and decides to go home. The second solution is an example of using a **coordinative rule** to solve a problem of redundancy.

Bernstein suggested that the problem of motor redundancy is solved using flexible relations (**synergies**) among control variables directed at individual elements that he called (see also chapter 19). This notion was further developed by two great Russian mathematicians, Israel Gelfand and Michael Tsetlin. They suggested that for any task, elements of the system for movement production (for example, individual joints or muscles) are assembled into task-specific **structural units.** Synergies represent purposes of structural units, while behaviors can be viewed as masks of synergies.

Structural units can be introduced for systems of differing complexity. For example, an organism, a subsystem within an organism, or a group of organisms can each be viewed as a structural unit. Gelfand and Tsetlin introduced three major axioms to describe the essential properties of structural units:

1. The internal structure of a structural unit is always more complex than its interaction with the environment (which may include other structural units).
2. Part of a structural unit cannot itself be a structural unit with respect to the same group of tasks.
3. Parts of a structural unit that do not work with respect to a task are either
   a. eliminated or
   b. find their own places within the task.

Axiom 3a illustrates the principle of economy when a minimal number of elements carry out each given group of tasks. This principle was viewed as typical of movement organization in insects. Axiom 3b illustrates the principle of abundance, when many more elements than necessary are participating in the activity of a structural unit. This principle was considered typical of movement organization in higher animals.

The notion of structural unit and the three major axioms can be illustrated using as an example the organization of a scientific laboratory. The laboratory can be viewed as a structural unit, while individual researchers are its elements. Let us assume that the laboratory has been organized to solve a specific group of problems. The role of each researcher within the laboratory can be described much more simply than the way the brain of each researcher functions (axiom 1). If the laboratory functions properly, half of it cannot solve the same group of problems, although it may be able to solve other problems, that is, form a new structural unit (axiom 2). The laboratory may be organized based on axiom 3a or axiom 3b. In the first case, each researcher is assigned a unique, specific function and cannot be replaced by another member of the team. In the second case, a large group of talented researchers is assembled and asked to deal with a complex problem. Each researcher is expected to find his or her own place in the team and contribute to the process.

Synergies can be formed at different levels of the central nervous system. For example, reflexes among muscles crossing different joints of a limb can be viewed as elements of synergies decreasing the system's redundancy. Tuning the interneuronal apparatus of the spinal cord by descending signals from the brain can be viewed as a mechanism organizing and modifying synergies according to particular motor tasks. According to the dynamic systems approach, synergies are emergent features of the neuromuscular system that can be tuned by both descending signals and sensory information from the effectors.

It becomes obvious that in order to move further one needs to guess what the central control variables used by the brain are, or, in other words, what internal language is used by the brain to communicate with spinal structures. A number of neurophysiological findings prompt an answer; these will be considered in the next few sections. Note, however, that neurophysiological data, by their very nature, are likely to suggest a reductionist answer. So these prompts should be taken with a grain of salt and be treated with caution. Particularly, it is always advisable to analyze a suggested answer based on the general properties of the system and to look for inconsistencies with experimental data and common sense.

Problem 21.3

Suggest an approach (a realistic or a hypothetical one) that would be able to help one guess the independently controlled variables.

21.3. SPINAL MECHANISMS OF MULTI-JOINT COORDINATION: INTERJOINT REFLEXES

A variety of reflex responses to a stimulus applied to a limb induce contractions of muscles controlling different joints of the limb or even muscles of another limb. Among the best-known examples are the flexor reflex and the crossed extensor reflex described in an earlier chapter. Remember that a pinch applied to the surface of a paw of an animal, or electrical stimulation of a skin nerve, may induce bursts of activity in virtually all the major flexor muscles of the limb. Simultaneously a burst of activity in extensor muscles of the contralateral limb may be seen. These responses come at a relatively long latency (between 50 and 100 ms) suggesting their polysynaptic nature. They originate from the activation of afferent fibers of relatively small receptors (nociceptors, free endings, and secondary muscle afferents) united under the name flexor reflex afferents (cf. discussion in chapter 9).

In an intact animal or human, a change in the length of a muscle of a limb necessarily leads to a joint motion and therefore to a change in the length of other muscles crossing the same joint. In addition, the presence of biarticular muscles makes purely single-joint motions impossible; that is, a movement in a joint leads to a change in the length of all the muscles crossing the joint, including the biarticular muscle(s), which may lead to a motion in an adjacent joint (figure 21.5). In animal experiments, however, it is possible to separate the distal tendon of a muscle from its place of attachment and to apply controlled changes in muscle length without changing the length of other muscles. Moreover, in such studies one can independently manipulate muscle force and length.

A series of such experiments was performed by T. Richard Nichols, who demonstrated a complex pattern of reflex effects among the muscles of a cat hindlimb. These effects could be induced by both length- and force-sensitive peripheral receptors. The "classical" pattern of these reflexes, described earlier, involves autogenic excitation and reciprocal inhibition induced by activity of muscle spindle afferents, as well as autogenic inhibition induced by the afferent fibers of the Golgi tendon organs. Nichols showed that reflex interaction among apparent agonists (in particular three heads to the triceps surae muscle) could be less "classical" and more asymmetrical. These patterns are sensible from the point of view of biomechanics and could provide the basis for organizing coordinated patterns of muscle activity (synergies) participating in functional multi-joint limb movements. However, by themselves, these findings do not prompt an answer to the big question: What are the control variables?

Problem 21.4

You want to perform a single-joint movement in a joint that is crossed by a uniarticular and a biarticular muscle. What kind of reflex effects would you expect there to be among peripheral receptors in the uniarticular muscle and α-motoneurons innervating the biarticular muscle?

21.4. SPINAL MECHANISMS OF MULTI-JOINT COORDINATION: CONTROL VARIABLES

There are a variety of exciting studies in multi-joint motor control using animal preparations. Let us look closely at one group, studies of the **wiping reflex** in the **spinal frog.** This choice is defined by the extremely intriguing performance of such a seemingly simple creature (a spinal frog) during such a complicated motor task (wiping a stimulus off the back with a hindlimb—try it and you will see that it is not easy!). The process of **spinalization** involves cutting the spinal cord at a cervical or high thoracic level so that impulses from the brain cannot reach segments of the spinal cord caudal to the place of transection. In contrast, the spinal neuronal mechanisms controlling hindlimb movements remain intact.

If an experimenter places a stimulus (a small piece of paper soaked in an acid solution) on the back of a sitting spinal frog (figure 21.6), the frog, after a certain latent period, performs a series of coordinated movements, wiping the stimulus off the back and sometimes throwing it away from the body. Wiping of the same skin area in successive cycles can be performed in various directions, and orientation of the foot relative to the stimulus (attack angle) can also change. If the stimulus is placed on the ipsilateral forelimb, accurate wiping movements are observed even if the position of the forelimb relative

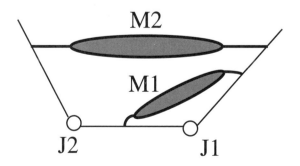

Figure 21.5 A change in the length of muscle M1 will lead to a motion in joint J1. As a result, the length of the biarticular muscle M2 will also change, leading to a motion in joint J2.

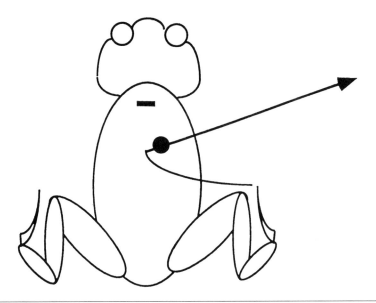

Figure 21.6 A spinal frog can remove an irritating stimulus from its back with a coordinated movement of the ipsilateral hindlimb.

Reprinted, by permission, from M.L. Latash, 1996, How does our brain make its choices? In *Dexterity and its development,* edited by M.L. Latash and M.T. Turvey (Mahwah, NJ: Lawrence Erlbaum Associates, Inc.), 286.

to the body changes. So, the spinal cord "knows" where the limbs are!

A series of experiments was performed to investigate the effects of unexpected "perturbations" on the wiping. In one series, a loose thread loop was placed on the hindlimb, preventing movements in the knee joint beyond a certain limit so that the maximal knee joint excursion was about 5°. The frog was able to remove the stimulus from its back in the first attempt! Then the knee was released and a cast was positioned to prevent movements in the next (more distal) joint. The frog once again wiped the stimulus at the first trial. Next a lead bracelet was placed on the distal part of the hindlimb; the weight of the bracelet was similar to the weight of the hindlimb itself. The frog still was able to wipe the stimulus accurately.

These experiments show that control signals, even on the spinal level, are not formulated in terms of contractions of individual muscles or even movements in individual joints. Otherwise, loading a segment or blocking a joint would have led to inaccurate movements. Second, the results imply the existence of very fast corrections of movement patterns, presumably built into the program for wiping.

21.5. SUPRASPINAL MECHANISMS

Earlier, several groups of studies were discussed that demonstrated a dependence between the activity of a population of neurons in a brain structure and the direction of a voluntary movement (chapters 8 and 9). The fact that neuronal populations in different anatomical

brain formations demonstrate basically the same behaviors underscores the limitations of these findings. These results suggest only that the activity of the studied neuronal groups is related to the studied movements—but not that there is a causal relation between the neuronal activity and movement generation. Although these studies, by themselves, fall short of proving that the neuronal populations control movements, they are in good agreement with the general idea that the central mechanisms are focused on certain parameters related to movement of a working point (commonly, the endpoint of a limb) rather than on parameters related to control of individual muscles or joints.

Other studies suggest that activity of the supraspinal structures during voluntary movements is related to characteristics of the endpoint trajectory. In particular, patterns of neuronal activity in the **supplementary motor area, motor cortex, putamen,** and **red nucleus** have suggested relations to characteristics of voluntary movement, at a rather **abstract kinematic level,** that are compatible with general ideas of working-point trajectory control during multi-joint movements. In particular, it has been shown that patterns of activity of cortical cells could code the trajectory independently of required muscle forces and patterns of muscle activation.

Jim Houk has suggested that the activity of red nucleus neurons can participate in motor control by coding properties of feedback reflex systems in the spinal cord. Earlier, Houk's group reported that the activity of separate red nucleus neurons could be related to initiation, speed, and amplitude of voluntary movements. These are the basic variables that are assumed to be used in limb endpoint control. Later, a more general model of control of endpoint position was suggested on the basis of interactions between the cerebellar and rubral nuclei. This model was based on positive feedback loops between the **nucleus interpositus** and **magnocellular red nucleus** and **nucleus reticularis tegmenti pontis** (figure 21.7). These loops were assumed to be under an inhibitory control from the Purkinje cells. Releasing of the feedback loops by switching off sets of Purkinje cells has been assumed to lead to emergence of adjustable pattern generators leading to a movement. Sets of Purkinje cells have been associated with "motor programs."

21.6. THE EQUILIBRIUM-TRAJECTORY HYPOTHESIS

The equilibrium-trajectory hypothesis, originally suggested by Neville Hogan and Tamar Flash, is a natural expansion of the single-joint **equilibrium-point hypothesis** (see chapter 10) to multi-joint movements. It implies that the central nervous system is able to shift an image of the working point along a desired trajectory expressed in external Cartesian coordinates. During a movement, this **virtual trajectory** is always ahead of the current actual position of the working point, and this disparity provides active forces driving the working point (figure 21.8). Note that the actual trajectory of a working point may be different from the virtual trajectory, because of a number of factors including the dynamic properties of the limb and changes in the external force field.

The equilibrium-trajectory approach avoids the computational problem of inverse dynamics and inverse kinematics, since muscle forces are not calculated by the central nervous system but emerge as a result of shifts of a central image of the working point that are accomplished in the external Cartesian space.

The equilibrium-trajectory hypothesis has been combined with an optimization approach called the **minimum jerk principle.** According to this approach, the central nervous system generates trajectories corresponding to a minimum of an integral of a function of jerk (the derivative of acceleration or the third derivative of displacement) of the limb endpoint. This approach has led to a number of theoretical predictions, which include straight paths of the working-point trajectories; smooth, unimodal velocity profiles (**bell-shaped velocity** profiles); and invariancy of the trajectory under translations, rotations, and its scaling with speed and/or amplitude. A number of these predictions correspond to experimental observations. In particular, nearly straight paths and bell-shaped velocity profiles have been observed for various initial and final working-point locations in external space, and for movements at different speeds, corresponding to the predictions concerning invariancy of the working-point trajectory.

Problem 21.5

What is (are) the independently controlled variable(s) used by the brain to control movements according to the equilibrium-trajectory hypothesis?

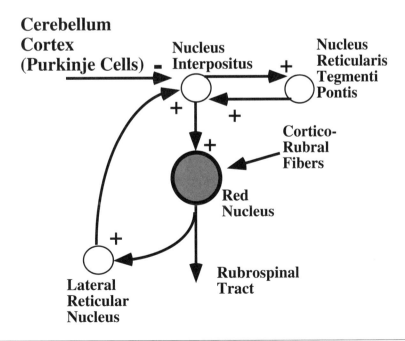

Figure 21.7   An interaction between the red nucleus and cerebellum is assumed to participate in the generation of "motor programs" by turning off sets of Purkinje cells, thus disinhibiting positive feedback loops shown in the scheme.

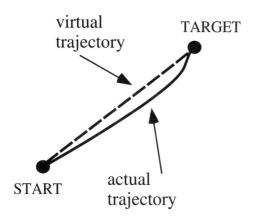

Figure 21.8   According to the equilibrium-trajectory hypothesis, the central nervous system plans a "virtual" trajectory of the working point, while its actual trajectory may be different because of dynamic factors.

21.7. WHAT IS CONTROLLED?

Presently, one can suggest only hypothetical answers to this question. But let us first try to answer another question: What is *not* controlled? I hope that all the preceding material has persuaded the reader that the following list *does not* contain viable candidates for the vacant positions of control variables for multi-joint movements:

1. Forces produced by individual muscles
2. Activation patterns (EMGs) of individual muscles
3. Torques in individual joints
4. Rotations in individual joints

In order to be able to assure accurate control over the trajectory of a working point, the central nervous system should use control variables related to functionally significant external variables, such as coordinates of the working point and/or force vector generated at the working point. These variables are what we care about during multi-joint movements because they are directly related to performance, whereas individual muscle forces and joint rotations are not so important as long as they do not lead to awkward limb configurations and postural problems. The fact that working-point trajectory is the most reproducible performance variable provides indirect support for this view. If we now remember that our muscles have spring properties, it becomes apparent that a working point has these properties as well; that is, if you "freeze" a motor command, coordinates of a working point in space will depend on the external force vector.

Perform a simple experiment. Ask a friend to push with a fist against your palm somewhere in front of his or her body (figure 21.9). Then ask the friend **not to intervene voluntarily,** and push his or her fist with your palm with smooth and quick pushes. You will feel that

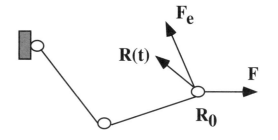

Figure 21.9   If a working point is in an equilibrium exerting a vector of force (F) in a certain location (R_0) in the work space, a change in the external force (F_e) will lead to a movement of the working point in a springlike fashion (R[t]).

the working point (the fist) resists attempts to move it from the original position in a springy fashion.

So the motor command of the subject does not define the position vector or the force vector of the fist, because these both change when you change the external force (all the EMGs would change as well if you cared to record them). Rather it defines spring parameters of the system that can be expressed with an **equilibrium vector** (similarly to the situation with equilibrium length of a regular, unidimensional spring) and properties of the **force field** in the vicinity of the equilibrium point generated by all the arm muscles (these properties, for a single muscle, can be associated with just one number, apparent stiffness). Actually there is an indirect link between this approach and neurophysiological observations by Donald Humphrey, who identified two groups of neurons in the motor cortex of a monkey. Stimulation of the neurons of the first group caused movement in a joint, while stimulation of the neurons of the other group caused co-contraction of antagonist muscles, thus modifying joint stiffness. This is exactly what we would expect from hypothetical cells controlling equilibrium position and matrix of stiffness.

You can visualize this approach by imagining a ball on an elastic membrane (figure 21.10). The ball will be in an equilibrium on the bottom of a potential well created by its weight. If you want to move the ball to a new point, you can either calculate and apply patterns of forces directly to the ball or change the shape of the elastic force field, for example by pressing near the ball with your finger and then moving your finger to a new position. Note that in the second case, possible errors in the estimation of the mass of the ball, as well as possible small perturbations during the ball movement, will not change the final position: the ball will eventually end up in the same spot, that is, on the bottom of a newly created potential well. This property is called **equifinality.** If the subject of this mental experiment applies force patterns directly to the ball, the same error factors may lead to different ball trajectories and different final positions. Recently, similar approaches have been developed by

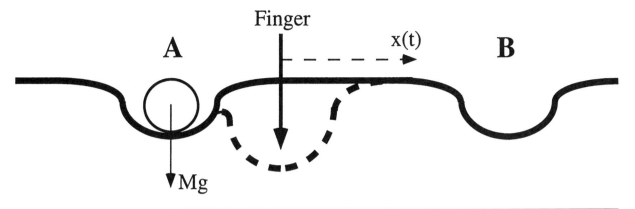

Figure 21.10 An illustration of equilibrium-point control. A ball on an elastic membrane can be moved from point A to point B by pressing with a finger on the membrane close to the ball and moving the finger to point B. No direct contact with the ball is required.

Anatol Feldman and Mindy Levin, who consider control of multi-joint movements with shifting positional frames of reference, and by a group including Emilio Bizzi, Ferdinando Mussa-Ivaldi, and Simon Giszter, who have proposed that multi-joint movements are controlled with combinations of force fields applied to the endpoint of a limb.

At the end of this chapter it is time for the confession that Bernstein's problem remains unsolved, and moreover, that researchers have failed to agree on a universally acceptable formulation for the problem. The author has a feeling that maybe the word "redundancy" is to blame because it means something that one would like to get rid of and therefore may not be appropriate for addressing this problem. Maybe a better word would be "abundance," which also implies the presence of choice and numerous solutions but does not necessarily suggest that they are sources of problems for the central nervous system; rather, abundance may be viewed as a luxury that allows human movements to be flexible, to be switchable, and to display adaptive properties.

Chapter 21 in a Nutshell

Reaching movements to a target are characterized by nearly straight endpoint trajectories, nearly symmetrical bell-shaped velocity profiles, and two-peak acceleration profiles. Movement trajectories vary across trials at the same motor task. Trajectory of the working point (endpoint) demonstrates lower variability than individual joint trajectories. The number of kinematic degrees of freedom (independent joint axes of rotation) in human limbs is typically higher than the number of parameters characterizing motor tasks. The problem of choosing a unique motor pattern from an infinite number of options is known as Bernstein's problem. Bernstein viewed as the main issue of motor control "the elimination of the redundant degrees of freedom." The equilibrium-trajectory hypothesis views control of a multi-joint limb as a process of shift of an equilibrium point defined by the properties of the motor apparatus and the external forces. Exact control variables for multi-joint movements are unknown; they are not muscle force patterns, patterns of muscle activation, or joint trajectories. The motor cortex, the cerebellum, and the red nucleus are likely to be very important for control of voluntary reaching movements.

CHAPTER 22

VISION

Key Terms

anatomy of the eye

light receptors

retina

optic nerve

oculomotor control

central mechanisms of vision

role of vision in movements

22.1. THE EYE

The human eye is a unique device that on the one hand represents a peripheral organ containing receptors sensitive to light and on the other hand, unlike other receptor systems that have been discussed up to now, is part of the central nervous system. The sensory structure of the eye, the retina, is derived during development from the neural ectoderm, which also gives rise to the brain. So, the retina can be considered a peripheral brain structure.

The structure of the human eye is illustrated in figure 22.1. Light entering the eye is focused by the **cornea** and the **lens.** Then it travels through the **vitreous humor** that fills the eye cavity and is absorbed by **photoreceptors** of the **retina.** Behind the retina is a layer of **pigment epithelium** whose cells are packed with a black substance, **melanin.** Melanin absorbs the light that is not captured by the retina and prevents it from being reflected off the back of the eye to the retina again. Pigment epithelium cells also play an important role in the metabolism of retinal cells.

The highest concentration of photoreceptors is in the **fovea,** which also receives the least-distorted light signals because there are relatively few cells between the photoreceptors of the fovea and the lens. The center of the fovea, called the **foveola,** provides the best reception of light signals, so that humans constantly move their eyes to focus the scene of interest on the foveola. Laterally (closer to the nose), with respect to fovea, is the so-

called **blind spot,** an area of the retina where the optic nerve leaves it and where there are thus no photoreceptors. If light reflected by an object falls onto the blind spot, it does not induce any sensory effects.

Problem 22.1

Why don't we perceive "holes" in the environment that could be brought about by the presence of the blind spot?

22.2 PHOTORECEPTORS

There are two types of photoreceptors, **cones** and **rods.** Cones are responsible for day vision when there is plenty of light. They mediate color vision and provide better spatial and temporal resolution than rods. The loss of cones is considered legal blindness. Rods function in dim light and thus provide night vision. The number of rods is 20 times higher than the number of cones; however, there are few rods in the fovea. In addition, signals from rods demonstrate a high degree of convergence; that is, signals from different rods come to the same interneuron. This organization facilitates detection of low stimuli (dim light) but decreases spatial and temporal resolution.

Rods and cones have similar internal structure (figure 22.2). They consist of the **outer segment,** which contains the light-transducing apparatus; the **inner seg-**

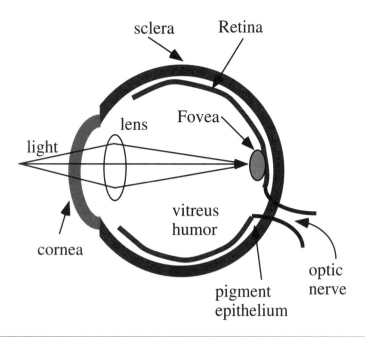

Figure 22.1   Light entering the eye is focused by the cornea and the lens. Then it travels through the vitreous humor and is absorbed by photoreceptors of the retina. Behind the retina is a layer of pigment epithelium whose cells absorb the light that is not captured by the retina.

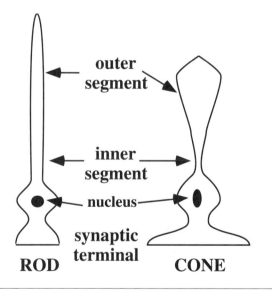

Figure 22.2   Rods and cones consist of an outer segment that contains the light-transducing apparatus, an inner segment containing the nucleus and much of the biochemical machinery, and the synaptic terminal, which makes connections with the receptor's target cells.

ment containing the nucleus and much of the biochemical machinery; and the **synaptic terminal,** which makes connections with the receptor's target cells. Phototransduction results from a series of biochemical events in the outer segment of photoreceptors. Light is absorbed by visual pigments (rhodopsin in rods and cone opsin in cones) leading to the closing of Na⁺ channels,

which blocks the flow of Na⁺ from the extracellular space and hyperpolarizes the receptor membrane.

Problem 22.2

What kind of a visual deficit can you expect in a person who has a much smaller-than-normal amount of rhodopsin?

22.3. RETINA AND OPTIC NERVE

Just below the photoreceptor level of the retina is an intermediate layer containing three types of cells—**bipolar neurons, amacrine cells,** and **horizontal cells** (figure 22.3). Amacrine and horizontal cells provide means for a lateral flow of information, while bipolar cells play the central role in transmitting information from photoreceptors to **ganglionic cells.** Ganglionic cells are located under the intermediate layer. Their round receptive fields are organized in such a way that bipolar neurons in the center of a receptive field are depolarized while bipolar neurons on the periphery are hyperpolarized, thus increasing the contrast of the stimulus (an **on-/off-center response**). As a result, the activity of a ganglionic cell depends not only on the intensity of a stimulus in its receptive area but also on the intensity of the stimuli in the neighboring areas. This explains why humans perceive gray-shaded areas as being darker on a white background than on a black background.

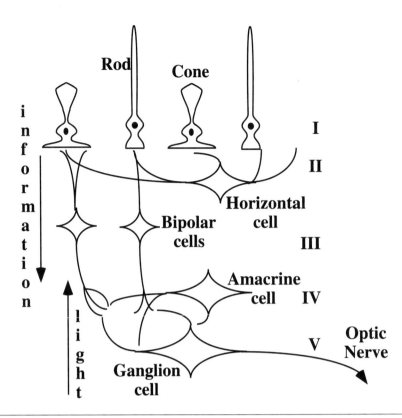

Figure 22.3   Below the photoreceptor level of the retina is an intermediate layer containing three types of cells: bipolar neurons, amacrine cells, and horizontal cells. Ganglionic cells are located under the intermediate layer. Their axons form the optic nerve. I: Outer nuclear layer; II: outer plexiform layer; III: inner nuclear layer; IV: inner plexiform layer; V: ganglion cell layer.

The axons of ganglionic cells form the **optic nerve,** which carries optical information to brain structures. The optic nerve contains one million fibers, more than all the dorsal root fibers entering the spinal cord and much more than the number of auditory fibers (about 30,000).

Two areas are identified in each retina. The **nasal hemiretina** lies medial to the fovea; the **temporal hemiretina** lies lateral to the fovea. If the foveas of both eyes are fixed on one point, it is possible to define a left and a right half of the visual field (the field that is seen without moving the head). The left (right) half of the visual field projects to the nasal hemiretina of the left (right) eye and to the temporal hemiretina of the right (left) eye. Light from the central region of the visual field is called the **binocular zone.** Note that images on the retina are inverted by the lens (figure 22.4).

22.4. OCULOMOTOR CONTROL

Eye movements were extensively studied by a great German physicist and physiologist, von Helmholtz, in the 19th century. In particular, von Helmholtz noticed that voluntary eye movements were associated with a feeling of a stationary visual field, while eye shifts created "artificially" (for example, when you press on your eyeball

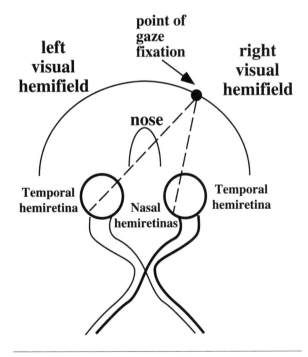

Figure 22.4   Definitions of the left and right visual hemifields. Note that the optic tracts convey information from the ipsilateral temporal hemiretina and contralateral nasal hemiretina, i.e., visual information about the contralateral visual hemifield.

with a finger) lead to the sensation of a moving environment. These observations led him to a hypothesis on an important role of motor command in perception in general and in visual perception in particular.

Each eye is controlled by six muscles that may produce five functionally different types of movement (figure 22.5). These muscles involve **four recti muscles** (superior, inferior, lateral, and medial) and **two oblique muscles** (superior and inferior) that can produce eye rotations around three major axes: **adduction/abduction** (horizontal movements), **elevation/depression** (movements up and down), and **intorsion/extorsion** (rotation without changing the direction of gaze). Torsional movements are not normally used in voluntary shifts of gaze.

Two types of reflex movements keep visual images fixed on the retina (fovea, to be precise) during head movements. The first mechanism is that of the **vestibulo-ocular reflex** (VOR), which acts at a relatively short latency (about 14 ms) at any time during head movements. It changes the activity of ocular muscles and the induced motion of the eyes during head rotations so that the retinal image of the visual field is stabilized. If head rotation continues after the eyes reach the edge of the orbit, the eyes do not stay at the extreme position but rapidly reverse the direction of their movement and jump quickly back. This entire phenomenon is called **vestibular nystagmus;** the rapid reversal is called the quick phase. The VOR is coordinated at the brainstem level. Vestibular receptors send signals about the velocity of head rotation to vestibular nuclei that project on the oculomotor nuclei. The cerebellum participates in modulation of the gain of the VOR.

The second mechanism is the **optokinetic system,** which uses visual information to complement the VOR. It also acts to keep stable features of the environment (faces, buildings, etc.) on the fovea during head movements. Its latency is longer and it takes time to build up. The loop of this reflex involves both cortical and subcortical structures. Both reflex systems demonstrate habituation and alter their gain adaptively, for example, if a person is wearing glasses.

If a person wants to shift gaze from one object of interest to another, his or her eyes will demonstrate a **saccade,** which is a very quick and accurate eye movement reaching a peak velocity of up to 900°/s. Actual peak velocity depends upon the angular distance between the objects and is higher for larger distances. Humans can control voluntarily the direction and amplitude of saccade movements, but not their velocity. Saccade velocity changes only under the influence of drugs, diseases, or fatigue. Saccades are typical examples of movements controlled in a feedforward manner because, apparently, there is no time for any feedback. Saccades are controlled by the **cerebral cortex** with participation of the **basal ganglia** and are generated in the **pontine** and **mesencephalic reticular centers.** Specifically, the pontine reticular formation is the place where horizontal saccades are generated, while the mesencephalic reticular formation generates vertical saccades.

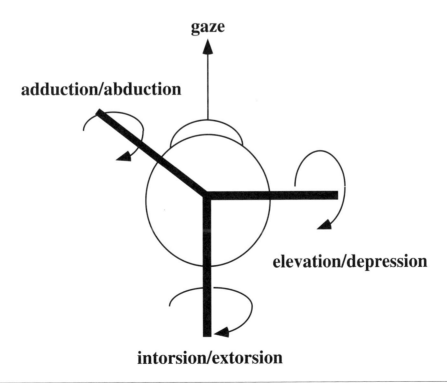

Figure 22.5 Major direction of eye movement.

If the image of an object is fixed on the fovea and the object starts to move, the person keeps its image in the fovea with the system of **smooth pursuit.** Smooth pursuit is a voluntary movement whose velocity can be changed (if there are several objects in the visual field, one can choose a slow one or a fast one to follow). Maximal velocity of smooth pursuit is about 100°/s. It is impossible, however, to make a smooth-pursuit movement without an object to follow. Try it and you will see that your eyes will make a saccade and jump to bring the image of another object into the fovea. Smooth pursuit has a very complex control system that involves the **striate cortex, prestriate motor areas, pons,** and **cerebellum.**

The fifth type of ocular movement is **vergence,** which is different from the first four types in that it induces disconjugate eye movements, that is, rotations in opposite directions. The purpose of these movements is to fix the gaze at targets with different depths. An important role in the organization of vergence is played by midbrain structures in the region of **oculomotor nuclei.**

The mechanism of eye control acts against very low inertia and never encounters unexpected perturbations. Also, fatigue is rarely an issue. As a result, the design of the oculomotor system is different from that of skeletal muscles controlling limb movements. In particular, ocular muscles are rich in muscle spindles but do not demonstrate a stretch reflex. Their motorneuronal pools do not demonstrate recurrent inhibition, and there are no special fast and slow muscles. The discharge frequency of ocular motor neurons is proportional to the position and velocity of the eye (just as with Ia-spindle afferents).

Problem 22.3

What can be the functions of muscle spindles in oculomotor muscles if these muscles do not demonstrate the stretch reflex?

22.5. CENTRAL MECHANISMS OF VISUAL PERCEPTION

The optic nerves from each eye join each other at the **optic chiasm** and form two **optic tracts** (left and right) that project to three subcortical regions (figure 22.6). Only one of the three areas, the **lateral geniculate nucleus,** participates in processes leading to visual perception. The **pretectal area of the midbrain** participates in producing **pupillary** reflexes, while the **superior colliculus** participates in the generation of eye movements.

If one eye receives a light input, its pupil is constricted (this is called the **direct response**) together with the pupil of the other eye (this is called the **consensual response**). These reflexes are mediated by retinal ganglionic neurons whose firing reflects overall changes in

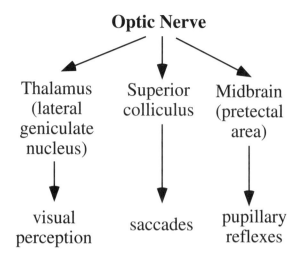

Figure 22.6   The optic nerve projects onto three subcortical areas: lateral geniculate nucleus of the thalamus, pretectal area of the midbrain, and superior colliculus. Projections to the superior colliculus control saccades; pretectal projections control pupillary reflexes; and projections to lateral geniculate nucleus participate in visual perception.

---

brightness. These neurons project to the **pretectal area,** which is located just rostral to the superior colliculi (figure 22.7). The neurons in the pretectal area project to parasympathetic neurons in the **accessory oculomotor nucleus,** which project to the brainstem and innervate the **ciliary ganglion.** This ganglion contains neurons that innervate the smooth muscle of the **pupillary sphincter.**

The **superior colliculi** (figure 22.8) coordinate information from a number of sources—including visual, au-

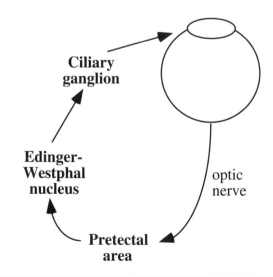

Figure 22.7   Neurons in the pretectal area receive an input from the optic nerve and project to the Edinger-Westphal nucleus, which in turn generates a parasympathetic input to oculomotor neurons in the ciliary ganglion. These neurons innervate the smooth muscle of the pupillary sphincter.

ditory, and somatosensory—and adjust movements of the head and the eyes toward a stimulus. The internal structure of the superior colliculi is rather complex, involving seven layers that contain three **sensory maps:** visual, auditory, and somatosensory. The maps are aligned spatially with respect to each other so that various sensory information about the location of a stimulus with respect to a part of the body is received by a common region of the superior colliculi. These sensory maps connect to a **motor map** located in the deeper layers of the superior colliculi. This organization allows the superior colliculi to use sensory information to participate in control of saccadic (very fast) eye movements together with the frontal eye fields of the cortex.

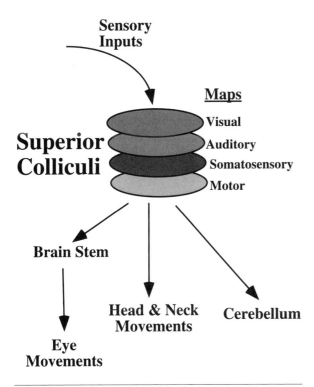

Figure 22.8 The superior colliculi integrate sensory information from different sources and contain three sensory maps and one motor map. The superior colliculi project to the regions of the brainstem that control eye movements and contribute to two descending tracts: the tectospinal tract, which is involved in the reflex control of head and neck movements, and the tectopontine tract, which delivers visual information to the cerebellum for further processing.

The superior colliculi project to the regions of the brainstem that control eye movements and also contribute to two descending tracts: the **tectospinal tract,** which is involved in the reflex control of head and neck movements, and the **tectopontine tract,** which conveys visual information to the cerebellum for further processing.

The majority of retinal axons project to the **lateral geniculate nucleus,** the most important subcortical re-

gion participating in visual perception, which in turn makes projections to the **primary visual cortex** (area 17). Note that the axons from the nasal hemiretinas cross the midline at the optic chiasm whereas the axons from the temporal hemiretinas do not. As a result, the left optic tract contains information from the right visual hemifield, while the right optic tract contains information from the left visual hemifield. The receptive fields of neurons in the lateral geniculate nucleus are similar to those of retinal cells: they are concentric with a diameter of about 1°. There is an on-/off-center response of these neurons, similar to that of the retinal neurons. As a result, neurons in the lateral geniculate nucleus respond best to small, contrasting spots of light and demonstrate a relatively low sensitivity to distributed dim light.

The next relay point in visual processing is the **primary visual cortex** (figure 22.9) or visual area 1 (it is also called the striate cortex, or Brodmann's area 17). The structure of the primary visual cortex is rather complex; an important and unexpected feature, though, is that its neurons are rather insensitive to spots of light (which are very effective stimuli for the retinal and lateral geniculate neurons). The neurons of the primary visual cortex respond best to linear stimuli such as a line or a bar. As a result, these neurons decompose the outlines of a visual image into short line segments of different orientations.

The primary visual cortex is organized into narrow vertical **columns** running from the surface to the white matter. Each column is approximately 30 to 100 μm wide and 2 mm deep. Note that cells with similar axes of orientation tend to be organized in one column. A detailed analysis of the columns reveals that there is an orderly shift in the axis of orientation from one column to its

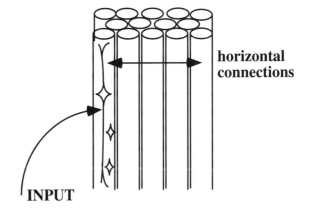

Figure 22.9 The primary visual cortex is organized into narrow vertical columns running from the surface to the white matter. Each column is approximately 30 to 100 μm wide and 2 mm deep. There is an orderly shift in the axis of gaze orientation from one column to its neighbors. There are horizontal connections among columns so that the activity of a neuron within a column may be influenced by stimuli corresponding to other gaze orientations.

neighbors. Occasionally the columns are interrupted by blobs, pear-shaped regions of cells that deal with color perception rather than with orientation. There are horizontal connections among columns so that the activity of a neuron within a column may be influenced by stimuli of other orientations. This may provide a contextual link among different visual stimuli.

Problem 22.4

Suggest a mechanism for the illusion in which one sees a round gray spot in the intersection of two black lines forming a cross.

22.6. THE ROLE OF VISUAL INFORMATION IN VOLUNTARY MOVEMENTS

Most of our movements are performed under visual control. Visual information is used to identify a target and its location in space, and also for corrections of ongoing movements. A crucial role in preparation for a movement toward a visual target is played by the **posterior parietal cortex** (in humans it occupies areas 5, 7, 39, and 40). Note that the posterior parietal cortex demonstrates a high degree of hemispheric specialization. The left posterior parietal cortex specializes in processing linguistic information, while the right posterior parietal cortex plays an important role in processing spatial information. Patients with lesions of this area demonstrate an inability to synthesize movements whose spatial coordinates would correspond to the spatial coordinates of a visual target. They also demonstrate spatial errors in drawing, typically ignoring the contralateral side of the visual field.

Note that area 5 receives its main input from the **somatosensory cortical areas** (1, 2, and 3) and also input from the **vestibular system,** from the **premotor areas,** and from the **limbic cortical structures.** Thus it is informed about limb and body position, head position, motor plans, and motivational state. This area projects to area 7 and to premotor areas.

Area 7 is involved in the processing of visual information related to the location of objects in space. It integrates this information with the somatosensory information from area 5 and auditory inputs from area 22. Area 7 projects to the premotor areas and to the lateral cerebellum and thus participates in directing movements.

The information about central connections of different cortical areas allows one to speculate about the integration of information of different modalities and its role in the control of voluntary movements. Most human everyday movements are planned using visual information about the environment, and many of them are monitored also using visual information. In chapter 19, we analyzed postural perturbations induced by high-frequency muscle vibration (vibration-induced fallings, VIFs). Note that VIFs are strong only when the subject is standing with eyes closed; they are much weaker and can disappear if the eyes are open. This observation suggests that visual information can "override" the artificially changed information from muscle spindles and other proprioceptors. However, we cannot look all the time at all moving body parts. Therefore visual information needs to be supplemented by information from other sensory sources. Projections of information from different sensory systems onto the same cortical areas may well be part of the mechanism of **sensory-motor integration.**

Chapter 22 in a Nutshell

The human eye is a peripheral organ that is also part of the central nervous system. The retina contains two types of sensory receptors, rods and cones, that are sensitive to visible light. Their concentrations are highest in the fovea. After processing by the neuronal apparatus of the retina, signals go to the brain in the optic nerve. At the chiasma, a portion of the fibers within each optic nerve cross to the other side so that two optic tracts are formed, carrying information about the left and right visual fields. Each eye is controlled by three pairs of muscles. These muscle have muscle spindles, but no stretch reflex. Eyes display reflex movements induced by signals from the vestibular receptors (VOR) and from optical receptors (optokinetic system), as well as very fast movements called saccades, slower smooth-pursuit movements, and vergence. The lateral geniculate nucleus participates in processes leading to visual perception. The pretectal area of the midbrain participates in producing pupillary reflexes, while the superior colliculi participate in control of eye movements. Superior colliculi contain several sensory and motor maps, including a visual map. The primary visual cortex is organized into narrow vertical columns running from the surface to the white matter. The posterior parietal cortex is likely to play a major role in the preparation of movements to visual targets.

CHAPTER 23

KINESTHESIA

Key Terms

proprioceptors

the role of motor command in kinesthetic perception

efferent copy

kinesthesia and the equilibrium-point hypothesis

central mechanisms of kinesthesia

vibration-induced illusions

pain

23.1. WHICH PHYSICAL VARIABLES ARE SENSED BY PROPRIOCEPTORS?

Each person is always aware of the position of the segments of his or her body in space and in relation to each other. This sensation is called **kinesthesia.** It allows humans to perform accurate movements without continuous visual control, to adjust motor control patterns with respect to the force field in which they move, to perform motor tasks that require multi-limb coordination, and so on. In a previous chapter, we considered the properties of some of the peripheral receptors whose firing level depends upon such parameters as muscle length, velocity, and force and upon joint angle, pressure on skin, and the like. All these parameters may be used to get kinesthetic information. However, a more careful analysis of the properties of all these receptors shows that the situation is much more complicated; in particular, the mechanical design of human muscles and tendons seems to make the information coming from receptors of each modality dependent on several of the physical parameters mentioned (table 23.1). Let us once again consider the properties of the most important proprioceptors; here, we will view their signals not as peripheral components of the reflex machinery, but as sources of kinesthetic information.

23.2. PERIPHERAL SOURCES OF KINESTHETIC INFORMATION

Muscle spindles and **articular receptors** look like perfect candidates for the role of getting information about the position of segments of the body, while **Golgi tendon organs** seem to be perfect detectors of muscle force.

Remember that muscle spindles are small structures scattered throughout the parent muscle in parallel to the power-producing (extrafusal) muscle fibers. Muscle spindles contain two types of sensory endings, primary and secondary spindle receptors. Primary spindle receptors are sensitive to both muscle length and velocity whereas secondary receptors are sensitive only to muscle length.

Up to this point, things are straightforward. Remember, however, that muscle spindles have a special system of innervation, the **gamma system,** which changes the sensitivity of both primary and secondary receptors. A number of experiments have demonstrated that γ-motoneurons are commonly activated together with α-motoneurons (**α–γ coactivation**), which leads to muscle activation and the development of muscle force and/or movement. This means that the level of activity of a spindle receptor depends not only upon actual muscle length (and velocity, for primary receptors) but also upon the level of muscle activation. For example,

Table 23.1

Receptor	What it measures	Complicating factors
Ia-spindle	Length, velocity	Sensitivity is modulated by gamma motoneurons; muscle fiber length differs from the muscle+tendon length.
II-spindle	Length	
Ib-Golgi tendon organs	Force	Measure force at the point of attachment between muscle fibers and tendons. Force is length and velocity dependent. Torque depends on the effective lever length.
Articular receptors	Joint angle	Show maximal sensitivity close to physiological limits of joint rotation. Rather insensitive in the midrange. Sensitive to joint capsule tension.
Cutaneous and subcutaneous receptors	Pressure on the skin, skin displacement	Skin pressure and displacement may depend on many factors.

consider a muscle in isometric conditions (figure 23.1). The average level of firing of its spindle receptors is proportional to muscle length.

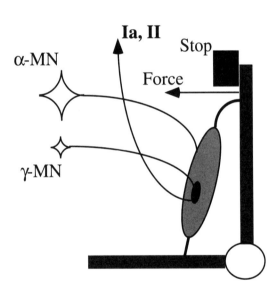

Figure 23.1 An increase in the level of activation of a muscle in isometric conditions leads to an increase in the activity of the gamma system and an increase in the firing level of muscle spindle sensory endings. This may be interpreted by the central nervous system as a joint motion corresponding to an increase in muscle length.

Now imagine that there is an increase in the level of muscle activation. Muscle length will not change, because the conditions are isometric. On the other hand, muscle activation is accompanied by an increase in the activity of the gamma system. So one may expect to see an increase in the activity of spindle endings, which can

be interpreted by the central nervous system as a movement even though the conditions are isometric. On the other hand, if the joint is released (nonisometric conditions, figure 23.2) and the muscle is allowed to shorten, there will be an increase in the level of activity of the γ-motoneurons, which may lead to the same average level of activity of spindle receptors at different values of muscle length. Since humans do not misjudge muscle length at different levels of muscle activation, there must be a mechanism that allows accurate assessment of muscle length in these conditions.

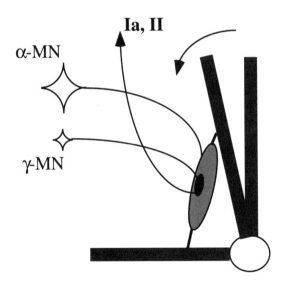

Figure 23.2 In nonisometric conditions, an increase in the level of muscle activation leads to muscle shortening accompanied by an increase in the activity of the gamma system. As a result, one may see the same average level of firing of muscle spindle sensory endings at different joint positions.

Another complicating factor is muscle and tendon **elasticity.** If a muscle is passive, its stiffness is lower than tendon stiffness. If the muscle is activated, its stiffness is considerably higher than tendon stiffness. Imagine again that a muscle is being activated in isometric conditions (figure 23.3). Although the total length of the muscle+tendon complex is unchanged, the length of muscle fibers will decrease during the activation, while the length of the tendon will increase. In order to accurately assess the position of a limb segment, the central nervous system needs to know the length of the muscle+tendon complex rather than the length of individual muscle fibers. However, the level of firing of muscle spindle receptors depends upon the length of muscle fibers and not upon the length of the tendon.

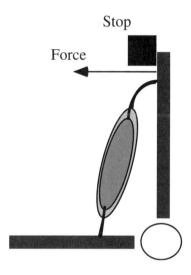

Figure 23.3 In isometric conditions, an increase in the level of muscle activation leads to an increase in the stiffness of muscle fibers, a relative shortening of muscle fibers, and stretching of the tendon.

What about articular receptors? In order to get reliable information about joint angle, it would be desirable to have a receptor whose level of activity is related to joint angle. At first glance, articular receptors seem to fulfil this requirement. However, if only the slowly adapting receptors are considered, that is, those that maintain their level of activity for a long time when there is no joint motion, one can notice that such receptors cover mostly the extremes of the range of joint motion and that they are rather sparse in the middle. This is a good feature for detecting when the joint is approaching the physiological limits of its rotations, but it is not very helpful if the task is to assess joint position somewhere in its midrange. Moreover, articular receptors change their level of firing when the tension of the articular capsule changes. This happens, in particular, when muscles acting at the joint change their force. Again, in isometric conditions

(figure 23.4) there are likely to be changes in the activity of articular receptors with changes in the level of muscle activation even though no movement occurs. It seems that for both articular and spindle receptors, the central nervous system needs to have information about the level of muscle activation and/or muscle forces (or joint torques) in order to calculate muscle length or joint angle. Let us look for sources that may provide this information.

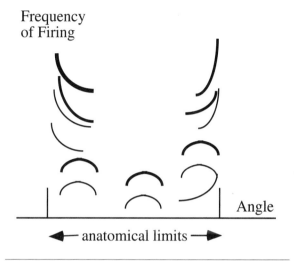

Figure 23.4 Articular receptors show maximal sensitivity to joint angle close to the physiological limits of joint rotation. Their firing level is also sensitive to joint capsule tension (bold curves).

Golgi tendon organs are nearly ideal force detectors that are located in series with muscle fibers. They are not sensitive to muscle length and do not have central innervation. However, calculating joint torques from signals from Golgi tendon organs is not simple, because the relation between muscle force and generated joint torque changes depending upon joint angle due to changes in the lever arm (figure 23.5).

Problem 23.1

Does muscle and tendon elasticity affect signals from Golgi tendon organs? Do these receptors always accurately monitor muscle force?

So the reader may end up with the seemingly pessimistic conclusion that there are no peripheral receptors signaling functionally significant posture and movement parameters such as joint torques and positions. Remember, though, the basic philosophical principle: *if a system within the human body looks imperfectly designed, it is likely that we have overlooked or misinterpreted something.* Accurate kinesthetic perception is likely to emerge with participation of signals

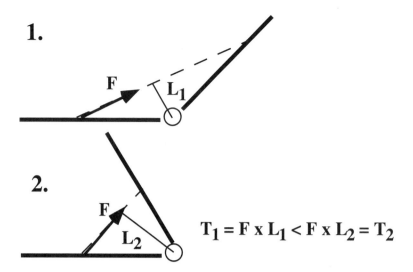

$$T_1 = F \times L_1 < F \times L_2 = T_2$$

Figure 23.5   Joint torque is the sum of products of muscle forces and corresponding lever arms. Joint movement leads to a change in the lever arm, and therefore joint torque is dependent on both muscle force and joint angle.

from various sensors, and this design has more positive features than potential problems. For example, if articular receptors were the only source of positional information and were absolute reliable, inflammation of a joint (which is unfortunately rather common) would cause a major deterioration of kinesthetic perception. If there is a mixture of kinesthetic information represented in receptors of different types, the system becomes less susceptible to a disorder of one of the receptor systems. Actually, even if a joint is replaced with an artificial one, position sense virtually does not suffer.

It is time now to turn to the role of motor command in kinesthetic perception. This issue was touched on briefly in the chapter on control of eye movements. Remember that if you displace your eye by pressing on it with a finger, you perceive a shift of the environment, whereas an active eye movement does not lead to a similar false perception.

23.3. THE ROLE OF THE MOTOR COMMAND IN KINESTHESIA

An important role of **voluntary motor command** in kinesthetic perception was hypothesized by von Holst, who introduced the notion of an **efferent copy** (sometimes called an "efference copy"). It is supposed that an efferent copy represents a copy of a voluntary motor command and participates in deciphering the mixed information from peripheral receptors. Its importance is particularly obvious in the case of spindle receptors, because the level of activity of these receptors depends on the activity of the gamma system, which in turn depends on the current descending motor command.

In order to discuss the role of central motor command in kinesthetic perception, one needs to specify what

the motor command is. Based on my personal views on motor control, I am going to accept the **equilibrium-point hypothesis** (see chapter 10). According to this hypothesis, a motor command to a muscle represents a value of the threshold of the tonic stretch reflex and may be described with a position of the tonic stretch reflex characteristic on the force-length plane (figure 23.6). As such, a given value of the motor command makes only certain combinations of muscle length and force stable (those corresponding to points on the force-length curve) and thus helps to solve the problem of position and force perception. In more formal terms, it cuts a single-dimensional subspace from the two-dimensional state-space of the muscle.

Actually, when a person chooses a motor command, half of the problem of perception is solved. Now it is necessary to cut another single-dimensional subspace in the muscle state-space, that is, to draw another line on the force-angle plane. This line can be derived from a weighted sum of afferent activities from all the available sources (figure 23.7). Note that each point on the tonic stretch reflex characteristic is characterized by different values of muscle force, muscle length, and joint angle. This means that each point has a unique combination of activity levels of the spindle, Golgi, and articular receptors. The information from these sources is redundant, but this redundancy (or shall we call it abundance?) helps to overcome potential problems if any one of the sources becomes unreliable, for example as a result of a disease.

Thus when a motor command to a muscle is specified, two characteristics emerge on the force-angle plane. One corresponds to a chosen value of the central command (λ, according to the equilibrium-point hypothesis), while the other corresponds to a certain level of activity of proprioceptors and signals the state of the peripheral

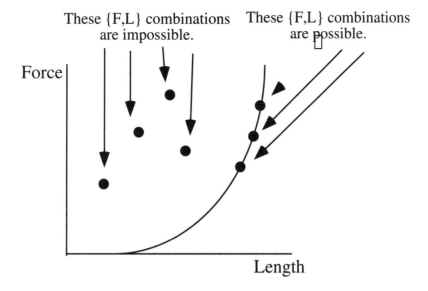

Figure 23.6 According to the equilibrium-point hypothesis, motor command to a muscle can be described as a fixed force-length characteristic (the tonic stretch reflex characteristic). As such, it allows only certain combinations of muscle force and length to occur in a static (equilibrium) state and solves half of the problem of muscle force and length perception.

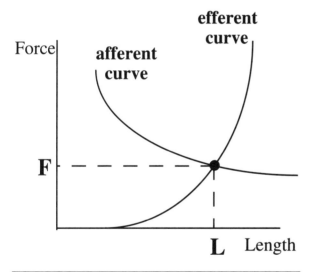

Figure 23.7 When we send a motor command, two characteristics emerge on the force-angle plane. The first corresponds to a chosen value of the central command (efferent curve), while the second corresponds to a certain level of activity of proprioceptors (afferent curve). The intersection of the characteristics defines current perceived values of muscle length and force.

apparatus. The intersection of the two characteristics defines current values of muscle length and force.

Problem 23.2

What kind of illusions can be expected from muscle vibration on the basis of the servo hypothesis of Merton and on the basis of direct force control?

23.4. WHERE DOES THE INFORMATION GO?

Signals from a peripheral receptor travel along the peripheral end of the **T-shaped axon** of a ganglionic neuron and then are transmitted along the central end of the sensory axon into the spinal cord (figure 23.8). Sensory axons from receptors of differing modality ascend into supraspinal structures within the **ipsilateral dorsal column** and make synapses in the dorsal column nuclei at the medullar level. Neurons within these nuclei cross the midline and ascend further on the contralateral side of the body to the **ventral posterior nucleus** of the thalamus in the **medial lemniscus pathway.** The **thalamus** is a major relay that transmits sensory information to the sensory cortical areas. **Thalamocortical** projections are made via a large bundle of fibers called the **internal capsule.**

There are two major types of thalamic nuclei. **Relay nuclei** process either a single sensory modality or information from a distinct part of the body; they project to a specific region of the cerebral cortex and receive recurrent input from the same cortical region. **Diffuse-projection nuclei** mostly deal with transmitting afferent inputs related to the functioning of the limbic structures and modulation of the thalamus' own activity. Their projections are more widespread. Somatosensory perception, which is presently the focus of our attention, is transmitted via a relay, the **ventral posterior nucleus.**

Thalamic inputs terminate in the parietal cortex, in the somatosensory areas. There they create sensory maps that look like distorted images of the body with a disproportionate representation of the face, tongue, hand, and particularly the thumb (figure 23.9). It is supposed that information processing within the cortex leads to

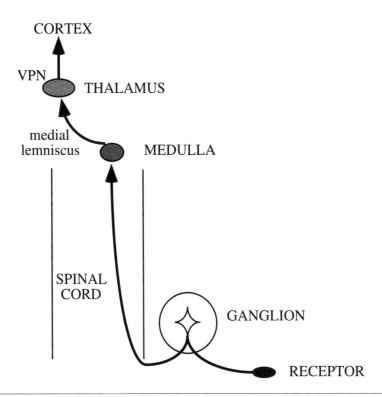

Figure 23.8   Sensory axons from receptors of different modalities ascend within the ipsilateral dorsal column and make synapses at the medullar level within the dorsal column nuclei. Neurons within these nuclei send their axons in the medial lemniscus pathway to the contralateral ventral posterior nucleus (VPN) of the thalamus.

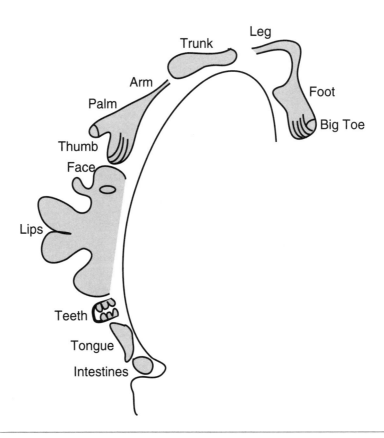

Figure 23.9   Thalamic inputs project to the somatosensory areas within the parietal cortex where touch receptors form distorted maps of the body surface (a sensory homunculus).

conscious perception and also participates in the use of kinesthetic information for purposes of control of voluntary movements.

23.5. KINESTHETIC ILLUSIONS

Under the term **kinesthetic illusions,** researchers imply misperceptions of the position or movement of a body segment or of the whole body. Since kinesthetic perception is based on an interaction of two processes, a control process (an efferent copy) and a sensory process, two kinds of kinesthetic illusions can theoretically occur. Illusions of the first type may result from distorted signals from peripheral receptors of a certain modality or distorted central processing of afferent signals, while illusions of the second type may result from a distorted efferent copy signal, that is, when a muscle receives a command that differs from what is expected by the brain based on the efferent copy.

Problem 23.3

Suggest an example of a kinesthetic illusion induced by an unusual activity of skin receptors.

Illusions of the first type have been most widely studied using **muscle vibration.** As already mentioned, muscle vibration is a very potent stimulus for muscle spindle receptors and induces an unusually high level of activity of these sensory endings. The central nervous system interprets these signals as a sign of an increase in the muscle length and, in the absence of other sources of information, generates an illusory perception of a new joint position that corresponds to an increased muscle length. For example, vibration of the biceps muscle induces the feeling of an elbow joint extension that corresponds to a longer biceps. Thus, if an experimenter asks a subject to match elbow joint angles of two arms during vibration of the biceps of one of the arms, the subject will extend the elbow joint on the side of the vibration less because the length of the biceps is overestimated (figure 23.10). These illusions may be very strong and may even lead to perception of anatomically impossible joint positions, for example a hyperextension in the elbow. If another source of information is available, for example if the subject looks at his/her arm, the illusion disappears.

Problem 23.4

Vibration of a muscle that is shortening during a movement is much less effective (or is even ineffective) for inducing kinesthetic illusions as compared to vibration of the same muscle during a movement corresponding to its stretch. Why?

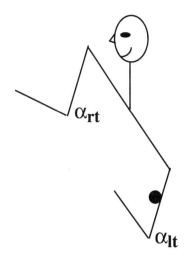

Figure 23.10   If a vibrator is placed on the biceps of one arm, the subject's central nervous system overestimates the length of the biceps because of the increased activity of spindle sensory endings. As a result, the subject perceives joint positions of the two elbows as being equal while the elbow joint on the side of vibration is more flexed (compare α_{lt} and α_{rt}).

Note, however, that the effects of muscle vibration are complex and may involve both sensory and motor effects (e.g., the tonic vibration reflex). As a result, vibration-induced illusions are sometimes not that simple and straightforward. In particular, the direction of an illusory joint motion may reverse if the subject is experiencing sensory stimulation of another modality (e.g., auditory or visual). These observations suggest that muscle vibration may distort the other, efferent component of kinesthetic perception, that is, the efferent copy as well.

It is theoretically possible to induce a motor illusion if muscle activation level is artificially changed. This can be done, for example, by a direct electrical muscle stimulation superimposed on a voluntarily induced contraction.

Problem 23.5

What kind of kinesthetic illusion can you expect if a joint flexor muscle is directly stimulated by an electrical stimulator?

23.6. PAIN

The sense of **pain** is a subjective feeling, an unpleasant sensation in a certain region of the body that represents an important defensive mechanism of the human body, frequently informing it about potentially damaging stimuli. The sense of pain may seem a nuisance;

however, patients who lack this sense are in constant danger of not noticing stimuli that may induce a major injury (e.g., a very hot iron, a burner, or a chemical that can damage skin).

The sense of pain has its own mechanism of peripheral receptors (**nociceptors**) and central neural structures. Nociceptors are scattered all over the body, both in the skin and in deep tissues, and represent small sensory endings that generate action potential in response to a potentially damaging stimulus of a certain modality, such as temperature, pressure, or certain chemicals. These signals are transmitted along thin, fibers of the Aδ and C type. The speed of action potential transmission along Aδ fibers is in the range from 5 to 30 m/s, while C fibers transmit impulses at speeds ranging from 0.5 to 2 m/s (see chapter 3). Activation of Aδ fibers by thermal or mechanical stimuli leads to the sensation of sharp, pricking pain. Activation of C fibers is associated with the sensation of long-lasting, burning pain.

The sensitivity of nociceptors may be increased by damage of peripheral tissues or inflammation (**hyperalgesia**), which may result in a decrease in the threshold of stimuli perceived as painful or an increase in the magnitude of pain without a change in the threshold.

Pain can emerge, however, in the absence of activity of nociceptors. Typical examples involve pain accompanying damage of a peripheral nerve or phantom pain after amputation of a limb. The worst possible scenario is **chronic pain** that may be felt in an area of the body even after a total transection of the spinal cord that does not allow signals from this area to reach the brain. The origins of chronic pain are not clear, and its therapy is commonly unsuccessful. One hypothesis is that the subjective feeling of pain is created by a disparity between signals from proprioceptors and signals from nociceptors (figure 23.11). This is called the **gate control theory of pain.** This theory predicts that a decrease in the activity of proprioceptors may be a strong enough factor to induce a feeling of chronic pain without any additional contribution from nociceptors. For example, in **ischemia** (block of blood flow into a limb), the first fibers to suffer and stop transmitting impulses are the fastest-conducting ones. These involve, in particular, Ia- and Ib-afferents from muscle spindles and Golgi tendon organs and also Aα fibers from large cutaneous receptors. If the blood flow in a person's arm is blocked, after a few minutes the person will report a burning pain in the arm, which will subside after some time. When the blood flow is restored, the pain returns again and disappears after a few minutes. Probably everyone has experienced a similar feeling when a limb "falls asleep" after prolonged maintenance of an uncomfortable posture and then "wakes up." These observations may be explained by the ordered blockade and restoration of conduction along afferent fibers of differing size.

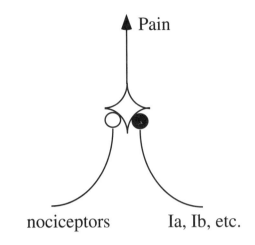

Figure 23.11 The gate control theory of pain is based on an interaction of afferent signals from nociceptors and proprioceptors. These signals converge on common interneurons that receive excitatory synapses from nociceptors and inhibitory synapses from proprioceptors. A decrease in the activity in proprioceptive afferents may lead to a disinhibition of the interneuron, leading to a feeling of persistent pain.

Problem 23.6

On the basis of the idea that pain equals signals in nociceptors minus signals in proprioceptors, suggest a method of treating chronic pain.

The afferent fibers of nociceptors enter the spinal cord through the dorsal roots and make synaptic connections with interneurons in laminae I to V. They also send branches in the **Lissauer tract** that make synaptic connections a few segments rostrally and a few segments caudally with respect to the dorsal root entrance. This mixture of information among several segments may underlie, in particular, the phenomenon of pain irradiation, that is, its spread beyond the apparent limits of the nociceptive stimulus.

Nociceptive information is transmitted to the brain structures along five major ascending pathways. These are the **spinothalamic tract,** the **spinoreticular tract,** the **spinomesencephalic tract** (going to the mesencephalic reticular formation), the **spinocervical tract** terminating in the lateral cervical nucleus, and the tract that runs in the dorsal column of the spinal cord to the cuneate and gracile nuclei of the medulla. The spinothalamic tract has been most extensively studied. The **thalamus** apparently relays the nociceptive information to the cerebral cortex; however, it is not clear how the cortex processes these signals. In particular, patients with extensive cortical lesions of the somatosensory areas do not lose the ability to perceive pain.

Pain can be controlled by central mechanisms. Specifically, electrical stimulation of certain brain areas, including the ventrobasal region of the thalamus and the internal capsule, can produce analgesia without affecting the sense of touch and temperature. The descending pathway mediating analgesia has been shown to involve medullar structures such as the **nucleus raphe magnus** and **nucleus paragiganto cellularis** and the **dorsolateral funiculus.** An increase in the activity along this pathway leads to suppression of activity of dorsal horn neurons that respond to noxious stimuli. Similar effects can be produced by the action of opiates (e.g., morphine) and are likely to be mediated by the same mechanism. Opioid and non-opioid mechanisms are likely to be involved in analgesia induced by stress, which is well known from anecdotal reports by athletes, soldiers, and explorers.

Chapter 23 in a Nutshell

Kinesthetic perception is based on signals from proprioceptors. Each type of proprioceptor provides information that is in itself insufficient to extract joint angle or torque. A copy of motor command signals (the efferent copy) is likely to play an important role in kinesthetic perception. Unusually high activity of proprioceptors (as during muscle vibration) can lead to kinesthetic illusions. Information from proprioceptors ascends in the ipsilateral dorsal column, crosses the midline at the medullar level, and ascends further in the contralateral side of the body to the ventral posterior nucleus of the thalamus and then to the cortex via thalamocortical projections. Somatosensory areas in the parietal cortex play a major role in kinesthetic perception. Pain is a safety mechanism; it is linked to activity in certain types of peripheral receptors (nociceptors). The subjective feeling of pain is likely to get a contribution from the disparity between signals from nociceptors and signals from proprioceptors (gate control theory of pain).

CHAPTER 24

FATIGUE

Key Terms

muscle mechanisms of
fatigue

spinal mechanisms of
fatigue

supraspinal mechanisms of
fatigue

adaptations during fatigue

abnormal fatigue

24.1. FATIGUE AND ITS CONTRIBUTORS

Human beings demonstrate a striking difference from machines in their reaction to prolonged use. Machines basically deteriorate with functioning, and the best machines are those that do not require repair for a long time. The situation with the "human machine" is the opposite, at least on a certain time scale. The longer a human being practices a certain activity, the better he or she performs it. Humans not only do not become worse with work but, quite the opposite, become stronger, quicker, more endurant, and more dexterous, particularly with respect to the type of activity that has been performed. This feature of living organisms has been termed **exercisability.**

However, on a short-term scale, humans can demonstrate machinelike behavior; their performance drops, and this drop may also spread to other types of activities. This phenomenon is commonly called **fatigue.** Among most apparent causes of fatigue, one can name **shortage of chemical fuel** for muscle work and the inability of the circulatory system to quickly remove the **products of muscle metabolism** (lactic acid being probably the best-known one). However, fatigue is a complex phenomenon that may involve factors at different levels contributing to the overall drop in performance. These may include

a. a decrease in the ability of muscle fibers to generate force,

b. a decrease in the efficacy of neuromuscular synapses,

c. changes in the activity of certain peripheral receptors leading to changes in their reflex effects,

d. changes in the patterns of firing (recruitment patterns) of α-motoneurons,

e. changes at any level of the hypothetical process of generation of a motor command, and

f. psychological factors, including, in particular, motivation.

For the purposes of the discussion I will address all changes that occur in the neuromuscular synapse and in the muscle as **peripheral,** and all changes that occur earlier (in the α-motoneurons, the spinal cord, and the brain) as **central.**

There are rather straightforward methods for studying the relative contribution of peripheral and central factors in fatigue. In particular, if a short episode of electrical stimulation is applied to a muscle or its motor nerve, a direct muscle contraction can be induced. If a fatigued muscle demonstrates contractions whose characteristics are different from those in nonfatigued muscles, apparently all these differences may be attributed to peripheral factors. On the other hand, if the response of a muscle to direct electrical stimulation is unchanged while its force during voluntary activation is decreased, the decrease in force may be attributed to central factors. Despite the existence of such seemingly direct methods, the relative contributions of central and peripheral factors to fatigue are still very much under discussion.

Not all the changes occurring in the muscle or the central nervous system with fatigue are detrimental. Some of them may actually be considered **adaptive,** that is, an attempt to counteract the drop in active force produced by a fatigued muscle.

24.2. MUSCULAR MECHANISMS OF FATIGUE

Some fatigue-induced changes occur within a muscle. These changes have been studied mostly in animal preparations in which fatigue has been induced by a prolonged direct electrical stimulation of a muscle. Among these changes are the following:

1. **Slowing of conduction velocity** of the muscle action potential leading to a decrease in its amplitude and an increase in its duration when recorded with surface electrodes (figure 24.1). Eventually, the action potential may stop propagating completely. Similar effects have been shown in experiments with an increase in the extracellular K^+ concentration. So the efflux of K^+ ions during muscle action potentials has been assumed to contribute to this effect.

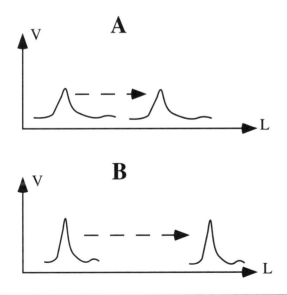

Figure 24.1   An action potential recorded in a fatigued muscle (A) by surface electrodes has a smaller amplitude, longer duration, and slower conduction speed than in a nonfatigued muscle (B).

Problem 24.1

Why does the slowing of conduction lead to a decrease in the amplitude and an increase in the duration of a potential recorded from the muscle surface?

---

2. Alteration of the **excitation threshold** of muscle fibers to external stimulation, which may contribute to the slowing of conduction of action potentials just mentioned.

3. **Slowing of the relaxation phase** after a twitch contraction. There may be a two- to threefold increase in the time from the peak of a contraction to the time when the force drops to 50% of the peak value (figure 24.2). Possible mechanisms for this phenomenon include the slowing of Ca^{++} removal following a decrease in the ATP concentration and changes in the time course of cross-bridge detachment after Ca^{++} ions are removed.

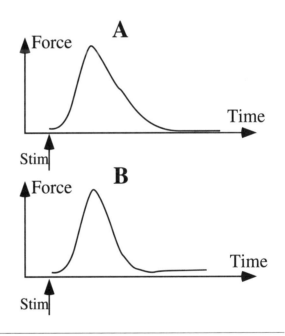

Figure 24.2   A twitch contraction of a fatigued muscle (A) is characterized by a longer relaxation phase than in nonfatigued muscle (B).

4. After a brief tetanic stimulation, twitch contraction force is commonly increased for a short time. This effect is called **post-tetanic potentiation.** However, an inverse effect has also been described after a longer tetanic contraction. The twitch peak becomes smaller and is prolonged mostly due to the prolongation of the relaxation phase (see figure 24.2).

Restoration of muscle characteristics after a fatiguing tetanic stimulation may take minutes or even hours.

24.3. SPINAL MECHANISMS OF FATIGUE

Maximal voluntary contraction force declines with prolonged contraction and has been used as the most common index of fatigue. The drop in muscle force is accompanied by a decrease in α-motoneuron excitability and a decrease in the frequency of firing of individual motor units. Individual motor units differ in their ability to maintain a constant level of firing during prolonged contractions (see chapter 6). Basically, smaller, slower motor units are less fatigable and are able to maintain a constant level of firing throughout a prolonged contraction. Larger, faster motor units are more likely to show a decrease in the level of firing and even to fail to maintain a sustained level of activity. According to the Henneman principle, larger motor units are likely to recruit last and to derecruit first during voluntary changes in muscle force. Both recruitment order and modulation of discharge rate can be changed by fatigue; in particular, the variability of the discharge frequency increases. However, the basic size principle holds in fatigued muscles as well. This principle also works for the pattern of derecruitment during a prolonged, fatiguing contraction at a constant level: larger motor units will show a decrease in the frequency of firing and derecruitment, while the induced drop in muscle force will be compensated by recruitment of new motor units or a change in the firing pattern of already recruited motor units.

Problem 24.2

Prolonged fatiguing contraction is frequently accompanied by tremor at a frequency of 4-6 Hz. Can you suggest a mechanism for this phenomenon?

A fatigue-induced decline in EMG has been shown to be central to the neuromuscular junction and has been suggested to result mainly from **autogenic reflex inhibition** of the α-motoneuronal pool (inhibition originating from receptors within a muscle and affecting motoneurons innervating the same muscle). In particular, a **decrease in the H-reflex** amplitude has been observed in fatigued muscles. However, the origin of the presumed reflex effects is unknown. One hypothesis favors a decline in spindle afferent firing rate during isometric contractions as the primary cause of the reflex-induced inhibition of α-motoneurons; an alternative hypothesis suggests that this inhibition originates from small afferents of groups III and IV (including free nerve endings) reacting to the products of muscle metabolism.

Problem 24.3

A decrease in apparent joint stiffness has been reported during fatigue. Suggest a mechanism for this finding.

If a subject is maintaining a constant level of isometric force, there is a gradual increase in the average level of interference EMG recorded by surface electrodes. This increase is mostly due to the recruitment of new motor units, which compensates for a decrease in the contribution of fatigued motor units to total muscle force. Discharge frequency of motor units changes only slightly.

Changes in various components of muscle reflexes to stretch have been described in fatigued muscles. Specifically, monosynaptic reflexes (in particular, the H-reflex) are suppressed. Conflicting results have been reported for the long-latency reflexes (sometimes called preprogrammed or triggered reactions; see chapter 12), including no changes or a decrease in gain. Moreover, the tonic stretch reflex is also likely to have a smaller gain in fatigued muscles.

24.4. SUPRASPINAL MECHANISMS OF FATIGUE

Basically, all the supraspinal structures involved in control of voluntary muscle activation can contribute to the decrease in muscle force during fatigue. In general, prolonged, fatiguing contractions in humans are accompanied by a gradual increase in the activity of cortical neurons, as well as by an increase in the *Bereitschaftpotential* (readiness potential; see chapter 14). Experiments on monkeys demonstrated changes in the activity of neurons in the primary motor area during prolonged muscle contraction. However, these changes could vary from animal to animal and from neuron to neuron. So at present it is impossible to identify supraspinal structures or mechanisms that can be blamed for playing a particularly important role in the fatigue-induced drop in voluntary muscle contraction force.

24.5. ADAPTIVE CHANGES DURING FATIGUE

First it is necessary to define what an "adaptive change" is (also see chapter 27). This term can be used with respect to all secondary changes that occur in an organism as a reaction to some phenomenon, for example, to fatigue. Some of these changes, however, may be forced upon the system and may not be helpful in counteracting the unwanted effects of the original cause. For example, if a stone hits a window, the glass may break.

This is apparently not an adaptive reaction. However, if the glass has an ability to change its mechanical properties in response to an impact, for example, to become viscous and absorb the energy of the stone without breaking, this would be a useful adaptive reaction. Unfortunately, in humans and animals, the problem of "usefulness" of a reaction may not have an unambiguous solution. For example, if a person co-contracts many limb and trunk muscles and stiffens all the joints in a certain situation, this reaction looks suboptimal if one considers energy expenditure. However, the reaction may serve a purpose, for example, if unexpected external perturbations can occur and the person does not want to change posture or lose balance. So I will consider all secondary reactions within the human body as "adaptive" if they are not obviously forced upon the body. In some cases, it will be possible to classify a reaction as useful or detrimental; in many cases, however, this is impossible to do with certainty.

A number of adaptive mechanisms to fatigue have been suggested. In particular, the **prolongation of the relaxation phase** (figure 24.2) may be considered adaptive and useful because it does not allow muscle force to drop quickly when the ability of the muscle to generate a new contraction is impaired and/or when action potentials are generated by α-motoneurons at a lower frequency. A negative correlation between prolongation of the relaxation phase and firing frequency of individual motor units has been reported. This finding makes sense, because the prolongation of the relaxation phase helps generate smooth muscle contractions in conditions of a low-frequency motoneuronal drive.

Synchronization of motor unit discharges is another adaptive mechanism. It leads to an increase in muscle force, although it may eventually lead to burstlike activity and to a sawtooth-like tetanus rather than smooth tetanus. Synchronization of motor units occurs not only in fatigue but also in motor disorders characterized by reduced muscle force (paresis) due to damage of the central nervous system. In conditions of an increased synchronization of motor unit discharges, the **spectrum** of an EMG recorded by surface electrodes demonstrates a shift toward the area of lower frequencies (figure 24.3).

Problem 24.4

Why does the EMG spectrum shift to lower frequencies in conditions of excessive motor unit synchronization? Can you suggest conditions under which a spectral shift toward high frequencies may be expected?

The central nervous system apparently makes use of the notorious **redundancy** of the motor apparatus at dif-

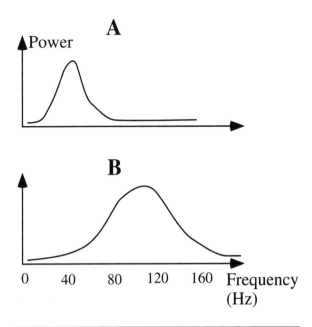

Figure 24.3 Spectrum of an EMG recorded by surface electrodes in a fatigued muscle (A) is shifted toward low frequencies as compared to the spectrum of an EMG recorded in a nonfatigued muscle (B).

ferent levels. For example, if there are several muscles that can contribute to joint torque in a certain direction, their relative contribution can be rotated during a prolonged fatiguing contraction, so that fatigued muscles get a rest period without a drop in total joint torque. Similar effects can apparently be seen at the level of motor unit recruitment when, during a prolonged contraction, a group of motor units can be derecruited (turned off) and replaced through recruitment of another group of motor units; at a later time, the second group may take a rest while the first will resume firing.

24.6. ABNORMAL FATIGUE

Patients with **multiple sclerosis** often demonstrate an abnormal sense of tiredness, out of proportion to the degree of daily effort or degree of disability, which represents a major disabling factor. This sense is commonly addressed as "fatigue," although patients with multiple sclerosis commonly regard it as a fundamentally different experience than ordinary fatigue. However, when tested in laboratory conditions requiring a prolonged, fatiguing contraction of one muscle group, patients with multiple sclerosis show a faster drop in muscle force suggesting a change in the "ordinary" muscle fatigue as well. A study of the relative contributions of central and peripheral factors to muscle fatigue in multiple sclerosis demonstrated an apparent role for the central factors that was not seen in healthy subjects. This is an expected result, because the primary underlying cause of all the symptoms in multiple sclerosis is demyelination of fast-conducting axons within the central nervous system.

Recently, much attention has been drawn to a state characterized by exhaustion and inability to be involved in virtually any kind of activity requiring even minimal motor effort. This condition has been termed **chronic fatigue syndrome.** The syndrome is of an unknown etiology, with a possible role played by an episode of viral infection or by a central neurological disorder. It is unclear whether changes in muscle fatigue contribute to this condition or whether it has an absolutely different, central nature. Unfortunately, there is no treatment.

Chapter 24 in a Nutshell

Fatigue is a complex phenomenon that receives contribution from peripheral, central neural, and psychological factors. Fatigued muscles show slower conduction velocity of action potentials and prolonged twitch contractions, primarily due to the prolongation of the relaxation phase. Fatigue-related reflex changes, particularly the suppression of the H-reflex, are likely to be mediated by changes in the activity of small receptors of groups III and IV. During voluntary contraction, there is a decline in the EMG level, while motor units show an increase in the synchronization of their firing patterns with fatigue. Prolonged, fatiguing contractions in humans are accompanied by a gradual increase in the activity of cortical neurons, as well as by an increase in the readiness potential. An unusual sense of fatigue (e.g., chronic fatigue and fatigue in multiple sclerosis) is likely to be mostly of a central nature.

Self-Test Problems

1. A person demonstrates normal ocular reflexes and no changes in the peripheral eye structures. What pathology can you suspect if the person reports no visual experiences (blindness)?

2. Suggest example(s) of kinesthetic illusions induced by distorted or inappropriate efferent copy signals.

3. A student is standing quietly. Unexpectedly, a friend pushes her from behind. Describe all the mechanisms that help the student not to fall down.

4. When a person increases the speed of walking, at some speed he/she will be forced to start running. Explain this observation based on the ideas of motor programming (CPG) and the ideas of dynamic pattern generation.

5. Describe changes in H-reflexes, M-responses, EMG patterns during fast single-joint movements, and corrective postural reactions that can be expected in fatigued muscles.

6. A standing person wants to initiate walking, that is, to take a first step with the right leg. What kind of anticipatory changes can you expect to see in the background activity of leg and trunk muscles prior to the step?

Recommended Additional Readings

Dietz V (1992). Human neuronal control of automatic functional movements: Interaction between central programs and afferent input. *Physiological Reviews* 72: 33-69.

Enoka RM (1994). *Neuromechanical Basis of Kinesiology.* 2nd ed. Champaign, IL: Human Kinetics. Chapters 7, 8.

Grillner S (1975). Locomotion in vertebrates: Central mechanisms and reflex interaction. *Physiological Reviews* 55: 247-304.

Latash ML (1993). *Control of Human Movement.* Champaign, IL: Human Kinetics. Chapter 7.

Massion J. (1992). Movement, posture and equilibrium: Interaction and coordination. *Progress of Neurobiology* 38: 35-56.

Meijer OG, Wagenaar RC, Blankendaal FCM (1988). The hierarchy debate: Tema con variazione. In: Meijer OG, Roth K (Eds.), *Complex Movement Behavior: The Motor-Action Controversy,* pp. 489-561. Amsterdam: Elsevier.

Nashner LM (1979). Organization and programming of motor activity during posture control. In: Granit R, Pompeiano O (Eds.), *Reflex Control of Posture and Movement,* pp. 177-184. Amsterdam: Elsevier.

Turvey MT, Carello C (1996). Dynamics of Bernstein's level of synergies. In: Latash ML, Turvey MT (Eds.), *Dexterity and Its Development,* pp. 339-376. Mahwah, NJ: Erlbaum.

WORLD V

DISORDERS

CHAPTER 25

SPASTICITY

Key Terms

spinal cord injury

signs and symptoms of spasticity

effects on voluntary movements

treatment

multiple sclerosis

25.1. CHALLENGES OF CLINICAL STUDIES

Clinical observations present a serious challenge to any neurophysiological analysis of motor behavior. First, the language of clinical reports differs substantially from the language of theoretical or experimental studies of movements and requires some kind of translation to make the data interpretable. For example, such commonly used clinical terms as **"hypotonia"** and **"rigidity"** do not have clear neurophysiological definitions and reflect an impression that an expert (a neurologist or physical therapist) gets during a clinical examination of a patient. Second, movement pathologies are usually defined in terms of signs and symptoms rather than in terms of neurophysiological mechanisms, in part because of the virtual lack of knowledge about the underlying mechanisms. At best, some of the commonly studied motor pathologies are associated with dysfunction of a relatively well-localized anatomical formation within the central nervous system, for example with pathological changes in basal ganglia as in Parkinson's disease and Huntington's chorea. Let us consider two very common causes for movement disorders whose consequences include impoverished control of voluntary movements and, frequently, increased involuntary movements.

25.2. SPINAL CORD INJURY

Injury of the spinal cord is, unfortunately, a not very rare consequence of auto accidents, diving accidents, and some athletic activities. Such an injury may have a number of very serious consequences. Only a fraction of these are directly related to the primary mechanical damage to tissues, including neural structures; the rest are induced by secondary phenomena such as edema, loss of presynaptic input to groups of neurons, and others.

Two major groups of consequences of a spinal cord injury may be identified. The first group is related to the destruction of the **intraspinal neuronal apparatus** including both interneurons and motoneurons. In particular, if all the α-motoneurons of a pool controlling a certain skeletal muscle are destroyed, it is impossible to restore normal voluntary control of the muscle. At the very best, it may be possible to substitute for the lost muscle control with artificial devices driven by voluntary effort generated by the subject, for example, using EMG signals from healthy muscles (or from other sources) to drive electrical stimulators applied to paralyzed muscles. This approach is addressed as **functional electrical stimulation.**

The second group of consequences includes those related to an injury of neural conduction pathways, both ascending and descending. Apparently, a total transection of the spinal cord leads to both complete paralysis and a lack of sensations below the level of trauma. To date, all attempts at restoring the function of the spinal cord after its total transection have been unsuccessful. As a result, therapies are frequently directed not at restoration of a lost function but at substituting for it, for example, by means of functional electrical stimulation or various assisting devices, with the ultimate goal of making life more comfortable for patients with such injuries.

The consequences of spinal cord injury are not limited to an impairment in control of movements and sensation. An equally or even more important group of consequences consists of those related to the functioning of internal organs, in particular, those of the bowels and the bladder, whose control centers are located in the spinal cord. Another important consequence is chronic pain, which may frequently be phantom. This means that a patient complains of a chronic pain in an area of the body that has no sensation with respect to either potentially painful or nonpainful stimuli. Chronic pain may persist even in cases of total transection of the spinal cord above the level where the patient localizes the pain, that is, may be of a purely central origin.

Note that the level of spinal cord injury is an important predictive factor for the prognosis. A trauma at a cervical level frequently leads to **quadriparesis,** or partial loss of voluntary motor function in all four extremities, or even to **quadriplegia,** that is, total loss of motor function, combined with impaired sensation below the level of trauma. A trauma at a thoracic level is commonly associated with a **paraparesis** or **paraplegia** (only the motor function of the legs is impaired). Both cervical and thoracic traumas are associated with a complex of signs and symptoms characteristic of damaged descending spinal tracts that is commonly termed **spasticity.** A trauma at the lumbar section of the spinal cord frequently leads to paraparesis of varying degrees of severity that is not accompanied by spasticity (so-called **flaccid paraparesis**).

Problem 25.1

Can you suggest why there is no spasticity in cases of lumbar spinal cord injuries?

Problem 25.2

What kinds of motor and sensory consequences can be expected from an injury of the sacral area of the spine?

25.3. SIGNS AND SYMPTOMS OF SPASTICITY

Spasticity is a common component of a variety of motor disorders resulting from **brain trauma** (including **cerebral palsy**), spinal cord injury, and certain systemic degenerative processes (including **multiple sclerosis**). It is sometimes addressed as an **upper motor neuron disease,** while spastic symptoms may be addressed as **pyramidal symptoms,** implying damaged transmission of signals along the pyramidal tract from cortical neurons to the spinal cord.

Problem 25.3

Do you like these terms? Why or why not?

Unfortunately, spasticity is a rather common disorder that in many cases does not permit patients to perform functionally significant voluntary movements or even occupy certain postures. Spastic spasms are frequently vigorous and painful. They may prevent patients from having normal sleep. If a patient sits in a wheelchair, the spasms may require strapping the limbs to the chair. Since spasticity is frequently associated with a total loss of sensation in the affected limbs, uncontrolled spastic movements may lead to a trauma without the patient's knowing about it. Spasticity is also sometimes associated with the chronic pain syndrome, which may lead to constant excruciating pain.

Clinicians have defined spasticity as a disorder of spinal proprioceptive reflexes manifested as profound **changes in reflexes to muscle stretch with a strong velocity-dependent component,** emergence of **pathological reflexes** and **uncontrolled spasms,** an increase in **muscle tone,** and **impairment of voluntary motor function.** This is a descriptive definition in terms of signs and symptoms rather than underlying mechanisms. Furthermore, it contains a couple of vague terms, such as "strong velocity-dependent component" (what is "strong"?), and one of the worst misnomers, "muscle tone." Clinicians define "increased muscle tone" as a "feeling of increased resistance when you try to move a joint."

Problem 25.4

Suggest a mechanism underlying increased "muscle tone"? What about decreased "muscle tone"?

Although it has been commonly assumed that spasticity is associated with a deficit in spinal inhibitory mechanisms including both postsynaptic and presynaptic inhibition, there is no consensus about what causes these deficits in the first place. To say that they are due to disruption of the normal functioning of certain descending systems does not help much, since these systems are not well defined and their role in voluntary motor control is unclear (see chapter 17).

The relations between spasticity and muscle reflexes are not as unambiguous as implied by the definition presented. Let us consider typical changes in muscle reflexes associated with spasticity.

1. Spasticity can be associated with exaggerated, unchanged, and even absent monosynaptic reflexes including the H-reflex, although an increase in monosynaptic reflexes is more typical.

2. A common correlate of spasticity is spasmlike bursts of activity in leg muscles in response to a tactile stimulation of the sole of the foot (figure 25.1). This response is sometimes imprecisely called the **Babinski**

reflex or a **defensive reaction.** It is quite variable across patients and may involve bursts of activity in all major flexor muscles or a sustained contraction of the flexor muscles, either with or without a comparable activation of extensor muscles. However, this reflex can be absent in certain patients with spasticity.

3. Another typical sign of spasticity is **clonus** (figure 25.2), which represents a series of alternating bursts of activity in the flexor and extensor muscles of a joint at a frequency of about 6-8 Hz in response to a single quick movement of the joint performed by the experimenter (passively) or by the patient (if there is enough voluntary motor control left). Clonus may last for only about a second or may continue for tens of seconds or even minutes until it is stopped mechanically, for example by clamping the joint and preventing it from moving. Clonus is likely to represent an auto-oscillation in the hyperexcitable monosynaptic stretch reflex loop: when a muscle is stretched, a monosynaptic stretch reflex leads to its phasic contraction, leading to a reversal of the joint movement direction. As a result, the antagonist muscle is stretched and demonstrates a monosynaptic stretch reflex. And so on. Remember that joint movements in healthy

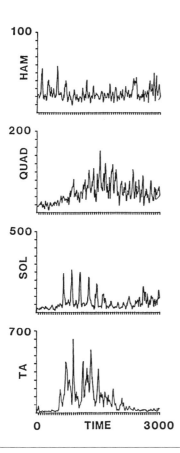

Figure 25.1   An example of a spasm in leg muscles induced by tactile stimulation of the sole of a foot in a spastic patient. This reaction is sometimes imprecisely addressed as the Babinski response.

Reprinted, by permission, from M.L. Latash, R.D. Penn, D.M. Corcos, and G.L. Gottlieb, 1989, "Short-term effects of intrathecal baclofen in spasticity," *Experimental Neurology,* 103: 167.

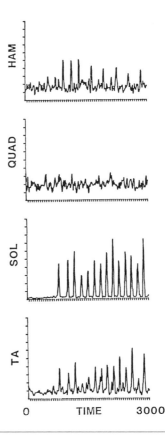

Figure 25.2   An example of electrical muscle activity during ankle clonus induced by a single rapid dorsiflexion of the foot.

persons do not normally induce monosynaptic reflexes. There is an alternative hypothesis claiming that clonus is a result of the functioning of a central generator.

Problem 25.5

What changes in the clonus frequency would you expect to see, based on these two conflicting hypotheses, if the limb is loaded inertially or if the strength of contractions is reduced by a drug?

---

4. A variety of changes in various components of muscle reactions to stretch have been reported. No reproducible differences have been found between gains of the long-latency reflexes to muscle stretch (including the tonic stretch reflex) in spastic and control subjects, and the increased resistance to muscle stretch has been partially attributed to peripheral changes in muscle and tendon stiffness. However, when spasticity was dramatically reduced in a patient by **intrathecal baclofen** (we will discuss this later), the gain in the tonic stretch reflex was also reduced.

5. **Suppression of monosynaptic reflexes by muscle vibration,** which is presumably mediated by presynaptic inhibitory mechanisms, has been suggested as a quantitative index for spasticity. This suppression is pronounced in healthy humans, leading, in particular, to a 3- to 10-fold decrease in the peak-to-peak amplitude of the H-reflex in the triceps surae muscle during vibration of the Achilles tendon. In spastic patients, however, this effect is much lower (less than 2-fold) or absent, or is even reversed, representing an increase in the amplitude of the H-reflex (figure 25.3). This index, however, does not reflect the state of postsynaptic inhibition and in some cases poorly correlates with clinical status. Also, monosynaptic reflexes are sometimes absent in spasticity, making this method inapplicable.

Two clinical scales have been successfully used for quantitative assessment of spasticity. The one employed most frequently is the **Ashworth scale,** which reflects the degree of muscle resistance to passive limb movements (table 25.1). The other is the so-called spasm scale, which reflects the frequency of spasms, their duration, and their general or local character (table 25.2).

Table 25.1 The Ashworth Scale

Score	Description of muscle tone
1	No increase in tone.
2	Slight increase in tone, giving a "catch" when affected segment is moved in flexion or extension.
3	More marked increase in tone, but affected segment is easily flexed and extended.
4	Considerable increase in tone; passive movement is difficult.
5	Affected part is rigid in flexion or extension.

Reprinted, by permission, from R.D. Penn, S. Savoy, D. Corcos, M. Latash, G. Gottlieb, B. Parke, and J. Kroin, 1989, "Intrathecal baclofen for severe spinal spasticity: A double-blind crossover study," *New England Journal of Medicine* 320: 1517-1521. © 1989 Massachusetts Medical Society. All rights reserved.

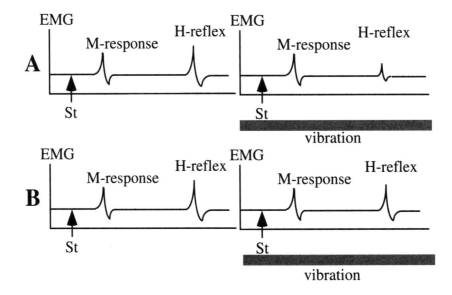

Figure 25.3 Changes in an H-reflex in the soleus muscle induced by vibration of the muscle tendon in a healthy person (A; note the suppression of the H-reflex) and in a person with spasticity (B; no suppression of the H-reflex).

Table 25.2   The Spasm Scale

Score	Frequency of Spasms
0	No spasms
1	Mild spasms induced by stimulation
2	Infrequent full spasms occuring less than once per hour
3	Spasms occurring more frequently than once per hour
4	Spasms occuring more frequently than ten times per hour

Reprinted, by permission, from R.D. Penn, S. Savoy, D. Corcos, M. Latash, G. Gottlieb, B. Parke, and J. Kroin, 1989, "Intrathecal baclofen for severe spinal spasticity: A double-blind crossover study," *New England Journal of Medicine* 320: 1517-1521. © 1989 Massachusetts Medical Society. All rights reserved.

Both scales are subjective and reflect the physician's general impression of the patient's state, which is likely to be important from the clinical view but is not very helpful for understanding the mechanisms of the disorder.

There is even more ambiguity in the relations between spasticity and voluntary motor control. A great British neurologist of the last century, Hughlings Jackson, classified the signs of spasticity into **positive** (an increase in muscle reflexes) and **negative** (the impaired control of movements). There has been a controversy concerning the relation between these two groups of symptoms: Are increased muscle reflexes and spasms interfering with voluntary motor control? Hughlings Jackson thought that eliminating the signs of spasticity should not be expected to help motor function. This view has been challenged by a number of studies in which hyperactive reflexes and co-contraction of antagonist muscles appeared to interfere with proper motor function. However, in order to solve this problem, an effective method of treating spasticity was necessary.

25.4. TREATMENT OF SPASTICITY

Treatment of spasticity, until recently, was rather unsuccessful. Attempts at reducing spastic signs and symptoms involved **drug therapies, physical therapy,** and in the worst cases, **destructive chemical** (e.g., permanent destruction of neuromuscular synapses with phenol) or **neurosurgical procedures** (e.g., cutting the dorsal roots of a number of segments, or even the spinal cord). Drugs taken orally were rather successful in a very small percentage of cases, marginally

successful in some cases, and virtually ineffective in most cases. The major problem was that taking a drug orally places it into the bloodstream so that the same concentration of the drug is achieved in the spinal cord (where it is needed) and in the brain (where it is not needed). As a result, a therapeutic concentration of a drug at the spinal level could lead to disorders of consciousness and even to coma.

A rather ingenious solution has been developed recently by a Chicago neurosurgeon, Richard Penn. It involves delivering a drug directly into the spinal canal (intrathecally), avoiding the systemic effects (figure 25.4). The drug is placed in a reservoir connected to an electronically controlled pump. The pump and the reservoir are placed under the skin and connected to the spinal canal with a thin catheter. In recent studies, intrathecal infusions of **baclofen,** an agonist of gamma-aminobutyric acid (GABA), have been shown to effectively reduce muscle spasms and exaggerated reflexes. The clinical effectiveness of this new, intrathecal method of drug delivery combined with its very fast action led to dramatic effects in many patients: virtually all the spastic signs were eliminated within 1 hour after the beginning of baclofen delivery. Figure 25.5 illustrates ankle clonus in a patient with a spinal cord injury prior to and after an intrathecal injection of baclofen. The difference is striking. At the same time, the scores for both Ashworth and spasm scales are reduced, accompanied by clear clinical gains. Intrathecal baclofen also provides a rare opportunity in clinical motor control studies to

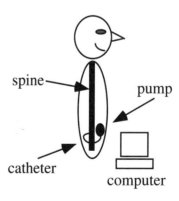

Figure 25.4   A scheme of intrathecal drug delivery with an implanted programmable pump.

use a spastic patient as his/her own control in two states, with and without spastic signs.

Most of these studies were carried out in patients with multiple sclerosis and spinal cord injury and spasticity resistant to all available nondestructive therapies, including oral baclofen. The effects, in some patients with residual voluntary movements in spastic limbs, were

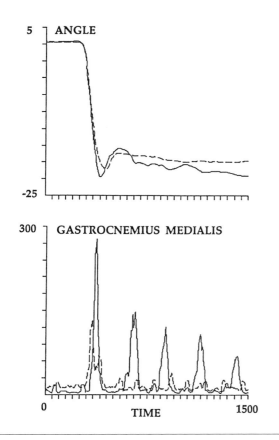

Figure 25.5   An example of ankle clonus in a spastic patient prior to the action of intrathecal baclofen (solid traces) and during administration of intrathecal baclofen (dashed traces). Note that the stimulus (ankle dorsiflexion) was the same during both tests (upper panel).
Adapted, by permission, from M.L. Latash and R.D. Penn, 1996, "Changes in voluntary motor control induced by intrathecal baclofen in patients with spasticity of different etiology," *Physiotherapy Research International* 1: 229-246.

accompanied by an improvement in movement patterns, including both movement kinematics and EMG patterns. Figure 25.6 shows an improvement in elbow flexion movements in a patient with spasticity after an injection of baclofen. Note that the improvement in movement kinematics (faster movement, fewer oscillations) is accompanied by a decrease in muscle co-contraction and fewer bursts of activity.

Some patients demonstrate spasticity in only one half of the body, left or right. These cases are called **hemisyndromes** and are rather common consequences of brain traumas, strokes, and cerebral palsy. A potentially very important and intriguing finding in the patients with hemisyndromes was that they did not notice any weakness in the unaffected limbs despite the high intrathecal baclofen doses. This apparent difference in the effects of baclofen upon pathological muscle reflexes and voluntary motor control suggests that intrathecal baclofen does not induce a nonspecific widespread inhibition throughout all spinal structures.

The site of action of baclofen in the spinal cord is not clear. As a GABA agonist, it binds to GABA receptor sites that occur widely in the central nervous system. In particular, baclofen-sensitive GABA receptors were found on primary afferent terminals. These findings suggest that probably most of the effects of baclofen are mediated through an increase in presynaptic inhibition. Thus, the observations in patients with hemisyndromes can be explained by either different numbers of baclofen-sensitive receptors on terminals of different descending systems or by their differing ability to bind to intrathecal baclofen due to anatomical and other factors (for example, diffusion of baclofen throughout spinal cord structures). The lack of apparent changes in intact muscles in the hemisyndrome cases suggests that one of the long-term reactions of spinal structures to a spasticity-inducing pathology can consist of an increase in the number of GABA-sensitive receptors or sensitization of the existent receptors on pathologically active reflex inputs.

Problem 25.6

What can you conclude from the observations of baclofen-induced similar suppression of monosynaptic reflexes on both sides of the body of a patient with a hemisyndrome, effective suppression of spastic signs, and no apparent changes in control of the intact side of the body?

Figure 25.7 shows schematically some of the possible consequences of a neural trauma. Any trauma is likely to lead to the lack of both descending inhibition and descending excitation to the segmental levels. The lack of excitatory inputs may be expected to lead to a decrease in the centrally induced levels of α-motoneuronal activity, and consequently to a decrease in voluntary muscle force (weakness or paresis). At the present level of our knowledge, it is impossible to adequately correct this deficiency. Functional electrical stimulation is a way to induce stronger muscle contractions, but it represents a substitution of the function rather than a correction.

The lack of descending inhibition has multiple consequences, including the characteristic features of spasticity, spasms, exaggerated reflexes, and increased "muscle tone" (whatever this is). According to our assumption, it may also lead to hypersensitivity to the lacking mediators, including GABA, below the level of trauma. The last reaction can probably be considered compensatory since it increases the effectiveness of remaining supplies of GABA and its agonists, including baclofen. It looks as if the central nervous system "knew" that intrathecal baclofen would be invented and made all the necessary preparations to increase its effectiveness!

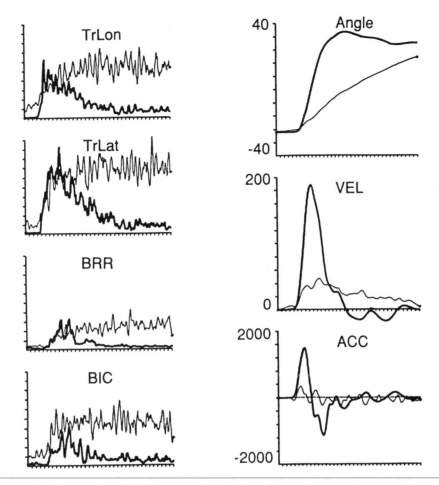

Figure 25.6 An example of kinematic and EMG patterns during elbow flexions by a spastic patient prior to the action of intrathecal baclofen (thin traces) and during administration of intrathecal baclofen (solid traces). Note an increase in movement velocity and a decrease in the level of muscle co-contraction. TrLon and TrLat: long and lateral heads of triceps; BRR: brachioradialis; BIC: biceps; VEL: velocity; ACC: acceleration.

Reprinted, by permission, from M.L. Latash, 1993, *Control of Human Movement* (Champaign, IL: Human Kinetics), 270.

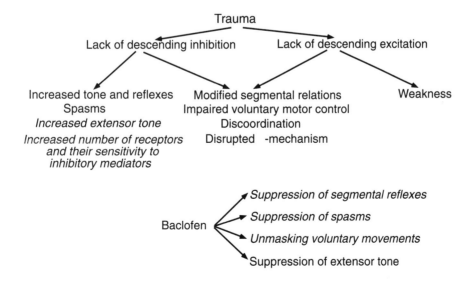

Figure 25.7 A scheme of possible consequences of a spinal cord injury and of baclofen action. Potentially useful consequences are italicized.

Reprinted, by permission, from M.L. Latash, 1993, *Control of Human Movement* (Champaign, IL: Human Kinetics), 273.

25.5. MULTIPLE SCLEROSIS

Multiple sclerosis is a degenerative disorder characterized by a loss of the **myelin sheath** by the axons of certain neural tracts. As a result, conduction along these tracts slows down, loses its regularity, and may even be totally interrupted. Saltatory transmission of action potentials becomes impossible because of the lack of the isolating myelin sheath that allows the local currents to reach the threshold for action potential generation in the next Ranvier node. On the other hand, the number of ion channels is disproportionally high in the Ranvier nodes and is disproportionally low under the myelin sheath, so that the "generic," unmyelinated transmission is also impossible when the sheath is destroyed.

The clinical picture of multiple sclerosis is rather variable and dependent on which tracts are affected. Frequently, the signs and symptoms of multiple sclerosis are similar to those seen in patients with an incomplete spinal injury at a cervical or thoracic level. These symptoms involve spasticity and paresis sometimes associated with changed somatosensory sensitivity in the lower spinal segments. Multiple sclerosis may lead to a partial or complete loss of vision (if the optic nerve is affected) and also to cognitive changes. Another prominent symptom of multiple sclerosis is the unusual sense of tiredness out of proportion to the degree of daily effort (see chapter 24). This feeling is frequently addressed as fatigue, although patients with multiple sclerosis report that it is a quite different feeling from ordinary fatigue.

Spasticity associated with multiple sclerosis can be treated with intrathecal baclofen, similarly to spasticity following a spinal cord injury. Unfortunately, there is no cure for the primary cause, that is, for demyelination. Therefore, treatment strategies include addressing specific symptoms of patients, such as spasticity, and using physical therapy and assisting devices.

Problem 25.7

Patients with multiple sclerosis frequently feel better in a cold room and worse in a hot room. Can you suggest an explanation?

Chapter 25 in a Nutshell

Spinal cord injury leads to sensory-motor consequences reflecting the disruption of transmission along ascending and descending neural pathways and the destruction of the spinal neuronal apparatus. Spasticity is a typical consequence of spinal cord injury; it is characterized by a partial or complete loss of voluntary control over muscles, partial or complete loss of sensation, uncontrolled spasms and increased reflexes, possibility of chronic pain, and disruption of functions of internal body organs below the level of trauma. Treatment of spasticity with intrathecal drug delivery, in particular by intrathecal baclofen, has been most successful. Suppression of spasms and reflexes can be accompanied by an unmasking of more normal voluntary movements while voluntary control of unaffected muscles does not change. Adaptive changes to the original trauma are likely to play an important role in the selective action of drugs. Multiple sclerosis is a progressive degenerative disease leading to a loss of myelin by fibers in central neural pathways. Many of its sensory and motor symptoms are similar to those typical of spinal cord injury. Treatment of multiple sclerosis has been unsatisfactory except for the elimination of spasticity by intrathecal drugs.

PARKINSON'S DISEASE AND DYSTONIA

Key Terms

clinical features of
    Parkinson's disease
the role of the basal ganglia

movement disorders
postural disorders
role of adaptive changes

treatment strategies
dystonia

26.1. CLINICAL FEATURES OF PARKINSON'S DISEASE

Parkinson's disease is a complex disorder reflecting malfunctioning of the basal ganglia. Patients with Parkinson's disease typically demonstrate a **poverty of movements** that is sometimes addressed as akinesia. Akinesia may involve a masklike expression of the face, stooped posture, shuffling gait, a lack of associated arm movements during walking, and "frozen" postures. Movements of these patients are slow and frequently ineffective. During many everyday tasks, they have problems switching from an apparently ineffective motor strategy to an alternative one. Hand trembling is another common disorder, making such activities as eating with a fork or a spoon and drinking from a cup very difficult.

Histological postmortem examination of the brains of patients with Parkinson's disease shows a **degeneration of neurons in the substantia nigra;** there is also a decrease in the dopamine content of the striatum (more pronounced in the putamen) due to the degeneration of the nigrostriatal connections. Degeneration may also be seen in other areas of the brain. It is believed that Parkinson's disease occurs because of a striatal dopamine deficiency, and this view is supported by the effectiveness of dopamine (L-dopa) therapy. On the basis of the connections

between the basal ganglia and other brain structures, one may conclude that removal of dopamine projections from the substantia nigra to the striatum may lead to two types of effects: (1) removal of dopaminergic excitation of the projection to the internal pallidum and (2) removal of dopaminergic inhibition of the projection to the external pallidum (figure 26.1). As a result, both direct and indirect pathways mediated by the basal ganglia (cf. chapter 16) lead to a decrease in the excitatory input to the brain cortex. This may explain some of the features of Parkinson's disease, such as poverty of movements.

The four basic clinical features of Parkinson's disease are **tremor, bradykinesia, rigidity,** and **deficit in postural reflexes** (figure 26.2):

- **Tremor** is characterized by 5-6 Hz alternating activity of antagonist muscles controlling a joint, leading to alternating joint movements that can be seen both at rest and during voluntary movements in the joint.

- **Bradykinesia** usually refers to slowness of voluntary movements and difficulty in their initiation, although deficits in spontaneous and/or automated movements are also sometimes addressed as bradykinesia. It can affect any part of the body and be more or less generalized.

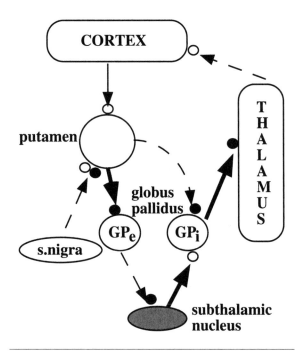

Figure 26.1 Weakening of both dopaminergic excitatory and inhibitory projections leads to a decrease in the excitatory input to the brain cortex through both direct and indirect pathways.

- **Rigidity** is a sustained increase in the resistance to externally imposed joint movements.
- **Deficits in postural reflexes** reveal themselves as decreased anticipatory postural adjustments and an increase in preprogrammed corrections in the activity of postural muscles associated with voluntary movements or in response to an external perturbation.

Problem 26.1

There are obvious similarities between symptoms of spasticity and those of Parkinson's disease. How would you differentiate between multiple sclerosis and Parkinson's disease?

For the purposes of this chapter, I am going to identify three functional levels related to the generation of voluntary motor command and peripheral characteristics of muscle activity (figure 26.3). The first level deals with generation of hypothetical control signals. The second level involves preprogramming and is responsible for corrections to possible perturbations. The third level includes segmental mechanisms (reflexes and intraspi-

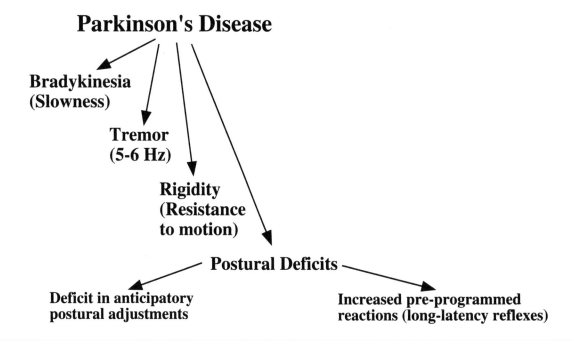

Figure 26.2 Four major symptoms of Parkinson's disease include tremor, rigidity, bradykinesia, and deficit in postural reactions. The latter deficit has two components: a deficit in anticipatory postural adjustments and a poorly controlled increase in later, preprogrammed reactions.

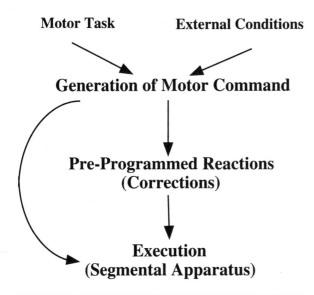

Figure 26.3 A scheme of the generation of a voluntary movement. Three levels are identified: generation of motor command, preprogrammed reactions (corrections), and execution.

nal connections) that normally act in a coordinated and predictable fashion. The major clinical features of Parkinson's disease are likely to reflect malfunctioning at different levels. For example, some are likely to be related to problems with preprogramming (deficits in postural reactions) and generation of hypothetical motor commands (bradykinesia). Rigidity and tremor can be observed at rest, when the patient is not trying to perform a voluntary movement, and therefore may be attributed to a dysfunction at the third level. Let me try to describe differences and similarities in motor phenomena in Parkinson's disease and control populations, relating them to one of the three functional levels.

26.2. VOLUNTARY MOVEMENTS IN PARKINSON'S DISEASE

Movement studies in Parkinson's disease have revealed a number of differences from healthy people. While performing a simple movement, when all the parameters of the movement are known in advance, patients with Parkinson's disease initiate and perform the movement more slowly. In particular, they demonstrate an **increase in reaction time** that is larger for more complex movements. An **increase in movement time** in Parkinson's

disease (bradykinesia) is accompanied by a considerable asymmetry of the acceleration and deceleration phases and is mostly due to a prolongation of the deceleration phase.

Both temporal and spatial **variability** of limb movements to a target have been shown to be higher in Parkinson's disease. Actually, increased variability is probably the most common feature of virtually all motor disorders. It has been suggested that bradykinesia in Parkinson's disease may in part result from the increased variability and the desire to preserve an acceptable level of accuracy, that is, be a result of a compensatory strategy adopted by the patient's brain rather than a primary deficit.

Fast movements of Parkinson's disease patients are typically **hypometric** (i.e., they undershoot the target), especially for movements of large amplitude. The entire targeted movement is frequently constructed of several discernible segments. Correspondingly, the EMG patterns demonstrate a number of repeated cycles of agonist-antagonist bursts (figure 26.4). Slow buildup of EMG during voluntary movements and the considerable amount of co-contraction of antagonist muscles can also be factors disrupting kinematic patterns during voluntary movements.

These findings allowed researchers to formulate a number of hypotheses about the origins of the deficit in voluntary motor control in Parkinson's disease. However, all these formulations imply that the EMGs and/or muscle forces are adequate measures of the voluntary motor command, which, as we know, is not true.

Problem 26.2

Why cannot muscle forces and EMGs be adequate reflections of a "central command" during normal voluntary movements?

In particular, it has been suggested that the mechanism controlling EMG magnitude during rapid movements is impaired. The failure to generate sufficient muscle forces has also been attributed to a basic failure to "sufficiently energize the muscles." It has also been concluded that although the overall form of motor programs in Parkinson's disease is preserved, the details of the number and frequency of activated motor units can be inaccurate. The last formulation suggests that the differences in voluntary motor patterns in Parkinson's disease are due to changes at the third (segmental) level of our hypothetical scheme (figure 26.3) rather than at the level of generation of motor command.

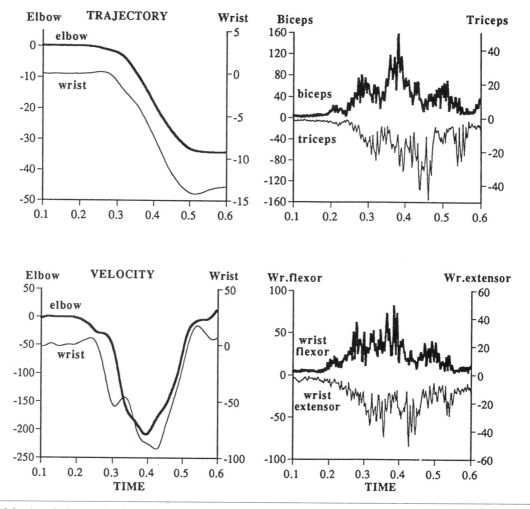

Figure 26.4 A typical example of muscle activation patterns during a fast voluntary flexion movement in the elbow joint by a patient with Parkinson's disease. Note the increased co-contraction and typical repeated bursts of activity. There was also an accompanying smaller wrist movement.

Reprinted from *Electroencephalography and clinical neurophysiology,* Volume 97, M.L. Latash, A.S. Aruin, I. Neyman, J.J. Nicholas, and M.B. Shapiro, "Feedforward postural adjustments in a simple two-joint synergy in patients with Parkinson's disease," 77-89, 1995, with kind permission from Elsevier Science Ireland Ltd., Bay 15K, Shannon Industrial Estate, Co. Clare. Ireland.

However, despite the slow buildup of EMGs during isometric voluntary contractions, patients with Parkinson's disease ultimately achieve the correct final level. These patients are able to produce accurate force levels, although the control of the rate of force increase and decrease seems to be more affected. This group of observations suggests that the problem is not in achieving absolute levels of EMGs but rather in the time pattern of muscle activation, which is likely to depend upon the action of reflex feedback loops and changes within the segmental spinal apparatus.

The deficits in motor performance in Parkinson's disease become especially pronounced for sequential multijoint movements. More specifically, the intervals between components of sequential movements are prolonged. These patients also have trouble integrating several components into one motor action.

26.3. DIFFERENCES IN ANTICIPATORY ADJUSTMENTS AND IN PREPROGRAMMED REACTIONS

Remember that postural control is based on two types of corrective reactions whose function is to assure postural stability in the presence of perturbations. Some of these reactions occur prior to a perturbation and are termed anticipatory adjustments. They are generated by the central nervous system in a feedforward manner and are attempts to alleviate the effects of a predictable perturbation. They are commonly seen as changes in the background activity of postural muscles when a person who is standing makes a fast arm movement. The second group involves reactions that are prepared by the central nervous system in advance and are triggered by a peripheral stimulus informing the central nervous system about a postural perturbation (feedback triggering). These preprogrammed corrections deal with actual perturbations that occur either because of the suboptimal performance of anticipatory adjustments or because the perturbation comes unexpectedly for the person. Reactions of both groups can be seen during standing as well as during postural tasks limited to a limb or joint.

Patients with Parkinson's disease demonstrate **profoundly different postural adjustments** suggesting an impairment in the hypothetical mechanism of preprogramming. Stretching of a quiescent or voluntarily activated muscle of a patient with Parkinson's disease leads to long-latency muscle responses whose amplitude has been shown to be considerably higher than in the control population. This increase has been attributed to an "overcompensation" in transmission in a hypothetical receptor—motor cortex—muscle loop (transcortical loop) and has been considered a possible mechanism of parkinsonian rigidity. Preprogrammed reactions induced by postural perturbations can be voluntarily modulated by healthy persons; this ability is impaired in Parkinson's disease. So it is fair to say that these patients demonstrate a poorly controlled increase in the feedback-triggered corrective postural reactions. On the other hand, anticipatory postural corrections before a voluntary movement are commonly smaller in amplitude in patients with Parkinson's disease. These patients more frequently demonstrate anticipatory **co-contraction** of antagonist muscles acting at a postural joint, which apparently stiffens the joint and stabilizes it against perturbations but is less efficient than the more typical pattern of alternating activity in couple of postural muscles of healthy persons.

The first group of observations suggests a poorly controlled increase in a group of preprogrammed reactions that are readily generated in conditions under which healthy humans do not usually demonstrate them; the second group indicates an impaired ability to generate appropriate anticipatory postural adjustments. The latter factor can be considered an example of the impaired ability of patients with Parkinson's disease to program and initiate movements.

It seems to be a good time to suggest to the reader a series of groundless speculations (figure 26.5). If the ability to preprogram motor corrections is impaired, most commonly used motor programs may become useless, since any external perturbation would lead to their disruption. Suppose that the central nervous system of such a patient still "wants" to use some of the programs that require continuous corrections, like walking and maintenance of the vertical posture. The necessary preprogrammed reactions are stored in memory, but the mechanism for triggering them adequately is defective. The central nervous system may try to compensate for the impaired ability to adequately preprogram by decreasing the triggering threshold for the preprogrammed corrections and/or increasing their gain. Overcompensation is likely to occur. One of its consequences can be a new perturbation, giving rise to a triggering signal leading to a preprogrammed reaction in the opposite direction. Several results can be expected from such a compensatory mechanism. First, the apparent stiffness of the system will increase (cf. rigidity). Second, oscillations can occur with a period corresponding to slightly more than

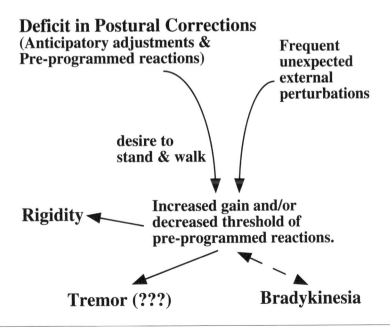

Figure 26.5 A scheme illustrating groundless speculations about the nature of various motor disorders in Parkinson's disease.

doubled latency of the preprogrammed reactions because of the time necessary for the peripheral receptors to react to a perturbation induced by a preceding preprogrammed reaction. This assessment corresponds to oscillations at about 5-6 Hz (cf. parkinsonian tremor). Third, walking and standing will be possible, although they are likely to look awkwardly "rigid." This is certainly not the ultimate truth about the origins of motor deficits in Parkinson's disease, but an example of how adaptive reactions can lead to nontrivial motor consequences.

Problem 26.3

Suggest an experiment that would test the hypothesis that tremor in Parkinson's disease is an oscillation in a long-latency reflex loop.

26.4. CHANGES IN SEGMENTAL REFLEXES

Since the primary cause of Parkinson's disease is undoubtedly supraspinal, it has been suggested that motor disorders in Parkinson's disease are due to changes in the descending motor commands while the segmental apparatus is generally intact. This view is supported by a number of observations, including unchanged tendon jerk reflexes and generally normal short-latency action of Ia-muscle afferents. However, a number of changes in presumably segmental mechanisms have been reported. These include a **deficit in reciprocal inhibition** that could, in particular, lead to a considerable co-contraction of antagonist muscles during voluntary movements, increased reflex activity during tracking phases in which the muscle is lengthening, and a "paradoxical" Westphal phenomenon. The Westphal phenomenon represents an abrupt reflex excitation of a muscle in response to an externally imposed muscle shortening. In a sense, it is the inverse of the stretch reflex.

Let me continue the line of speculations started in the previous section. It has been suggested that in the presence of a hypothetical deficit in preprogramming, some functions may benefit from an "overcompensation," that is, make the system generally more rigid. One of the possible mechanisms is an increase in the gain and/or decrease in the threshold of the preprogrammed reactions (as discussed earlier). A decrease in reciprocal inhibition may be another way to promote simultaneous activation of antagonist muscles, thus increasing apparent joint stiffness and making the joint less responsive to external perturbations. The Westphal phenomenon may represent a preprogrammed reaction in a shortening muscle that can sometimes be seen in control subjects. A general increase in the preprogrammed reactions in Parkinson's disease can lead to increased observation of the Westphal reaction.

26.5. POSSIBLE MECHANISMS

Basal ganglia are a part of the brain whose dysfunction leads to Parkinson's disease. The function of basal ganglia in control of voluntary movements, as well as in other brain activities, is virtually unknown. Many of the hypotheses related to the role of basal ganglia are based on observations in Parkinson's disease. The general scheme according to which such hypotheses are drawn is as follows. If something is different in the motor performance of patients with Parkinson's disease as compared to healthy people, this difference is assumed to be a reflection of a dysfunction of basal ganglia; therefore, basal ganglia take part in this aspect of motor behavior in healthy people. Following this line of reasoning, it has been hypothesized that basal ganglia are involved in assembling sequences of movements, in integration of several simultaneous motor programs, and in the transfer of information across a period of time before a response is initiated. Studies of primates have suggested that the activity of basal ganglia neurons is also related to the direction of an intended or executed movement and/or to the "amount" of voluntary muscle activity. Correspondingly, central theories of motor abnormalities in Parkinson's disease include faulty transmission of motor commands from the "decision-making" level and a loss of the ability to generate preprogrammed and ballistic movements. Peripheral theories complement the description of motor disorders in Parkinson's disease with a delay in the proprioceptive feedback and an overcompensating transcortical long-latency loop.

I have already discussed the possibility that some of the motor disorders in Parkinson's disease may reflect a process of **adaptation** rather than be direct consequences of the "primary disorder." From this view, disorders of motor performance in these patients must be first classified (at least, tentatively) into **primary** and **compensatory.** The latter group can hardly even be considered "motor disorders" but are rather reflections of a new order introduced in an attempt to minimize the consequences of the primary dysfunction or injury.

26.6. DYSTONIA

Dystonia is a disorder of voluntary movements characterized by twisted, sustained postures of the limb segments, limbs, neck, and/or trunk. Dystonic symptoms may be limited to a group of joints within a limb and be related to professional activities of patients. A typical example is the so-called **writer's cramp** or **typist's**

cramp occurring in the dominant hand muscles of persons whose profession involves prolonged usage of the hand in coordinated motor activities. Similar symptoms may be seen in musicians. In contrast, dystonia may affect movements of the whole body and the head. When neck muscles are involved, the disorder is called **torticollis.**

In most cases, even in most severe disorders involving the whole body, dystonia is not associated with any gross neurological abnormality. In some cases dystonia has been associated with a disorder of the basal ganglia; however, similar symptoms may be observed in the absence of any discernible pathology of the basal ganglia. Attempts at understanding the mechanisms of dystonia

have been unsuccessful, largely because patients with dystonia typically present rather different clinical pictures.

Increased movement **variability** is probably the most general feature of all disordered voluntary movements. This is particularly true for dystonic movements whose distinctive features include **irregularity** (figure 26.6). Therefore, qualitative analysis of single trials by individual patients remains the only method of analysis. Among common features typical for dystonic movements, there are oscillations, hesitations, temporary reversals of the trajectory, and multiple EMG bursts (in contrast to the commonly seen triphasic burst; see chapter 11). Another typical feature of dystonic movements,

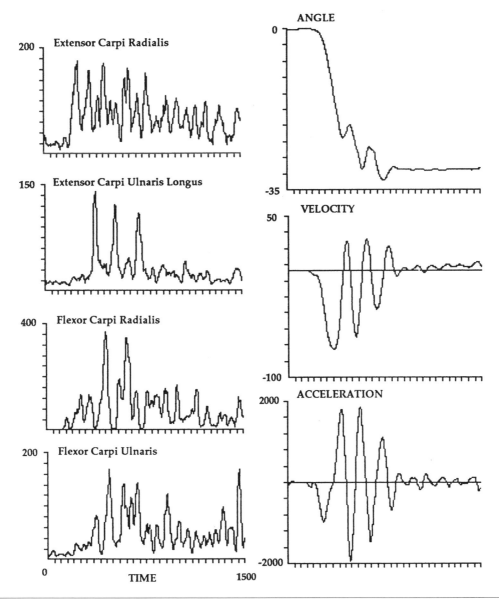

Figure 26.6 Typical patterns of a voluntary wrist flexion movement in a person with dystonia. EMG patterns are characterized by multiple, irregular bursts. The trajectory is "bumpy" and may have hesitations and reversals.

Reprinted, by permission, from M.L. Latash and S.R. Gutman, 1995, "Abnormal motor patterns in the framework of the equilibrium-point hypothesis: A cause for dystonic movements?" *Biological Cybernetics* 71: 87-94. © 1995 Springer-Verlag.

although it does not occur in all patients, is **coactivation** of antagonist muscles and frequently also of distant muscles during attempts at unidirectional fast movements.

Dystonia is apparently a problem of **control,** a problem of disbalance among the descending signals that may not be correlated with any discernible pathology in the supraspinal or spinal structures. A number of segmental abnormalities have been described in dystonia, in particular a deficit in Ia-mediated inhibition and the Westphal phenomenon. These, however, are not seen in all the patients and may represent secondary changes in the system in response to a long-lasting primary **disorder of motor control.**

Chapter 26 in a Nutshell

Parkinson's disease is a consequence of a loss of dopamine-producing neurons in the substantia nigra. Its symptoms include poverty of movements, tremor at about 5-6 Hz, rigidity, bradykinesia (slowness), and deficits in postural control. A deficit in anticipatory postural adjustment and a poorly controlled increase in corrective postural reactions have been reported as contributing to postural deficits. Problems with movement initiation and sequencing can be related to a decrease in the functioning of both direct and indirect cortico-thalamocortical loops involving the basal ganglia. Segmental changes, including a deficit in reciprocal inhibition and the Westphal phenomenon, have been described. The most common treatment of Parkinson's disease is a precursor of dopamine (dopa). Some of the typical motor symptoms may be consequences of adaptive changes within the central nervous system to a primary disorder. Dystonia is a disorder that in some cases is linked to a dysfunction of the basal ganglia. Voluntary movements in dystonia are characterized by twisted, sustained postures of the limb segments, limbs, neck, and/or trunk. Both Parkinson's disease and dystonia (as well as many other motor disorders) are characterized by an increase in the variability of voluntary movements.

IMPLICATIONS FOR MOTOR REHABILITATION

Key Terms

variability and choice in movements

CNS priorities

CNS plasticity

adaptive changes in motor patterns

adaptation at a control level

limb amputation

Down syndrome

practical considerations

Studies of populations whose ability to perform voluntary movements is impaired due to natural causes (e.g., **aging**), inborn deficiency (e.g., **Down syndrome**), trauma (e.g., **spinal cord injury**), or illness (e.g., **Parkinson's disease**) frequently result in a basic question: Are observed motor patterns, which may be rather different from those seen in healthy persons, actually abnormal, and should they be corrected? Analysis of this question is important not only for deeper understanding of the mechanisms of control of normal and disordered movements, but also to help us assess the effectiveness of existing therapeutic approaches and to provide a focus within which development of new therapies can be considered.

A common misconception is that any major deviation from motor patterns seen in the general unimpaired population is bad. This misconception is revealed in the way the research findings are presented and interpreted, and in the prescriptions to correct the "wrong" motor patterns. Let me suggest an alternative to this view and illustrate it with a few examples.

27.1. SOURCES OF VARIABILITY OF VOLUNTARY MOVEMENTS

Take a look at the schematic drawing representing the process of generation of a voluntary movement (figure 27.1). This scheme identifies three steps in the process: understanding of the motor task, generation of time patterns of control variables, and execution. The last step is assumed to involve neural mechanisms that are commonly addressed as "reflex," as well as mechanical properties of muscles, tendons, and joints and their interaction with the external force field. Assume that the subject participating in a mental experiment understands the instruction and correctly identifies the explicit motor goal. This assumption leaves room for variability at the first step: for example, a person with a cognitive disorder may understand the explicit motor task but at the same time be equally concerned with other factors that are not perceived as significant by unimpaired subjects (e.g., personal safety, not breaking the experimental setup, etc.). This may lead to the generation of different time

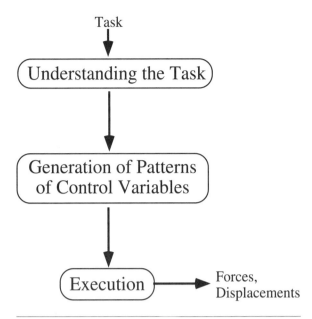

Task

Understanding the Task

Generation of Patterns
of Control Variables

Execution ——→ Forces,
Displacements

Figure 27.1   Three basic steps of the process of generation
of voluntary movements.

functions of control variables at the next level and consequently to different movement patterns.

However, even if there is no variability at the first step, the variability and flexibility of movement patterns during repetition of the same motor task by control (unimpaired) subjects (see chapter 21) suggests that the second step (generation of control patterns) virtually always involves choice. In other words, the central nervous system (CNS) engages in multiple strategies of muscle coordination to achieve a single movement outcome. This property of natural human movements is sometimes addressed as **motor equivalence** (in chapter 21, we illustrated motor equivalence with the various strategies used by the spinal frog during the wiping reflex). Thus, one may assume that the number of control variables at the second step is larger than the number of parameters defining a typical motor task. The problem of generation of appropriate values or time patterns of control variables becomes similar, for example, to solving a system of two equations with four unknowns. This problem is an example of a whole class of similar problems occurring at different levels of movement analysis. Such problems are commonly addressed as **redundancy problems** (or the **Bernstein problem;** for more details see chapter 21). They belong to a larger class of **"ill-posed" problems** that cannot be solved without the addition of other equations that are not explicitly imposed upon the system and can be chosen by the CNS based on some secondary considerations. I am going to use the term **priorities of the CNS** for sets of rules that help to solve redundancy problems during voluntary movements. Within the suggested scheme, CNS priorities participate in the

process of generation of the hypothetical control functions.

A few attempts at deciphering CNS priorities have been made. Most frequently, researchers try to guess the internal solutions of the CNS by investigating the consequences of **optimization** of certain functions of performance. Attempts at minimizing or maximizing certain **cost functions** based on movement kinematics (peak velocity, peak acceleration, jerk), movement dynamics (joint torques), energy, or functions related to such notions as "comfort" and "effort" have not led to a breakthrough in understanding how natural movements are actually controlled. Some of these approaches have demonstrated an impressive correspondence to the actual movement kinematics observed in experiments. But this fit, in itself, does not mean that the intact CNS is minimizing a function of jerk or joint torque, or calculating a "comfort" function, or doing something else of this kind. It rather suggests that the solutions preferred by the CNS do not violate any of these principles too much. Thus, the actual CNS priorities still remain unknown.

27.2. CHANGES IN THE CENTRAL NERVOUS SYSTEM PRIORITIES

The existence of choice (theoretically, at least) suggests that *the CNS may "wish" to reconsider its priorities* in certain situations in which the components of the system for movement production are grossly changed, or the task is atypical, or the external conditions are unusual. A change in the priorities may lead to a corresponding change in the externally observed patterns of voluntary movements. For example, the Fosbury flop is apparently not a coordinative pattern the CNS prefers to use for jumping on an everyday basis. But in the artificial conditions of track-and-field competition, when there are no unexpected changes in the external force field and no hidden obstacles and there is just one priority (to clear the bar at the greatest height possible), the CNS may be "persuaded" to use a new, quite unusual pattern of coordination. So, by changing the external conditions of movement execution (the context of a motor task in a broad sense) in combination with extensive practice, it may be possible to alter the CNS priorities in healthy persons and force the CNS to demonstrate movement patterns quite different from those commonly seen in the general population; compare, for example, walking patterns in ballet dancers and sumo wrestlers.

Changes in the CNS priorities are likely to occur during the early stages of human life. These **developmental jumps** seem to follow the discovery by the CNS of the biomechanics of its own effectors and the basic physical properties of the external force fields. For example, crawling may be considered a temporary solution for the problem of locomotion by babies, whose system of balance control is immature and does not allow "adult" bipedal walking. Later, new solutions are discovered by the CNS, and crawling is replaced by walking and running.

Consider now the system of motor control of a chronically impaired or otherwise atypical person. His or her lifetime experience is filled with everyday voluntary movements in conditions of frequently changing goals and external forces. If the differences between this person and an average "control subject" are large enough, there is a fair chance that his or her CNS will reconsider its priorities and elaborate, for everyday motor tasks, movement patterns that will look different from those observed in the majority of healthy persons. I certainly do not mean that changed CNS priorities are the only important factor defining abnormal motor patterns. An impaired system may well be genuinely unable to display movement patterns seen in the general population, for example, after a limb amputation or after a complete spinal cord injury. However, let me focus on possible changes in movement patterns that are not forced upon the system by a major chronic impairment but instead result from a person's reaction to a primary impairment.

A car with a broken engine does not reconsider its priorities and does not switch to alternative strategies. The ability of the body to adapt to pathological changes is a reflection of the basic differences between the design of a car and that of the body. First, the design of the car does not involve redundancy, so there is no room for such things as priorities, choice, and strategies. Second, the car does not have a brain. Brain plus redundancy makes the design of the human body—including the system for production of voluntary movements—flexible and gives it the ability to adapt not only to changes in external conditions but also, at least to some extent, to changes within the body itself.

Figure 27.2 illustrates the approach. "Normal movement patterns" (Average person) represent a spectrum that merges at one end with **clumsiness** and **impaired movements** and at the other end with **perfection** and uniquely specified movements. Central nervous system priorities are assumed to be the same for all the people within the central part of the spectrum. Clumsy children and elite athletes are at the opposite ends of the spectrum.

When one moves beyond these limits into an area that may be considered pathological or otherwise special, the CNS priorities may change and lead to apparently atypical motor patterns. This may happen in the absence of any gross neurological or motor pathology, for example, due to changes in cognition and/or intelligence (as in Down syndrome or schizophrenia). Further to the left there are morphological, biochemical, or structural CNS changes that may induce differences in motor patterns in themselves and also through changes in the CNS priorities, for example, in Parkinson's disease and spinal cord injury. Toward the left end of the axis, one sees peripheral changes, as in cases of amputation, that certainly limit motor patterns by themselves, but may also lead to a reorganization within the CNS and to resultant changes in CNS priorities.

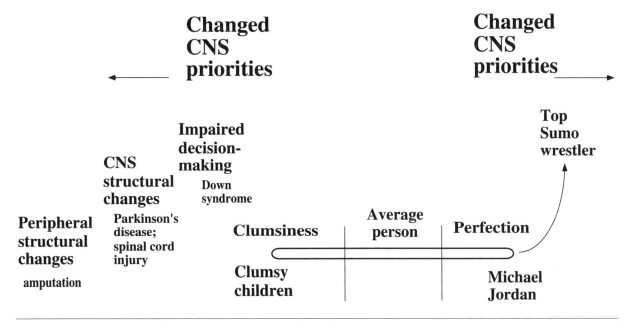

Figure 27.2 The spectrum of typical movement patterns (Average person) merges at one end with clumsiness and impaired movements and, at the other end, with perfection and uniquely specified movements. Beyond the spectrum, in the area that may be considered pathological, CNS priorities are changed, potentially leading to atypical movement patterns.

Reprinted, by permission of Cambridge University Press, from M.L. Latash and J.G. Anson, 1996, "What are normal movements in atypical populations," *Behavioral and Brain Science* 19: 55-106. © 1996 Cambridge University Press.

27.3. CENTRAL NERVOUS SYSTEM PLASTICITY

Central nervous system reorganization is likely to result from the ability of the CNS to display **plasticity,** in particular, changes in neural projections among its structures. Central nervous system plasticity represents one of its most remarkable features and is likely to contribute to the processes of motor learning and adaptation to trauma. Since the classical works of Lashley in the 1930s, it has been proposed that an injury of the brain cortex may lead to a dramatic **topographic reorganization** in adjacent cortical areas that may, in particular, significantly contribute to recovery after stroke. Changes in peripheral afferent flow have been shown to induce **changes in the receptor field** sizes and locations in brain cortex of the cat. Changes in somatosensory cortical representations in monkeys have been shown after specific training of one hand, and after digit amputation or fusion (figure 27.3). Plasticity of the CNS is not limited to grossly changed pathological states and supraspinal structures. Remember the studies by Wolpaw's group (chapter 18), who demonstrated alterations in the H-reflex excitability during prolonged operant conditioning in monkeys.

27.4. ADAPTIVE CHANGES IN MOTOR PATTERNS OF ATYPICAL INDIVIDUALS

Any major stable difference between impaired and unimpaired groups of human beings (e.g., changed cognition in Down syndrome, changed biomechanics and afferent sources in amputees, changed reflexes in spasticity, changed preprogramming in Parkinson's disease) makes the whole system of movement generation different so that its priorities are likely to be reconsidered and the patterns that were optimal for an unimpaired system are no longer optimal.

For any apparently abnormal motor pattern, the first question to be asked is: *What does the CNS perceive to be its primary goal during the execution of this particular motor task?* A straightforward answer—for example, following the exact instruction by the experimenter—may be true for motivated, healthy subjects, although even in healthy subjects, considerations such as minimizing discomfort, or making sure that the experimental setup does not break, may be as important as optimizing the performance.

Other, frequently ignored components of a motor task that may be considered important by the CNS are, for example, those related to maintaining **gaze fixation, equilibrium** of the head and body, and **posture** of the limbs with respect to the trunk during the required movements. In particular, control of a voluntary movement requires

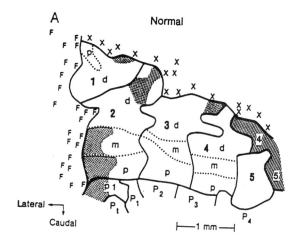

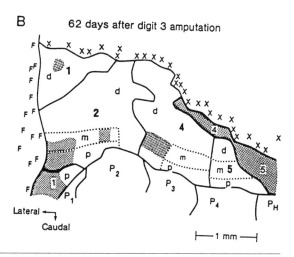

Figure 27.3 Changes in the somatosensory cortical representation in a monkey after amputation of one of the digits (digit 3). Note that after the amputation, representations of digits 2 and 4 expanded and occupied the area that previously represented digit 3.
Reprinted, by permission, from M.M. Merzenich, R.J. Nelson, M.P. Stryker, M.S. Cynader, A. Schoppmann, and J.M. Zook, 1984, "Somatosensory cortical map changes following digit amputation in adult monkeys," *The Journal of Comparative Neurology* 224: 591-605. Reprinted by permission of Wiley-Liss, Inc., a subsidiary of John Wiley & Sons, Inc.

maintaining a **reference frame** in conditions of possible external and internal perturbations. This reference frame may relate to the position of a segment, or an extremity, or the whole body. It may also relate to a more general notion of equilibrium, that is, keeping the projection of the body center of gravity within the support area.

In impaired subjects, one may expect less obvious factors to play an important role in making a choice of movement strategy. I will discuss in more detail two examples of changed movements in which some of the apparent abnormalities in motor patterns are likely to be consequences of adaptive changes within the CNS (also see the discussion of motor disorders in Parkinson's disease, chapter 26).

27.5. AMPUTATION

Amputation of a part of a limb is probably the most straightforward example. Here, the primary cause of the apparent motor disorders is unambiguously clear. Limb amputation leads to a major change in the biomechanical and neurophysiological relations developed during the lifetime. There is evidence, however, that the consequences of limb amputation may involve a major reorganization of both afferent (sensory) and efferent (motor) projections that by themselves may contribute to the difference in the motor patterns as compared to those seen in unimpaired persons.

Considerable changes in the **biomechanics of walking** occur after a leg amputation. In healthy subjects, ankle plantarflexors are the major energy generators. The role of hip extensors is relatively small. In below-the-knee amputees, ankle plantarflexors are obviously unavailable, and hip extensors become the main source of energy absorption and generation. This rearrangement should be considered adaptive since it allows amputees to walk even though the gait may be less energetically efficient.

Consequences of amputation also involve **neurological reorganization** at both segmental and suprasegmental levels. Obviously, the elimination of a considerable number of proprioceptors residing in the amputated portion of the leg leads to an abrupt change in the patterns of afferent inflow and is likely to lead to changes in the relative weight of the contribution of other, seemingly unaffected reflex projections. Remember that reflex contribution is considered an important factor in natural patterns of voluntary movements. Descending motor commands should apparently take into account the existing state of reflex connections. Moreover, proprioceptive inflow is used in the process of generation of automatic, preprogrammed adjustments in the activity of muscles providing postural stability during voluntary movements. Thus, amputation of a distal portion of a leg may be expected to lead to a rearrangement of descending motor commands and a shift of postural control from predominantly proprioception-based modalities to other modalities such as visual and vestibular signals.

Neurological reorganization of descending control signals after a below-knee amputation in humans was studied with **transcranial magnetic stimulation.** In these studies, stimuli at optimal positions of the coil recruited a larger percentage of α-motoneurons controlling the muscles in the residual leg. These muscles could also be activated from larger areas of the scalp than could the muscles at the intact side. Similar results, also in human subjects, have been reported after upper limb amputa-

tion. Thus, descending corticospinal projections are likely to be reorganized after an amputation.

The next example represents a condition not accompanied by any apparent peripheral or central injury or neurophysiological dysfunction. However, movements of these persons look different, and this impression of clumsiness correlates with changed performance in standardized laboratory tests.

27.6. DOWN SYNDROME

Movements by persons with Down syndrome are frequently addressed as **clumsy.** The word "clumsiness" is used to indicate movements that look different from and less efficient than those observed in the general population. Two major components of clumsiness in Down syndrome include **slowness** of the movements and the **inability to rapidly respond** to the changing environment. The latter factor can be seen in laboratory studies as a **deficit in preprogramming** (see chapters 12 and 19) and **longer reaction time** (the time from the presentation of a stimulus to a motor reaction). Other differences in motor performance of persons with Down syndrome include low **muscle tone** (we have already encountered this commonly used misnomer) and low voluntary muscle contraction force. Variability in various aspects of motor performance is increased in persons with Down syndrome (which is typical of a number of motor disorders), and they lack adequate adaptation to changes in sensory information.

Discrete, single-joint movements of individuals with Down syndrome are typically slow and frequently consist of several distinct submovements. In some trials, movement kinematics may be characterized by a normal-looking bell-shaped velocity profile (see chapter 11). Other trials in the same series, however, can demonstrate irregular trajectories with visible "bumps" and possible reversals of movement direction accompanied by multiple bursts of activity in the agonist and antagonist muscles (figure 27.4). Despite being slow and "clumsy," persons with Down syndrome are typically *very accurate* in achieving the prescribed target.

Prolonged practice of single-joint movements leads to a striking improvement in the performance of persons with Down syndrome: the movements become much faster and smoother without a decline in their accuracy (figure 27.5). This improvement can be **transferred** to different distances and different initial and final positions. The question of whether an improvement acquired in a standardized laboratory environment may benefit everyday movements performed in much less reproducible conditions remains open. There are enough reasons to be cautiously pessimistic. When the CNS of such a person for the first time encounters an unpredictable

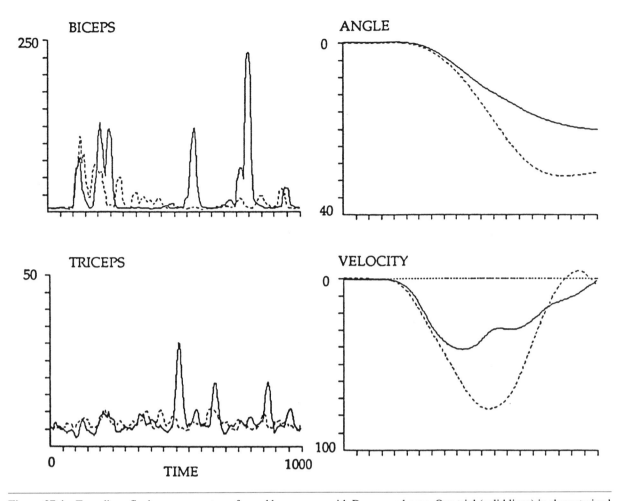

Figure 27.4 Two elbow flexion movements performed by a person with Down syndrome. One trial (solid lines) is characterized by a bumpy trajectory and numerous irregular EMG bursts, while the other trial (dashed lines) is much smoother and does not show many irregular EMG bursts.

Reprinted, by permission, from M.L. Latash and D.M. Corcos, 1991, "Kinematic and electromyographic characteristics of single-joint movements individuals with Down syndrome," *American Journal of Mental Retardation* 96: 189-201.

perturbation (which occurs abundantly in "real life"), it may quickly return to the old, reliable, and safe patterns. It is possible, however, that practice with an element of uncertainty may be successful in persuading the CNS that it is able to reconsider its priorities and shift to more effective, albeit more challenging, modes of control.

Mental retardation, which is almost always associated with Down syndrome, could affect **decision making** by delaying the accumulation and translation of information specific to the stimulus and motor response. During a lifetime, the CNS of such a person accumulates experiences that would allow it to predict that unexpected changes in external conditions occur rather frequently. Therefore, if the CNS is aware of its impaired ability to make quick, adequate decisions, it may be reluctant to produce motor commands leading to very fast movements in order to have more time for evasive actions or corrections in response to a change in the environment (perturbation) and/or to attenuate potentially damaging effects of the perturbation.

Remember that preprogramming during unidirectional single-joint movements in unimpaired control subjects usually involves a **reciprocal pattern** of muscle activation (chapter 12); that is, an unexpected loading leads to an increase in the agonist activity, while an unexpected unloading leads to a decrease in the agonist activity with a possible increase in the activity of the antagonist. Subjects with Down syndrome frequently demonstrate a coactivation pattern of preprogramming that involves an increase in the activity of both agonist and antagonist muscles irrespective of the direction of a perturbation (figure 27.6). Should this difference be considered a sign of an inability of the system of preprogramming to behave "correctly," or is it a sign of the preferred strategy for a changed CNS?

If the reciprocal strategy is used, preprogramming an increase in activity of a "wrong" muscle group can lead to exacerbation of the effects of the perturbation. The **coactivation** strategy is more universal in the sense that it stiffens the joint and hence leads to an attenuation

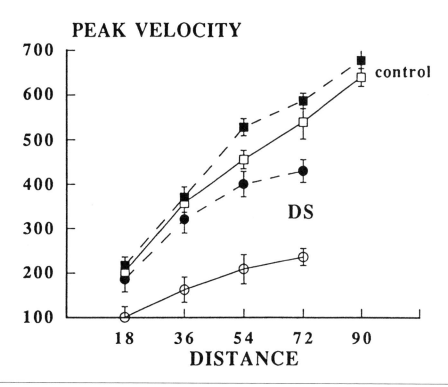

Figure 27.5 Prolonged practice can lead to a dramatic improvement in the performance of a simple motor task (fast elbow flexion movements) by persons with Down syndrome. Originally, their peak velocities were very low (open circles); they then increased (filled circles) to near to the level of performance of control subjects (open squares). Control subjects also benefitted from practice (filled squares) but to a much lesser extent.

Reprinted, by permission, from M.L. Latash, 1992, "Motor control in Down Syndrome: The role of adaptation and practice," *Journal of Developmental and Physical Disabilities* 4: 227-261.

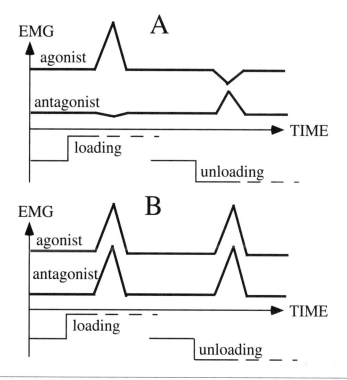

Figure 27.6 Here, the subject is holding a position in a joint against an external load. The upper drawing illustrates a typical reciprocal pattern of changes in the background EMG of an agonist and an antagonist muscle in response to an unexpected loading and an unexpected unloading. The lower drawing illustrates a typical coactivation pattern in response to the same perturbations.

of the effects of perturbations independently of the perturbation direction. On the other hand, it is always suboptimal, since it cannot in principle lead to total compensation of the effects of perturbation. This may be the reason this strategy has not been seen in highly practiced control subjects who prefer to use the more effective, although more challenging, reciprocal strategy. Apparently, this strategy is within a safety zone established by their unimpaired CNS.

Coactivation could represent the consequence of an impaired mechanism of preprogramming or it could represent a "safety catch" imposed by the CNS to allow movement to be controlled within the constraints of its impaired operating capacity. Novices in the early stages of acquiring a new motor skill frequently demonstrate greater-than-optimal levels of co-contraction that appear to increase stability and reduce the likelihood of error. This co-contraction often disappears after the skill is well learned. Co-contraction is also typical of movements of patients with Parkinson's disease and those of healthy elderly persons. Thus, it may well be that muscle coactivation is likely to reflect active intervention by the CNS rather than its inability to use "more normal" patterns of muscle activation. In the reproducible and friendly conditions of the laboratory, these internal restrictions may be lifted, leading to virtually normal performance in motor tests. In particular, subjects with Down syndrome who are well practiced frequently demonstrate a mixture of reciprocal and coactivation patterns of preprogramming in different trials within the same block of trials.

27.7. PRACTICAL CONSIDERATIONS

The purpose of this chapter has been to stress the potential role of **adaptive changes** within the CNS. More specifically, practitioners should be warned against jumping to quick conclusions on the inability of a patient's CNS to produce "correct movements" on the basis of observations of "wrong" peripheral motor patterns. Thus, the notion of **normality** with respect to peripheral motor pattern should be treated very cautiously, possibly as another frequently used misnomer.

Let me go through the most important practical conclusions based on this and the previous chapters:

1. Adaptive changes within the CNS can play an important role in shaping the patient's behavior (motor patterns).
2. Therapy should be directed at optimizing functional behavior, not movement patterns (this can be called a **pragmatic approach**). Therapists should take advantage of the adaptive abilities of the CNS; in other words, they should identify the goals, provide the tools, and allow the CNS to find a solution.
3. An important role in rehabilitation should be played by procedures that stimulate learning processes. For example, practicing a task in conditions of uncertainty may be a promising procedure.
4. Correcting the primary cause of a disorder must certainly be the first priority; unfortunately, this can very rarely be done.

Actually, physical and occupational therapists have important advantages as compared to the CNS of a patient. These include an ability to predict long-term outcomes and an ability to understand that exercise through pain may be necessary to achieve a functional optimum. If the CNS is allowed to generate adaptive patterns without any supervision, it may have a tendency to settle down in a local optimum with respect to a function because any exploratory activity leads away from this optimum, that is, to a deterioration of the function. It might never discover that there is a much more global optimum just behind a nearby ridge. Pain is another factor that the CNS does not like to experience. Thus, exercise through pain or through temporary functional deterioration may never be "discovered" by the CNS, but it may be prescribed by a therapist, leading to an optimization of long-term functional goals.

Chapter 27 in a Nutshell

The presence of choice during human voluntary movements, and plasticity within the CNS, allow for adaptive changes in movement patterns in persons with a cognitive, central neural, or peripheral disorder. Movement patterns in atypical persons may differ from those seen in healthy people but still be optimal for the given state of the system for movement production. Adaptive changes are likely to dominate in movement patterns of persons with cognitive disorders, may play an important role in patients with central neural disorders, and may contribute to motor patterns in patients after a limb amputation. Rehabilitation strategies should be directed at functional optimization rather than at bringing movement patterns as close to "normal" as possible. A therapist should provide the patient's CNS with tools and functional goals and supervise the process of rehabilitation to make sure that the patient does not settle down in a local optimum because of pain and lack of the ability to make long-term predictions.

Self-Test Problems

1. Describe the types of oscillatory, involuntary motor behavior that you know. Which structures/mechanisms can bring about these behaviors?

2. Persons with Parkinson's disease have marked difficulties in initiating walking. Suggest a hypothetical explanation for this deficit. Suggest methods of helping such patients based on your explanation.

3. You are a neurosurgeon and have perfect access to brain structures of a patient with a basal ganglia disorder. You can only destroy certain pathways (or structures) or stimulate them. What would you do to alleviate the symptoms of Parkinson's disease? What about Huntington's chorea?

4. Formulate principles for special physical education of persons with Down syndrome to optimize their motor performance, that is, make their movements more smooth and fast.

5. A person after a unilateral below-the-knee amputation is standing on the prosthetic leg without any additional support. This person makes a fast bilateral shoulder flexion (arm movement forward). What pattern of anticipatory changes in the leg and trunk muscle activity do you expect to see?

6. A person with spasticity resulting from multiple sclerosis is brought into a very cold room. What changes in spastic signs and voluntary movements do you expect to see? Explain.

Recommended Additional Readings

Burke D (1988). Spasticity as an adaptation to pyramidal tract injury. In: Waxman SG (Ed.), *Functional Recovery in Neurological Disease,* pp. 401-423. New York: Raven Press.

Fahn S, Marsden CD, Calne DB (Eds.) (1988). *Dystonia 2, Advances in Neurology* 50. New York: Raven Press.

Hallett M, Khoshbin S (1980). A physiological mechanism of bradykinesia. *Brain* 103: 301-314.

Latash ML (1993). *Control of Human Movement.* Champaign, IL: Human Kinetics. Chapter 9.

Latash ML, Anson JG. (1996). What are normal movements in atypical populations? *Behavioral and Brain Sciences* 19: 55-106.

Muller H, Zierski J, Penn RD (Eds). (1988). *Local-Spinal Therapy of Spasticity.* Berlin: Springer-Verlag.

Stelmach GE, Worringham CJ, Strand EA (1986). Movement preparation in Parkinson's disease: The use of advance information. *Brain* 109: 1179-1194.

LABORATORIES

INTRODUCTION

The purpose of the following six laboratory studies is to illustrate certain elements of the material covered in the book and to provide hands-on experience. Each study is designed so as to resemble an actual experimental neurophysiological study addressing a certain group of research problems covered in the main body of the textbook. Each of the described laboratory studies involves too much work to be done within a typical 1- to 1.5-hour session. Depending on the availability of equipment, time constraints, level of preparation of students, and other factors, some of the studies may be shortened while others may be performed within two or three sessions. For each study, an outline is presented addressing the following major components:

- Purpose
- Design
- Equipment
- Procedure
- Data analysis and presentation
- Expected findings
- Interpretation

Since students will be asked to write an interpretation of the findings themselves, only a brief outline is offered in the following description. Students should perform the experimental studies in groups; the size of each group will apparently be limited by the total number of enrolled students and the availability of experimental setups. Our experience suggests that optimal group size ranges from 3 to 5, so that one student is acting as the subject of the study while others perform the roles of the experimenters. If time allows, the roles should be rotated. Each group (or each student) is later required to produce a minipaper following the general structure outlined, pooling all the data generated within the group and performing statistical analysis.

The laboratory studies described imply that a minimal set of equipment is available. The following components are essential for running the sessions:

1. At least two electromyographic (EMG) amplifiers with electrodes, leads, and cables. In our laboratory, EMG signals are recorded with the aid of a specially designed system that includes disposable, self-adhesive pediatric electrocardiographic electrodes (one of these is used as a grounding electrode), leads with connectors that clip on the electrodes, miniature potted preamplifiers located about 10 cm from the electrodes, long leads to the main amplifier box, and the main amplifiers (total gain is 3000).

2. An electrical stimulator with stimulating electrodes and an isolation unit. In our laboratory, a Grass stimulator S48 is used with an SIU5 isolation unit. Recommended design of stimulation electrodes is illustrated in figure L.1; note that one electrode is flat while the other has a typical mushroom shape. These electrodes are designed to provide stimulation of n. tibialis in the popliteal fossa in order to induce M-responses and H-reflexes in triceps surae muscles.

3. A vibrator. A handheld massager can be used to provide low-amplitude vibration at 60 Hz.

4. A set of goniometers. Joint angle measuring devices can be either purchased or built using, for example, an external power source (a battery) and a rotational potentiometer.

5. A recording system. A storage oscilloscope can be used to display records that can subsequently be measured directly on the screen. A computer-based data acquisition system can be used as a more versatile alternative. We use a Macintosh computer with National Instruments data acquisition boards and software written using the LabView package.

The following equipment is desirable:

6. An accelerometer. A miniature device measuring acceleration with amplifiers can be purchased from a number of companies; we use accelerometers produced by Sensotec.

7. A force platform. In our laboratory, an AMTI OR-6 platform has been used.

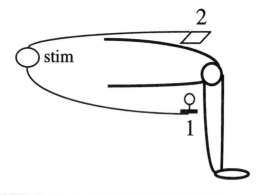

Figure L.1   Recommended design of stimulation electrodes for studies of the H-reflex and M-response in the triceps surae muscle. The mushroom-type electrode (1) is placed under the knee while the flat electrode (2) is placed on the distal, upper part of the thigh. The electrodes can be attached with a velcro strap.

LABORATORY 1

L1. Muscle Responses to Electrical Stimulation of the Muscle Nerve (see chapter 8)

L1.1. Purpose

To record and analyze the behavior of muscle responses to brief pulses of electrical stimulation applied to the muscle nerve; to suggest interpretations for various aspects of the behavior of muscle responses.

L1.2. Design

Brief electrical pulses are applied to n. tibialis in the popliteal fossa, and muscle responses in m. soleus are recorded. Two responses are expected, a direct response (M-response) and a monosynaptic reflex (H-reflex). The latency and the peak-to-peak amplitude of both responses are measured. Parameters of the electrical stimulation (such as its amplitude, frequency, and pulse duration) are changed in a systematic manner. Changes in the latencies and amplitudes of the muscle responses are analyzed.

L1.3. Equipment

An electrical stimulator with an isolation unit and stimulating electrodes; an EMG amplifier; a recording and

measuring system. The experimental setup is illustrated in figure L.2.

L1.4. Procedure

The subject sits comfortably in a chair with feet firmly on the floor. Hip, knee, and ankle joint angles are close to 110° each (full joint extension corresponds to 180°). EMG recording electrodes are placed on the belly of the right m. soleus at a distance of about 4 cm. A grounding electrode may be placed on the other leg. Rub the skin under the electrodes with a cotton ball or a small wiping cloth soaked in rubbing alcohol, wait until the alcohol on the skin evaporates, and then place the recording electrodes on the skin and press them firmly. Use adhesive tape to secure the electrodes in place if necessary. Connect the leads to the electrodes. Ask the subject to contract the muscle voluntarily a few times (to plantarflex the ankle) and watch the signal on your recording device. When the muscle is relaxed, a very low noise level should be seen. When the muscle contracts, a clear burst of activity should be observed.

Turn on the stimulator and make the pulse duration 1 ms, the frequency of stimulation 0.5 Hz, and the

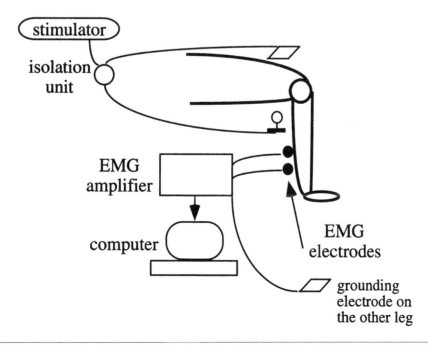

Figure L.2 Design of the experiments in Laboratory 1.

amplitude of stimulation 10 V. Place the flat stimulating electrode (see figure L.1) on top of the subject's thigh, just above the knee. Place the "mushroom" stimulating electrode into the lateral portion of the popliteal fossa. Start increasing the amplitude of the stimulation in small steps. At each step, try to move the mushroom electrode slightly and look for signs of muscle contraction. When the muscle starts to contract in response to the stimulation, try to move the mushroom electrode to induce a maximal response. After an optimal position of the stimulation electrodes has been chosen, fix them with a rubber band. Turn off the stimulation.

Now you are ready to run the experiment. Make the frequency of the stimulation 0.1 Hz (one stimulus every 10 s). Increase the amplitude of the stimulation in steps of 5 V. At first, no muscle reaction will be seen. Then, a slight contraction will emerge. Typically, the earliest contraction is induced through the monosynaptic reflex loop. So you should expect the first muscle response to represent the H-reflex and to emerge at a latency (time delay from the stimulus) of about 35 ms. Continue to increase the amplitude of the stimulation and observe the emergence of an earlier response (M-response at a latency of about 8 ms). Continue to increase the amplitude and observe the suppression and disappearance of the H-reflex. An illustration of changes in the M-response and H-reflex is presented in figure L.3.

Now, find an amplitude of stimulation at which both M-response and H-reflex are approximately of the same amplitude. Make the duration of the stimulation pulse 0.1 ms. Increase the duration of the pulse in steps of 0.1 ms up to 2 ms. Observe changes in the amplitude of the M-response and H-reflex.

Make the pulse duration 1 ms. Start increasing the frequency of the stimulation from 0.1 Hz to 0.3 Hz, 0.5 Hz, 1 Hz, 2 Hz, 5 Hz, and 10 Hz. Observe changes in the amplitude of the M-response and H-reflex. Note that for each condition, you need to analyze only one record, for example, muscle responses to the fifth stimulus.

L1.5. Data Analysis and Presentation

Measure peak-to-peak amplitude of both M-response (A_M) and H-reflex (A_H) in each record. Plot graphs showing the dependencies of A_M and A_H on the manipulated variables such as the amplitude of the stimulation, pulse duration, and frequency of the stimulation. For each condition, and for each subject, calculate two ratios: A_H/A_M and $A_H/A_{H.max}$ where $A_{H.max}$ is the maximal value of the amplitude of the H-reflex observed in a given subject. Plot graphs showing the dependences of $A_H/A_{H.max}$ on the parameters of the stimulation.

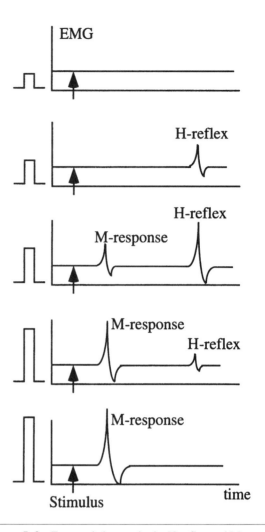

Figure L.3 Expected changes in the H-reflex and M-response with an increase in the amplitude of the electrical stimulus.

L1.6. Expected Findings

You expect to observe the following general dependencies:

1. An increase in the amplitude of the stimulation leads to a monotonic increase in the amplitude of the M-response reaching plateau at some level.
2. An increase in the amplitude of the stimulation initially leads to an increase in the amplitude of the H-reflex, then to its suppression, and then to total disappearance.
3. The A_H/A_M ratio shows a nearly monotonic decrease with the amplitude of the stimulation, from a very high value to zero.
4. Very short pulses of stimulation may be unable to induce any of the responses; an increase in the width of the pulse leads to an increase in both M-response and H-reflex.

5. An increase in the frequency of the stimulation does not affect the M-response; the amplitude of the H-reflex decreases with an increase in the frequency, and at a high frequency, H-reflex can disappear altogether.

L1.7. Interpretations

Electrical stimulation at a low strength is expected, first, to excite the largest neural fibers (axons) in the nerve. These are Ia-afferent fibers whose excitation leads to a monosynaptic H-reflex in the muscle. An increase in the amplitude of the stimulation leads to an increase in the H-reflex amplitude as more and more fibers are excited by each stimulus. Simultaneously, efferent axons of α-motoneurons become excited by the stimulation, leading to a shorter-latency, direct muscle response (M-response). Further increase in the strength of the stimulation leads to an increase in the M-response; H-response, however, begins to get smaller because of the antidromic conduction in the efferent axons. Antidromic volleys render motoneurons nonexcitable by the afferent volleys because the membrane of the motoneurons is in a refractory state when the afferent stimuli come.

An increase in the frequency of stimulation does not affect the M-response but leads to an inhibition of the H-reflex, indicating the presence of a synapse in the H-reflex but not in the M-response, because synapses are less able to conduct high-frequency stimuli.

Shorter pulses of stimulation lead to smaller total charges passing through the membrane. As a result, both afferent and efferent fibers are less likely to be excited by a shorter pulse of the same amplitude.

LABORATORY 2

L2. Phenomena of Excitation and Postsynaptic and Presynaptic Inhibition (see chapters 7, 8, and 9)

L2.1. Purpose

To observe and record the effects of excitation during activation of a motoneuronal pool and the effects of postsynaptic and presynaptic inhibition using, as a test, monosynaptic reflexes.

L2.2. Design

Brief electrical pulses are applied to n. tibialis in the popliteal fossa, and muscle responses in m. soleus are recorded. Parameters of stimulation are chosen that induce both an M-response and an H-reflex. Peak-to-peak amplitude of both responses is recorded when the subject is relaxed. Then the subject is asked to voluntarily activate the triceps surae muscle or its antagonist, m. tibialis anterior. Peak-to-peak amplitudes of the M-response and the H-reflex are recorded. Then, high-frequency vibration is applied to the Achilles tendon, and again peak-to-peak amplitudes of the M-response and the H-reflex are recorded.

L2.3. Equipment

The experimental setup should include an electrical stimulator with an isolation unit and stimulating electrodes, two EMG amplifiers, a vibrator (handheld massager), and a recording and measuring system. The experimental setup is illustrated in figure L.4.

L2.4. Procedure

Subject position and location of electrodes should be the same as described for Laboratory 1. Place recording EMG electrodes on both m. soleus and m. tibialis anterior (two EMG amplifiers are required). At the beginning of this experiment, an optimal position of the stimulation electrodes should be found. The electrodes should be fixed. Use the same parameters of electrical stimulation as described for Laboratory 1. Find an amplitude of stimulation that induces both a visible M-response and a large H-reflex. Do not change the parameters of the stimulation during the entire experiment.

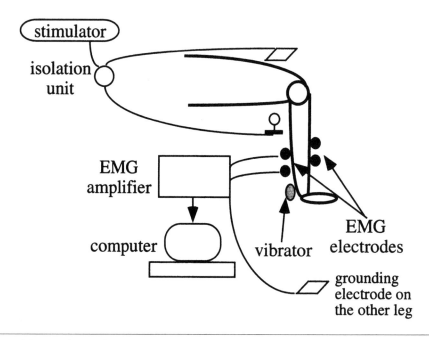

Figure L.4 Design of the experiments in Laboratory 2.

Record muscle responses to the stimulation when the subject is relaxed. Ask the subject to increase the level of activation of the triceps muscle (to lift the heel off the floor just a little bit). Monitor the increase in the soleus activity with the EMG signal. Record muscle responses to the electrical nerve stimulation. Ask the subject to relax again. After 10 s, ask the subject to lift the front part of the foot just off the floor (to activate m. tibialis anterior). Monitor the increase in the tibialis activity with the corresponding EMG signal. Again record the M-response and H-reflex in m. soleus. Repeat the experiments with soleus and tibialis activation three times.

Ask the subject to relax again. Apply electrical stimulation every 10 s. After the second stimulus, apply the vibration to the Achilles tendon. Watch a decrease in the H-reflex amplitude while the amplitude of the M-response remains unchanged. Keep the vibrator on for 30 s (three stimuli). During vibration, watch for tonic vibration reflex (TVR) that can occur in m. triceps surae on the background of vibration. If it occurs, ask the subject to relax the muscles. After 30 s, turn the vibrator off. Watch the process of restoration of the H-reflex for 30 s (three stimuli). Repeat the same experiment in the presence of a TVR. If no TVR occurs, ask the subject to activate the soleus muscle on the background of the vibration by lifting the heel just off the floor.

L2.5. Data Analysis and Presentation

Calculate average values of the peak-to-peak amplitude of the M-response and of the H-reflex across trials when the subject was relaxed and no vibration was applied. Calculate average values of the peak-to-peak amplitude of both responses for conditions of activation of the soleus and for conditions of activation of the tibialis separately. Plot column graphs, for the three conditions mentioned, for M-response and H-reflex.

Plot a graph of changes with time of the peak-to-peak amplitude of the M-response and the H-reflex during the experiment with vibration in the presence and in the absence of tonic muscle activity. Indicate the time of vibration application with a solid bar under the graph.

L2.6. Expected Findings

On the background of soleus activity, the amplitude of the H-reflex is expected to increase, while the amplitude of the M-response should not change. On the background of tibialis activity, the amplitude of the H-reflex is expected to decrease, while the amplitude of the M-response should not change.

On the background of vibration, a gradual decrease in the amplitude of the H-reflex is expected, with a slow restoration after termination of the vibration. This suppression should also be seen on the background of muscle activation (voluntary or reflex).

L2.7. Interpretation

Voluntary activation of a muscle is associated with an increase in the excitability of the motoneuronal pool innervating the muscle. Thus, an increase in the H-reflex amplitude is observed. If an antagonist muscle is activated voluntarily, the system of reciprocal inhibition leads to a postsynaptic inhibition of the motoneuronal pool, leading to a suppression of the amplitude of the H-reflex.

Tendon vibration leads to an increase in the presynaptic inhibition of Ia-afferent terminals, bringing about suppression of the H-reflex (no changes are expected in the M-response). These effects may be stronger than the postsynaptic excitation associated with reflex or voluntary activation of the muscle.

LABORATORY 3

L3. Preprogrammed Reactions (Long-Latency Reflexes) (see chapter 12)

L3.1. Purpose

To observe, record, and analyze the effects of different instructions, predictability of perturbation, and amplitude of expected perturbation upon preprogrammed reactions in different muscles.

L3.2. Design

Preprogrammed reactions in EMGs of arm muscles and body muscles are studied during load perturbations. The subjects are asked either not to interfere with the effects of perturbations or to counteract them as quickly as possible. Perturbation magnitude and direction are varied so that they are either known or unknown to the subject in advance.

L3.3. Equipment

The experimental setup should include two EMG amplifiers, a goniometer, a force platform, a set of loads, and a recording and measuring system. An accelerometer is desirable.

L3.4. Procedure

Experiment 1: The subject sits on a chair and places the right elbow on a table in front of the subject (figure L.5). The forearm and the hand should be vertical; the palm faces the subject. Place EMG electrodes on the biceps and lateral head of triceps (don't forget about the ground electrode!). Tape the accelerometer onto a fingertip or the palm. Signals from the accelerometer will be used to detect the exact timing of the perturbation. Ask the subject to close his/her eyes. First, instruct the subject not to correct arm position if it changes. Apply a few brief pushes/pulls to the forearm, moving it over approximately 45°. Record the EMGs and joint angle changes. Now, instruct the subject to try to always return to the original position "as quickly as possible." Apply similar pushes/pulls unexpectedly for the subject. Then, prior to each perturbation, tell the subject which direction the perturbation will be in (a push or a pull). Again, record joint angle changes and EMGs.

Experiment 2: The subject stands on a force platform (figure L.6; if no force platform is available, the subject can stand on the floor; in this case, only EMGs will be analyzed). Place electrodes on tibialis anterior and so-

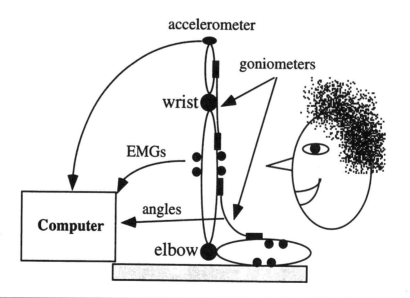

Figure L.5 Design of experiment 1 in Laboratory 3.

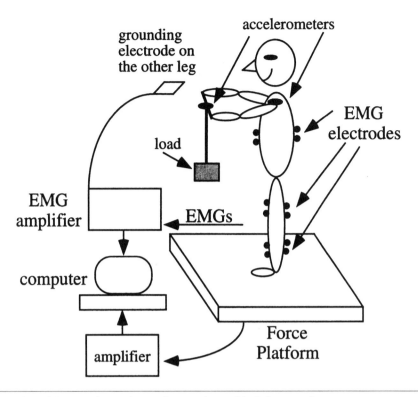

Figure L.6 An illustration of the experimental setup for experiment 2 in Laboratory 3.

leus (if more EMG channels are available, also place EMG electrodes on rectus femoris, biceps femoris, rectus abdominis, and erector spinae). Ask the subject to stand, with eyes closed, holding the bar with the load suspended on a short cord in extended arms. Tape the accelerometer onto the bar. Signals from the accelerometer will be used to detect the exact timing of the perturbation. Unexpectedly cut the cord so that the load drops down. Use loads of different weights. Record EMG and force-platform signals. Then, ask the subject to stand quietly with the hands down along the sides and eyes closed. The accelerometer should be placed on a shoulder. Push the subject slightly forward or backward a few times. In one series, do not give the subject advance information about the direction of an upcoming push. In another series, always tell the subject in advance which direction the push will come in.

L3.5. Data Analysis and Presentation

In order to characterize EMG bursts, the following parameters need to be measured: (1) the latency of each EMG response, that is, the delay between the first visible sign of a perturbation (you can use signal from the accelerometer or signals from the platform as markers) and the beginning of a clear EMG burst; (2) the ampli-

tude of each EMG burst; (3) the duration of each EMG burst; and (4) if possible, the integral under the rectified EMG trace within time limits when you expect preprogrammed reactions to occur (e.g., from 50 ms to 120 ms after the perturbation). Note that we are interested in EMG bursts that start not later than 150 ms after the perturbation.

For each recorded muscle, plot a graph showing the dependence of the specified EMG parameters on the instruction (resist vs. let go, in Experiment 1), the availability of preliminary information about the direction of the perturbation, and magnitude of the perturbation (Experiment 2). Look for differences in the latency and magnitude of preprogrammed responses. Also look for differences in the characteristics of the preprogrammed responses in the distal (soleus and tibialis anterior) and proximal (rectus femoris, biceps femoris, erector spinae, rectus abdominis) muscles.

L3.6. Expected Findings

Preprogrammed responses will be seen in all conditions at a latency of about 50 to 70 ms. Longer latencies can be expected in distal muscles (soleus and tibialis anterior), while shorter latencies can be expected in proximal muscles (rectus abdominis and erector spinae).

The magnitude of the preprogrammed responses will depend crucially on the instruction. In Experiment 1, strong responses will be seen under the instruction "return back as quickly as possible" as compared to the "let go" instruction. The availability of preliminary information about the direction of an upcoming perturbation may lead to changes in both the magnitude of the responses and their pattern. In particular, if the direction of a perturbation is known in advance, a reciprocal pattern of preprogramming can be expected, that is, an increase in the background activity of one muscle and a decrease in the activity of the other muscle of an agonist-antagonist pair. If the direction of the perturbation is unknown, a coactivation pattern may be observed (an increase in the levels of activation of both muscles). An increase in the magnitude of an expected perturbation (Experiment 2, dropping loads of different magnitude) can be expected to lead to an increase in the preprogrammed reaction.

L3.7. Interpretation

Preprogrammed reactions come at an intermediate latency defined by both travel time in the peripheral nerves and central processing time. The magnitude and pattern of a preprogrammed reaction to a perturbation are determined prior to the perturbation. In particular, these reactions can be scaled according to the magnitude of a perturbation. Typically, a reciprocal pattern of preprogramming is used. If a subject does not know exactly in which direction a perturbation will occur, he/she may use an alternative, coactivation pattern of preprogramming.

LABORATORY 4

L4. Kinematic and Electromyographic Patterns During Single-Joint Movements
(see chapter 11)

L4.1. Purpose

To study the properties of EMG patterns during single-joint voluntary movements over different distances, at different velocities, against different inertial loads, and under different accuracy requirements.

L4.2. Design

Record EMG patterns of the biceps and triceps muscles and joint kinematics during single-joint elbow movements while the subjects are asked to move over prescribed distances, at prescribed velocities, with or without an additional load in the hand, and with or without explicit accuracy constraints.

L4.3. Equipment

The experimental setup should include two EMG amplifiers, a goniometer, a set of loads, and a recording and measuring system. An accelerometer is desirable. The experimental setup is illustrated in figure L.7.

L4.4. Procedure

It is better to have a manipulandum moving in a horizontal plane (to avoid possible effects of gravity; figure L.7A). If no manipulandum is available, movements in a sagittal plane can be studied (figure L.7B). Place recording EMG electrodes on the biceps and triceps of the subject's dominant arm. Attach a goniometer so that it

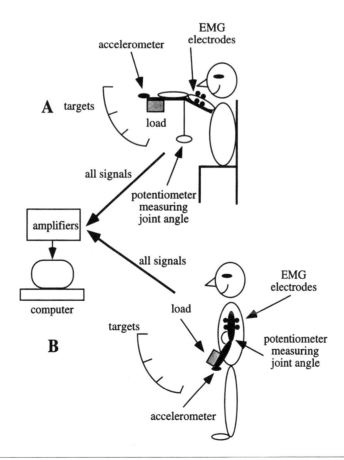

Figure L.7 An illustration of the experimental setup for Laboratory 4.

measures angle in the elbow joint. Tape an accelerometer on a fingertip or on the palm. Prepare a set of loads (e.g., 0.5, 1, 2, and 5 lb) that can be fixed on the wrist (exercise loads with Velcro straps can be used). Prepare a system for presentation of spatial targets. Targets can be drawn on a wall or fixed on a free-standing stand. Recommended target sizes are 1 in., 2 in., and 5 in.

Ask the subject to stand facing the wall with the targets (or near the stand), both arms hanging loosely by the sides, the right index finger extended (it will be used as a pointer), and all other fingers and the thumb flexed. Present the largest target (5 in.) at about 40° of flexion. Ask the subject to make a series of movements (e.g., six movements) from the initial position to the target "at a comfortable speed." Always insist that the subject is accurate in 90% of the trials. Record each movement. Then instruct the subject to perform a series of "fast" movements. Then ask the subject to move "as fast as possible."

Next, tell the subject that in all the trials to follow, the movements should be "as fast and accurate as possible." Change the position of the target so that it corresponds to movement distances of 20°, 40°, and 60°. Record series of movements to each target location.

Then, present the target at 40° and ask the subject to perform movements with different additional loads attached to the wrist. Record a series of movements for each load value. Next, remove the load and replace the target with the smallest one. Insist that the subject preserve the accepted level of accuracy and still move "as fast as possible." Record series of movements to targets of different sizes.

L4.5. Data Analysis and Presentation

To analyze the data, you will need to do trial alignment and data averaging across trials within each series. (Alternatively, to save time, analysis may be restricted to single, representative trials for each condition. In this case, measurements can be done directly on the screen of the monitor or a storage oscilloscope.) Trial alignment can be done with respect to a certain point in time related to movement initiation, for example by the first visible deviation of the signal from the accelerometer or the first visible increase in the background EMG of the prime mover muscle (biceps, in our case). Prior to averaging, it is necessary to filter and rectify the EMG signals. Low-pass filtering at 50 Hz is recommended. After the trials of each series are aligned and averaged, measure the following indexes for each series:

- Peak velocity
- Movement time
- Peak value of the first biceps (agonist) EMG burst
- Peak value of the triceps (antagonist) EMG burst
- Time delay between the beginning of the first biceps EMG burst and the beginning of the delayed triceps burst (antagonist latency)

Plot graphs showing the dependence of each of the measured indexes on task parameters such as movement distance, velocity ("comfortable" vs. "fast" vs. "as fast as possible"), target size, and additional load.

L4.6. Expected Findings

Peak velocity is expected to show an increase with movement velocity, distance, and target size. It is expected to decrease with an increase in the additional load.

Movement time is expected to decrease with an increase in movement velocity and with an increase in target size. It is expected to increase with distance and with additional load.

Peak value of the first agonist burst is expected to increase with movement velocity, distance, target size, and maybe load. Peak value of the antagonist burst is expected to increase with movement velocity, load, and target size; it may show nonmonotonic changes with movement distance. Antagonist latency is expected to increase with movement distance and load; it is expected to decrease with movement velocity and target size.

L4.7. Interpretation

The findings can be described within more than one theoretical framework. You may assume that the central nervous system prescribes certain patterns of muscle activation to match required patterns of muscle torque. In this case the original language of the dual-strategy hypothesis can be used, implying that movements are controlled with rectangular pulses of excitation sent to motoneuronal pools such that the width and amplitude of each pulse, and the delay between the pulses to the agonist and antagonist pools, are modulated according to the task parameters.

Alternatively, EMGs may be considered consequences of both central commands and reflex effects from receptors sensitive to movement kinematics, and the language of the equilibrium-point hypothesis can be used.

LABORATORY 5

L5. Postural Control
(see chapter 19)

L5.1. Purpose

To study different mechanisms involved in maintenance of vertical posture in the field of gravity; to study the dependence of these mechanisms on parameters of postural perturbations, actions by the subject, availability of vision, and adequacy of peripheral kinesthetic information.

L5.2. Design

In standing subjects, record force-platform signals and EMGs of postural muscles and of certain arm muscles during fast voluntary arm movements and load dropping induced either voluntarily by the subject or by an experimenter. During quiet standing with the eyes open or closed, apply vibration to a major leg muscle tendon. Observe and measure changes in posture.

L5.3. Equipment

The experimental setup should include at least two EMG amplifiers (better to have eight), a force platform, a set

of loads, a vibrator, and a recording and measuring system. An accelerometer is desirable. The experimental setup is illustrated in figure L.8.

L5.4. Procedure

Place EMG electrodes on the bellies of the following muscles on one side of the body: soleus, tibialis anterior, rectus femoris, biceps femoris, rectus abdominis, erector spinae, and posterior and anterior heads of the deltoid muscle. Tape an accelerometer to the right wrist or palm; always choose a position of the accelerometer such that its axis of maximal sensitivity is in the direction of a planned action.

Experiment 1: Ask the subject to stand quietly on the platform and to perform fast shoulder flexions of both arms so that both arms are horizontal in the final position. In another series, ask the subject to perform fast bilateral shoulder extensions (movements of both arms backward) within a comfortable range. In the last series, ask the subject to perform fast bilateral shoulder abductions (movement sideways) so that both arms are horizontal in the final position.

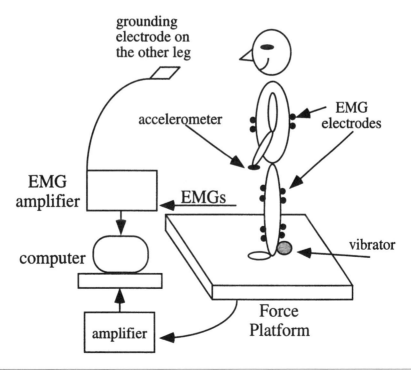

Figure L.8 An illustration of the experimental setup for Laboratory 5.

Experiment 2: Ask the subject to stand on the platform and hold a load in extended arms. In one series, the subject is required to drop the load by an arm movement, for example, by a fast, low-amplitude bilateral shoulder abduction. In another experiment, unloading will be done by an experimenter (for example, if the load is hanging on a rope from a bar held by the subject, the experimenter may cut the rope with scissors) in two conditions: when the subject does not look at the load (e.g., has eyes closed) and when the subject watches how the experimenter induces the unloading. In the last experiment, you can help the subject by having a metronome and warning the subject that the load will drop at the third beat.

Experiment 3: Ask the subject to stand quietly, and apply vibration to the right Achilles tendon or to the right patellar tendon. Observe changes in posture in two conditions: when the subject is standing with eyes open and with eyes closed.

In all experiments, record changes in the background activity of postural muscles and displacements in the center of pressure in both anterior-posterior and lateral directions, which can be calculated from platform signals as (M_x/F_y) and (M_y/F_x) where $M_{x,y}$ are force moment components and $F_{x,y}$ are horizontal force components measured by the platform.

L5.5. Data Analysis and Presentation

You will need to have quantitative indexes of changes in the background EMG activity in postural muscles. Depending on the methods of measurement available, EMG integrals during appropriate time intervals, EMG peak amplitudes, and/or EMG burst durations may be used. Note that you will need to have separate indexes of EMG changes for anticipatory postural adjustments (APAs) and for later, corrective reactions (CRs). Hence, you will need to define the time of subject's action (or unloading) initiation, which can be done with the aid of the signal from the accelerometer or, in cases of the subject's voluntary movement, with the aid of EMG signal from the prime mover (posterior or anterior deltoid muscle). After this time (t_0) is defined, APAs can be quantified using EMG changes that occur prior to t_0 or a few tens of milliseconds after t_0 (so that no feedback effect on EMG could possibly occur). Corrective reactions can be quantified using time intervals starting about 50 ms after t_0 and until about 150 ms after t_0. Displacements of the center of pressure during APAs can also be assessed, for example by comparing the position of the center of pressure at t_0 with its position a few hundred milliseconds (e.g., 300 ms) prior to this time.

For the data collected in Experiment 1, plot indexes of changes in the EMGs during APAs and during CRs as functions of the direction of arm movement. Also, plot displacements of the center of pressure as functions of movement direction.

For Experiment 2, compare changes in the background EMG of postural muscles and displacements of the center of pressure during APAs associated with self-induced unloadings, unexpected experimenter-induced unloadings, and expected experimenter-induced unloadings.

During experiments with muscle vibration (Experiment 3), you will need to assess displacements of the center of pressure in both directions (anterior-posterior and lateral) during the course of vibration and plot them as functions of time. Compare these dependencies during vibration of different tendons (Achilles and patellar tendons) and during standing with open eyes and with closed eyes.

L5.6. Expected Findings

In Experiment 1, you expect to see APAs in both EMGs and center-of-pressure displacements during arm movements forward and backward, and virtually no APAs during arm movements sideways. Direction of the APAs should depend on the direction of the movement. The APAs should be followed by CRs whose pattern should also depend on movement direction.

In Experiment 2, you expect to see clear APAs during self-initiated unloadings, and no APAs during experimenter-initiated unloading, even when the subject is able to predict the timing of the perturbation (in the series that involves watching how the experimenter induces the unloading and/or assistance with the metronome). Corrective reactions are expected to be present in all the series but to be larger in the series with experimenter-induced unloadings.

In Experiment 3, vibration of the Achilles tendon is expected to lead to a displacement of the body backward, while vibration of the patellar tendon is expected to lead to a displacement of the body forward. Note that a lateral body displacement is also expected because the vibration is applied only to one leg. All the effects of vibration are expected to be larger when the subject stands with the eyes closed.

L5.7. Interpretation

Experiments 1 and 2 suggest that there are two types of defensive postural reactions to perturbations. Reactions of the first type (APAs) are generated by the subject in anticipation of a perturbation only if the perturbation is generated by the subject's own action. The magnitude and direction of APAs are adjusted corresponding to anticipated mechanical effects of an expected perturbation. Note that APAs are always suboptimal and cannot compensate for the perturbation ideally, so they are followed by feedback-based reactions of the second type (CRs).

Experiment 3 illustrates the role of visual and kinesthetic information for postural control. In particular, vibration of a muscle leads to an unusually high level of activity of spindle afferents, which is interpreted by the central nervous system as an increase in muscle length. In turn, the increase in muscle length is interpreted as a change in joint position, and a correction for this illusory change is introduced, leading to an actual movement of the whole body. Availability of visual information makes the system less susceptible to illusions introduced by distorted kinesthetic information, and vibration-induced violations of vertical posture become smaller.

LABORATORY 6

L6. Organization of Multi-Joint Movements (see chapter 21)

L6.1. Purpose

To analyze the organization of targeted movement of a multi-joint limb, in particular, properties of joint and endpoint trajectories and patterns of muscle activation.

L6.2. Design

Sitting or standing subjects are asked to perform fast pointing movements of the right arm to a visual target. Joint trajectories and EMG patterns of major muscles are recorded. Subjects are also asked to use one hand to manipulate objects held by the other hand.

L6.3. Equipment

The experimental setup should include four EMG amplifiers, three goniometers, and a recording and measuring system. An accelerometer is desirable. Experimental setup is illustrated in figure L.9.

L6.4. Procedure

Experiment 1: Ask the subject to sit on a low chair close to a table and place the upper arm on the table in front of him/her. The forearm and the hand should be vertical with the palm facing the subject. Place EMG electrodes on the biceps, triceps, wrist flexor (flexor carpi radialis), and wrist extensor (extensor carpi ulnaris); place two goniometers so that they measure changes in the elbow and the wrist joint in the flexion-extension plane. Tape an accelerometer on a fingertip. Ask the subject to perform series of the following "very fast" movements: elbow flexions, elbow extensions, wrist flexions, and wrist extensions—each movement over about 40°.

Experiment 2: Ask the subject to stand up. Place three goniometers to measure abduction-adduction movements in the shoulder and flexion-extension movements in the elbow and the wrist. Ask the subject to perform a series of "very fast" movements starting from the fully extended and abducted right arm (the whole arm is horizontal, in a frontal plane).

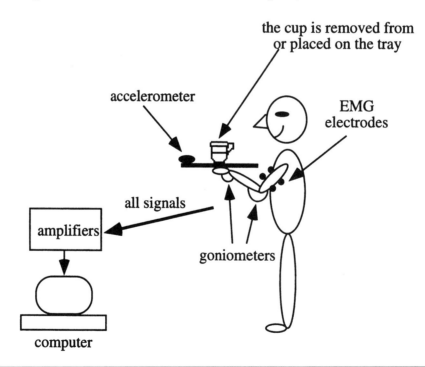

Figure L.9   An illustration of the experimental setup for Laboratory 6, experiment 3.

Experiment 3: Place EMG electrodes on the biceps and triceps muscles of the right arm. Ask the subject to stand up and hold a tray with a load (e.g., a pitcher) in a horizontal position with the left hand. Place an accelerometer on the tray; place goniometers so that they measure wrist and elbow flexion-extension angles of the left arm. One task is to pick up the load from the tray with the right hand. Another task is to place the load back on the tray. Then the same tasks are performed by an experimenter while the subject observes the experimenter's actions.

L6.5. Data Analysis and Presentation

Experiment 1: Plot time series for the EMG signals and joint angles for each task separately. Compare the timing and shape of the EMG bursts in the flexor-extensor muscle pairs controlling the two joints. You can use EMG burst durations, amplitudes, integrals, or even cross-correlations of the EMG curves, depending on the available equipment. Compare the timing of the antagonist burst for each joint with actual joint kinematics.

Experiment 2: Plot time series for angle joints and for the trajectory of the endpoint (calculated from joint angle curves and the length of arm segments measured in the subject). For a series of trials, calculate the standard deviation of each joint angle and of the endpoint coordinates for "special points" on the trajectory, for example, for the time of peak acceleration, time of peak velocity of the endpoint, and time of peak deceleration of the endpoint, as well as time of movement termination. Predict standard deviation of the endpoint coordinates at each point from the standard deviations of angles and actual limb configuration. Compare the predicted values with the measured ones.

Experiment 3: Align the trials with respect to the time of tray unloading (defined using the signal from the accelerometer; alternative methods are acceptable, for example using an electrical switch and breaking or establishing a contact between the load and the tray). Calculate changes in the background muscle activity with respect to the time of alignment (similarly to the way it was done in Laboratory 5). Do this separately for loading and unloading trials performed by the subject or by the experimenter.

L6.6. Expected Findings

Experiment 1: A synergy among control signals to the wrist and the elbow joints is expected to lead to a close relation between the EMG patterns of the two flexor-extensor pairs. This relation can be revealed in a correlation between parameters characterizing corresponding EMG bursts. Since this relation is assumed to be of central origin, EMG patterns are not expected to correlate closely with joint kinematics, particularly for the joint whose movement was not prescribed by the instruction (such a correlation could be expected if EMG patterns were of a reflex nature).

Experiment 2: Individual joints are expected to show larger relative variability than the endpoint trajectory. Standard deviations by themselves, however, are not adequate measures from which to draw such a conclusion. Thus, predicted endpoint variability (calculated based on the limb geometry and variabilities of individual joints) at certain "special times" is expected to be larger than actually measured variability.

Experiment 3: Anticipatory adjustments in the activity of muscles of the arm holding the tray are expected during both taking the load off the tray and placing the load back onto the tray by the other hand. These adjustments will not be seen when load manipulations are done by an experimenter, even when the subject watches what the experimenter does.

L6.7. Interpretation

Multi-joint movements are controlled using combinations of control signals to individual joints and muscles that are related to each other by a rule (a synergy) such that a common goal is successfully achieved. The existence of synergies can lead, in particular, to error compensation among joints if a movement is performed in conditions of motor redundancy.

Anticipatory changes in the activity of limb muscles can be seen if the muscles are involved in a postural task and the person performs an action that brings about a perturbation of the posture. Such anticipatory adjustments are not seen when a postural perturbation is predictable but not associated with an action by the subject. Thus, anticipatory adjustments may be viewed as distinct peripheral patterns associated with a motor action that is always directed at both apparently "focal" and appently "postural" muscles.

GLOSSARY

Acetylcholine—a **neurotransmitter;** the mediator of neuromuscular excitation.

Actin—a molecule; a major force-generating element within a skeletal muscle.

Action potential—a standard, brief pattern of changes in the **membrane potential;** a unit of information transmission within and among excitable tissues.

Afferent (fiber)—an axon transmitting signals from a "more peripheral" structure to a "more central" structure; commonly, a sensory fiber, i.e., the peripheral axon branch of a **proprioceptor** neuron.

Agonist—a muscle whose activation leads to a required motor effect.

"All-or-none" law—a law describing the generation of a standard, nongraded response to a stimulus exceeding a certain threshold.

Alpha-gamma coactivation—simultaneous activation of **α- and γ-motoneurons** during voluntary muscle activation.

Alpha motoneuron—a neuron innervating power-producing, extrafusal muscle fibers.

Amnesia—loss of memories.

Ampulla—a dilated area of a semicircular duct where vestibular receptor cells (hair cells) are located; innervated by the ampullary nerve.

Antagonist—a muscle whose activation apparently counteracts a required motor effect.

Anticipatory postural adjustments—changes in the activity of postural muscles seen prior to a self-generated postural perturbation (e.g., prior to a fast voluntary movement).

Antidromic conduction—conduction of **action potentials** along the **axon** to the **soma.**

Articular receptors—**receptor** endings located in and around the joint capsule sensitive to joint angle (typically, close to the anatomical limits of joint motion) and to tension of the joint capsule.

Ascending tracts—neural tracts carrying information from the peripheral receptors and from the spinal cord to the brain (major tracts include spinothalamic tract, spinocerebellar tracts, spinoreticular tract, spinovestibular tract, and spinotectal tract).

Asynergia—an impairment in interjoint coordination.

Axon—the output fiber of a neuron; commonly, the longest fiber originating from the **axon hillock.**

Axon hillock—an area where the **axon** exits the **soma,** characterized by the increased ability to generate **action potentials.**

Babinski reflex—a response in leg muscles to a tactile stimulation of the sole of the foot.

Baclofen—a drug used to treat **spasticity;** an agonist of **gamma-aminobutyric acid.**

Ballism—a disorder of the **basal ganglia** characterized by fast, large-amplitude, irregular, involuntary movements.

Basal ganglia—several paired structures within the brain playing an important role in voluntary movement generation and coordination.

Bernstein problem (redundancy problem)—an ill-posed problem of choice; a problem of how the central nervous system chooses a pattern of variables at a certain level of analysis based on a required summed effect at a "higher" level of analysis.

Blind spot—an area on the **retina** where the optic nerve exits the eye; this area lacks **photoreceptors.**

Bradykinesia—slowness of movements typical of **Parkinson's disease.**

Caudate nucleus—a neural structure; part of the **basal ganglia.**

Central pattern generator (CPG)—a hypothetical neural structure that generates a rhythmic neural activity later transformed into a rhythmic muscle activity leading to a rhythmic behavior, such as **locomotion.**

Cerebellar nuclei (dentate, fastigial, interpositus)—brain structures mediating most of the cerebellar output.

Cerebellar peduncles—six neural tracts connecting the **cerebellum** with the rest of the central nervous system.

Cerebellar tremor—a low-frequency **tremor** (3-5 Hz) seen in patients with cerebellar disorders.

Cerebellum—a large brain structure that lies just behind the **medulla** and the **pons.**

Chorea (Huntington's disease)—a disorder of the **basal ganglia** characterized by excessive, irregular, involuntary movements.

Chronic fatigue syndrome—a sustained feeling of exhaustion and inability to be involved in virtually any kind of activity requiring even minimal motor effort.

Clonus—a series of alternating bursts of activity in the flexor and extensor muscles of a joint at a frequency of about 6-8 Hz; may be induced by a quick joint movement.

Colliculus—a structure in the **midbrain** playing an important role in processing of visual and auditory information.

Complex system—a system whose properties cannot be derived from properties of its elements.

Computer tomography (CT)—a method of reconstruction of three-dimensional images of tissues based on a series of two-dimensional images.

Conditioned reflex—a **reflex** to a new stimulus developed as a result of simultaneous presentations of the new stimulus and an old stimulus associated with the reflex.

Consolidation (of memory)—a process of transferring information from the **short-term memory** into the **long-term memory.**

Convection—movement of a solvent (e.g., water) and dissolved particles under the influence of a difference in hydrostatic pressure.

Corpus callosum—a major neural tract connecting two large **cortical hemispheres.**

Corrective postural reactions—**preprogrammed reactions** in postural muscles to external perturbations.

Corrective stumbling reaction—a **reflex**-like response to a mechanical or electrical stimulation of a paw leading to a coordinated limb movement "stepping over" the fictitious obstacle.

Cortex (cerebral, cerebellar)—the external, thin layer densely packed with neuron bodies.

Cost function—a rather arbitrary function introduced to solve a problem of redundancy (**Bernstein problem**).

Cross-bridge—a molecular connection between an **actin** molecule and a **myosin** molecule that generates force during muscle contractions.

Cutaneous receptors—**receptor** endings sensitive to skin displacement, pressure on the skin, temperature, etc., including, in particular, pacinian corpuscles, Merkel disks, Meissner corpuscles, and Ruffini endings.

Dendrite—a relatively short fiber connected to the neuron body; commonly serves as a site of input signals to the **neuron.**

Depolarization—a decrease in the absolute value of the negative **membrane** potential.

Descending tracts—neural tracts carrying information from the brain to the spinal cord (major tracts include corticospinal tract, corticobulbar tract, pyramidal tract, rubrospinal tract, vestibulospinal tract, reticulospinal tracts, and tectospinal tract).

Diffusion—movement of dissolved particles under the influence of a difference in particle concentrations.

Dopamine—an important **neurotransmitter** whose deficit leads to **Parkinson's disease.**

Dorsal root (spinal)—a set of neural fibers carrying peripheral information into the spinal cord.

Dual-strategy hypothesis—a hypothesis assuming the existence of two strategies during voluntary movements, with and without explicit or implicit control over movement time.

Dynamic pattern generation (dynamic systems approach)—a mathematical modeling approach that uses nonlinear differential equations to describe the behavior of a complex system.

Dysdiadochokinesia—an inability to perform movements at a certain constant rhythm.

Dysmetria—an inability to achieve a required final position.

Dystonia—a complex neural disorder characterized by involuntary movements with clear rotational components.

Efferent (fiber)—an **axon** transmitting signals from a "more central" structure to a "more peripheral" structure; commonly, an axon of a **motoneuron.**

Efferent copy (efference copy)—a hypothetical copy of motor command signals participating in **kinesthetic** perception.

Elastic element—a mechanical element that deforms under the influence of an external force, generates force against the deformation, and can store and release potential energy of the deformation.

Electroencephalography (EEG)—a method of registration of waves of brain activity with electrodes placed over the skull.

Electrolyte—a fragment of a molecule with a non-zero total electric charge.

Electromyography (EMG)—a method of registration of compound **action potentials** generated by muscle fibers.

Emergent feature—a feature that emerges during an activity without being explicitly programmed.

Equilibrium-point hypothesis—a hypothesis of motor control that assumes that the central nervous system manipulates equilibrium states of the system effector+load.

Equilibrium potential (of an ion)—a potential for which there is no net passive movement of the ion across the **membrane.**

Equilibrium potential (of a membrane)—a potential on a **membrane** that is maintained in the absence of external stimuli.

Evoked potential—a potential synchronized with an external event (e.g., a stimulus).

Excitatory postsynaptic potential (EPSP)—a brief **depolarizing** change in the potential of the **postsynaptic membrane.**

Exteroceptor—a **receptor** transducing information from the environment.

Extrafusal fibers—power-producing muscle fibers external with respect to muscle **spindles.**

F-wave—a muscle response not involving central **synaptic** transmission, induced by an electrical stimulation of the muscle nerve; the stimulus induces an **antidromic** volley in the motor **axons,** leading to an **orthodromic** volley.

Feedback control—a principle of control according to which a controller changes command signals based on their outcome.

Feedforward control—a principle of control according to which a controller generates command variables independently of the outcome.

Flexor reflex—a **polysynaptic reflex** seen in several major flexor muscles in response to a mechanical or electrical stimulation of flexor reflex afferents.

Fovea—an area of the **retina** with the highest density of photoreceptors.

Foveola—the central area of the **fovea** providing for the best perception of light stimuli.

Functional electrical stimulation—a method of substituting for a lost motor function using EMG signals from healthy muscles (or other signals) to drive electrical stimulators applied to paralyzed muscles.

Gamma-aminobutyric acid (GABA)—a common **neurotransmitter** within the central nervous system.

Gamma-motoneurons—small motoneurons innervating **intrafusal fibers** and changing the sensitivity of **spindle endings** to muscle length (static γ-motoneurons) and to velocity (dynamic γ-motoneurons).

Ganglion—a group of neurons united by a common function.

Gate control theory of pain—a theory suggesting that the subjective feeling of pain is created by a disparity between signals from **proprioceptors** and signals from **nociceptors.**

Globus pallidus—a neural structure; part of the **basal ganglia.**

Golgi tendon organ—a **receptor** ending located at the muscle-tendon junction and sensitive to changes in muscle force.

Gray matter—neural tissue containing mostly neuron bodies.

H-reflex (Hoffman reflex)—a monosynaptic **reflex** induced by an electrical stimulation of the muscle nerve.

Habituation—a decrease in a response to a stimulus seen with repetitive presentations of the stimulus.

Henneman principle (size principle)—the principle of an orderly recruitment of **motor units,** from the smallest ones to the largest ones.

Hill's equation—an equation describing the relation between muscle force and velocity of muscle shortening.

Hippocampus—a large brain structure that is suspected of playing a major role in memory **consolidation,** storage, and retrieval.

Homunculus—a fictitious "little person" sitting in one's brain and making decisions with respect to appropriate actions to be taken.

Hyperpolarization—an increase in the absolute value of the negative **membrane** potential.

Hypometria—a tendency to undershoot the target that is typical of **Parkinson's disease.**

Hypothalamus—a structure in the diencephalon playing an important role in the autonomic and emotional functions; part of the **limbic circle.**

Hypotonia—a decrease in the resistance of a joint to an external movement.

Inactivation (of sodium channels)—phenomenon of a drop in the membrane conductance for sodium ions leading to **absolute refractory period** and preventing backfiring of **action potentials.**

Independently controlled variable—a hypothetical variable whose pattern can be preserved or modified by the central nervous system independently of possible changes in the environment.

Inhibitory postsynaptic potential (IPSP)—a brief **hyperpolarizing** change in the potential of the **postsynaptic membrane.**

Innervation ratio—the number of muscle fibers innervated by a single α-motoneuron; can vary from a few to over a thousand.

Interneurons—**neurons** receiving information from and transmitting it to other neurons; (a) Ia-interneurons mediate reciprocal inhibition; (b) Renshaw cells mediate recurrent inhibition; (c) Ib-interneurons mediate inhibitory effects from Golgi tendon organs.

Interoceptor—a **receptor** transducing information from within the body.

Intrafusal fibers—muscle fibers inside muscle spindles; innervated by a special system of fusimotor neurons (γ-**motoneurons).**

Ischemia—block of blood flow into an area of the body leading to a disruption of transmission of **action potentials** along neural fibers.

Isometric conditions—(a) conditions of muscle contraction when the length of muscle fibers does not change, typically unattainable in experiments; (b) conditions of muscle contraction when the length of the muscle+tendon system does not change.

Isotonic conditions—conditions of muscle contraction when the apparent external load on the muscle does not change; typically unattainable in experiments.

Kinesthesia—the awareness of the position of segments of our body in space and in relation to one another.

Latency—the delay between a stimulus and a reaction.

Lateral geniculate nucleus—the most important subcortical region participating in visual perception; makes projections to the primary visual **cortex.**

Limbic circle—brain structures (the **hypothalamus,** the fornix, the **hippocampus,** the amygdaloid nucleus, and the cingulate gyrus of the **cerebral cortex**) participating in particular in the generation of emotional reactions.

Lobes—parts of the large brain hemispheres (frontal, parietal, occipital, temporal, and insula).

Locomotion—a motor action during which the location of the whole body in the environment changes.

Locomotor area (mesencephalic)—an area in the **medulla** and in the **midbrain** whose electrical stimulation can induce **locomotion** in an animal.

Long-term memory—a memory that lasts for the lifetime.

M-response—a direct muscle response (contraction) to an electrical stimulation of the muscle nerve.

Medulla—part of the central nervous system connecting the spinal cord and the brain; contains, among other vital structures, the cardiac center, the respiratory center, and the vasomotor center.

Membrane—a biological, partially permeable structure separating the inside structures of a cell from the environment.

Membrane threshold—a value of **membrane potential** leading to the generation of an **action potential.**

Minimum jerk principle—an optimization principle based on minimization of an integral measure of jerk (derivative of acceleration) during voluntary movement.

Motor unit—an α-**motoneuron** and all the muscle fibers it innervates; a unit of force production in skeletal muscles.

Multiple sclerosis—a systemic disease leading to a loss of the **myelin** sheath by myelinated tracts within the central nervous system.

Myelin—a substance made of glial cells that forms a protective shield around **axons,** leading to an increase in the conduction speed of **action potentials.**

Myosin—a molecule; a major force-generating element within a skeletal muscle.

Negative feedback—feedback that leads to a decrease in the magnitude of an original stimulus.

Nernst equation—an equation for the **equilibrium potential** for an ion in the presence of an electrical field and a difference in ion concentrations.

Neuromuscular synapse—a place where an **action potential** on the **presynaptic membrane** of a motor **axon** excites the **postsynaptic** muscle membrane.

Neuron—an excitable cell, a unit of the nervous system.

Neurotransmitter (mediator)—a substance released through the **presynaptic membrane** that can **depolarize** or **hyperpolarize** the **postsynaptic membrane** of a **synapse.**

Nociceptors—small sensory endings that generate **action potential** in response to potentially damaging stimuli such as temperature, pressure, or certain chemicals; participate in the creation of the sense of pain.

Nonelectrolyte—a molecule or a fragment of a molecule with a net zero electric charge.

Operant conditioning—an experimental situation in which a relation between an action by the animal and an external stimulus is being learned.

Optic chiasm—the place where two optic nerves join each other.

Orthodromic conduction—conduction of **action potentials** along the **axon** from the soma.

Osmosis—movement of water induced by a difference in the concentrations of water measured as the total concentration of all particles.

Otoliths—crystals of calcium carbonate in the inner ear; participate in detection of linear acceleration.

Paresis—partial loss of voluntary control over muscles within an area of the body.

Parkinson's disease—a complex disorder with a clear motor component associated with an impairment of the functioning of the **basal ganglia.**

Pavlov's theory of conditioned reflexes—a theory assuming that behavior represents a combination of unconditioned (inborn) and **conditioned reflexes.**

Phasic stretch reflex—a monosynaptic **reflex** to quick muscle stretch (same as **T-reflex**).

Photoreceptors (cones and rods)—specialized neurons in the eye generating **action potentials** in response to visible light.

Physiology of initiative (physiology of activity)—a theory advanced by Bernstein suggesting that voluntary movements are initiated by active processes within the central nervous system.

Plasticity (neural)—an ability to modify neural connections in response to an injury or to specific training.

Plegia—total loss of voluntary control over muscles within an area of the body.

Pons—part of the brain, just rostral to the **medulla.**

Positive feedback—feedback that leads to an increase in the magnitude of an original stimulus.

Postsynaptic inhibition—an inhibitory influence acting on the **postsynaptic membrane** of a **neuron.**

Postsynaptic membrane—an area of the membrane of an excitable cell receiving excitatory or inhibitory stimuli through a **synapse.**

Post-tetanic potentiation—a short-lasting increase in the twitch contraction force after a brief tetanic stimulation.

Premotor cortex—part of the premotor area (area 6) of the cerebral **cortex.**

Preprogrammed reactions (long-latency reflexes, functional stretch-reflex, M_2-M_3, or triggered reactions)—muscle reactions to external signals (e.g., perturbations) prepared by the central nervous system in advance and triggered by an appropriate peripheral stimulus.

Presynaptic inhibition—an inhibitory influence acting on the **presynaptic membrane** of a synapse; selective with respect to the involved synapse(s).

Presynaptic membrane—an area of the membrane of a neural fiber transmitting information through a **synapse.**

Primary motor area—area 4 of the precentral **cortex;** requires low-stimulation currents to induce visible movement.

Proprioceptor—a **receptor** transducing information about the relative configuration and state of body segments.

Propriospinal tracts—neural tracts carrying information from one segment of the spinal cord to another.

Pupillary reflex—a reflex adaptation of the size of the pupil to light mediated by the pretectal area of the **midbrain.**

Purkinje cells—large inhibitory cells in the **cerebellum** providing its only output.

Putamen—a neural structure; part of the **basal ganglia.**

Pyramidal cells—large neurons of the **cerebral cortex;** the origin of the pyramidal tract.

Ranvier nodes—breaks in the **myelin** sheath with a high concentration of sodium channels; places where **action potential** can be generated during transmission along myelinated fibers.

Readiness potential *(Bereitschaftpotential)*—a slow, negative shift of the **EEG** seen as early as 1.5 s prior to a voluntary movement.

Receptor—a specialized neuron or a subcellular structure generating **action potentials** in response to specific sources of energy.

Reciprocal inhibition—a system using inhibitory Ia-interneurons, suppressing the activity of a motoneuronal pool when an antagonistic pool is being excited.

Red nucleus—a structure within the **midbrain;** the source of the rubrospinal tract.

Reductionism—an approach that attempts to describe properties of a system based on properties of its elements; it is, by definition, inapplicable to analysis of **complex systems.**

Reflex—a misnomer implying a relatively stereotypic, relatively standardized reaction to an external stimulus; (a) monosynaptic reflexes involve only one central synapse; (b) oligosynaptic reflexes involve a few central synapses; (c) polysynaptic reflexes involve many central synapses.

Reflex arc—a loop typically involving a **receptor,** a central processing unit (neural structures), and an output structure (a muscle).

Refractory period (absolute)—a period when an excitable structure cannot be excited even by a very strong external stimulus.

Refractory period (relative)—a period when an excitable structure needs a stronger-than-usual stimulus to generate a response.

Reinnervation—a process of the emergence of new synapses between terminals of an axon and target cells (neural or muscle) that have lost their original source of excitation.

Renshaw cell—an inhibitory **interneuron** excited by signals from **motoneurons** of a pool and inhibiting the activity of the same motoneuronal pool (recurrent inhibition).

Reticular formation—a structure containing numerous small neurons occupying areas of the **medulla** and of the **midbrain;** the source of the reticulospinal tract.

Retina—a layer with **photoreceptors** within the internal structures of the eye.

Rheobase—the lowest stimulus amplitude that can lead to the generation of an **action potential** for a stimulus of a very long (infinite) duration.

Rigidity—an increased resistance of a limb segment to attempts at moving it by an external force; typical of **Parkinson's disease.**

Saccade—a very quick and accurate eye movement used to shift the gaze from object to object.

Sarcolemma—the **membrane** of a muscle cell.

Sarcomere—a force-producing unit of a muscle filament.

Sarcoplasmic reticulum—a system of cisternae containing Ca^{++} ions within a muscle fiber.

Sensory ending—part of a **receptor** cell able to generate **action potentials** in response to specific influences (sources of energy).

Servo—a **feedback control** system providing for perfect generation of a desired value of an output parameter.

Servo hypothesis—a hypothesis of motor control according to which the mechanism of the **tonic stretch reflex** is considered a perfect **servo** keeping muscle length at a centrally programmed value.

Short-term memory—a memory that lasts for a few minutes or hours.

Sliding-filament theory—a theory of muscle force production based on molecular interactions, mostly between **actin** and **myosin** molecules.

Smooth pursuit—a relatively slow eye movement whose purpose is to keep the image of an object within the fovea.

Sodium-potassium pump—an active mechanism maintaining the difference of ion concentrations across biological **membranes.**

Soma—the body of a **neuron** containing organelles; commonly, the site of input signals.

Somatosensory cortical areas—areas 1, 2, 3a, and 3b in the parietal cortex receiving inputs from the **thalamus;** contain sensory maps that look like distorted images of the body.

Spasticity—a complex of symptoms associated with disruption of transmission along **descending spinal tracts;** involves uncontrolled spasms, increased muscle **"tone,"** and increased muscle **reflexes** to stretch with a pronounced velocity-dependent component.

Spatial summation—an increase in the combined effect of two (or more) stimuli when they come simultaneously to different sites belonging to the same excitable structure (e.g., a **neuron**).

Spindle (muscle)—a spindlelike structure located in parallel to power-producing muscle fibers containing **primary** and **secondary endings** sensitive to changes in muscle length and velocity.

Spindle endings—(a) primary: **receptors** sensitive to changes in muscle length and velocity; (b) secondary: **receptors** sensitive to muscle length but not to velocity.

Structural unit—a task-specific assembly of elements of a **complex system** whose purpose is to assure a **synergy.**

Substantia nigra—a structure in the **midbrain;** part of the **basal ganglia.**

Subthalamic nucleus—a neural structure; part of the **basal ganglia.**

Supplementary motor area—a **cortical** area (area 6) whose stimulation requires higher currents and induces more complex movements as compared to the **primary motor area.**

Synapse—a place where signals are transmitted from one excitable cell (a **neuron**) to another excitable cell (a neuron or a muscle fiber).

Synaptic cleft—a gap between the **presynaptic membrane** and the **postsynaptic membrane.**

Synergy (postural or movement)—a combination of control signals to a number of muscles and joints whose purpose is to assure a certain movement or preserve a certain posture.

T-reflex—a **monosynaptic reflex** to a quick muscle stretch (e.g., to a tendon tap).

T-tubule—an invagination of the **sarcolemma** where it comes close to the cisternae within the **sarcoplasmic reticulum.**

Taxonomy—a set of notions used to describe and analyze a **complex system.**

Temporal summation—an increase in the effect of a stimulus when it follows another stimulus after a brief delay.

Tetanus—a sustained muscle contraction commonly produced by a sequence of **action potentials** in the motor **axons.**

Thalamus—a large structure in the diencephalon playing an important role in sensory-motor coordination.

Tone (muscle)—a misnomer implying a feeling of resistance experienced by an examiner when he or she tries to move a limb segment of another person or to press on the muscle belly.

Tonic stretch reflex—a **polysynaptic reflex** leading to an increase in the level of muscle activation with slow muscle stretch.

Tonic vibration reflex—a **polysynaptic reflex** leading to an increase in the level of muscle activation induced by a low-amplitude, high-frequency muscle or tendon vibration.

Torticollis—**dystonia** affecting neck muscles.

Tremor—alternating activity of antagonist muscles controlling a joint, leading to alternating joint movements; 3-5 Hz in **cerebellar** disorders; about 6 Hz in **Parkinson's disease;** 8-12 Hz in healthy persons (physiological tremor).

Triphasic pattern—an EMG pattern typically accompanying voluntary movements that consists of an **agonist** burst, followed by an **antagonist** burst and by a second agonist burst.

Tropomyosin—a long molecule that lies parallel to an **actin** molecule.

Troponin—a molecule blocking a site for **cross-bridge** formation; it is inactivated by Ca^{++} ions during muscle contraction.

Twitch (contraction)—a brief muscle contraction in response to a single presynaptic **action potential** or a single, synchronized volley of action potentials.

Unloading reflex—a decrease in the muscle activity when the load is suddenly decreased.

Ventral root (spinal)—a set of neural fibers carrying output (motor) signals from motoneurons to their innervated structures.

Ventricles (brain)—hollow spaces within the brain filled with cerebrospinal fluid.

Vergence—an eye movement whose purpose is to fix the gaze at targets with different depths.

Vestibular ganglion (Scarpa's ganglion)—the **ganglion** innervating vestibular receptors.

Vestibular nuclei (lateral vestibular or Deiters', medial vestibular, superior vestibular, and inferior vestibular)—sources of the **vestibulospinal tracts;** located in the **medulla.**

Vestibulo-ocular reflex (VOR)—a **reflex** coordinating eye and head movements, helping to maintain constant visual field.

Vibration-induced fallings (VIFs)—postural disturbances introduced by a low-amplitude, high-frequency vibration applied to a postural muscle or to its tendon.

Westphal phenomenon—an abrupt **reflex** excitation of a muscle in response to an externally imposed muscle shortening.

White matter—neural tissue consisting mostly of conduction pathways.

Wiping reflex—a **reflex,** coordinated movement of a spinal animal leading to the removal of an irritating stimulus from the animal's skin.

Working point—the "most important" point whose trajectory is crucial for success during a multi-joint movement.

INDEX

ABOUT THE AUTHOR

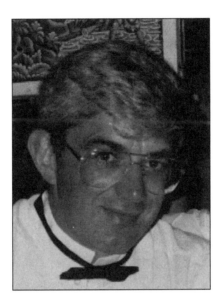

Mark L. Latash, PhD, is an associate professor of kinesiology at Penn State University. Since the 1970s, he has worked extensively in the areas of normal and disordered motor control. His work has included animal studies, human experiments, modeling, and clinical studies.

He has taught physiology in both Russia and the United States. Since 1995, he has taught a graduate course at Penn State titled, Neurophysiological Basis of Movement, from which he developed the material for this text.

He is the author of *Control of Human Movement*, published by Human Kinetics in 1993. He also translated Bernstein's classic, *On Dexterity and its Development* (Erlbaum), in 1996.

Latash earned a master's degree in physics of living systems from the Moscow Physico-Technical Institute in 1976 and a PhD in physiology from Rush University in 1989. He is a member of the Society for Neuroscience and the American Society of Biomechanics.

Latash lives in State College, Pennsylvania. His leisure activities include spending time with friends, playing guitar and singing, and reading.

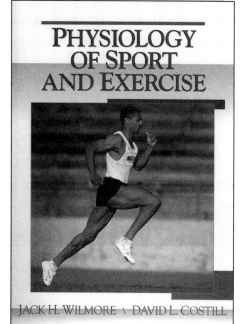